HANDBOOK OF
In Vitro Fertilization

Alan Trounson • David K. Gardner
Centre for Early Human Development
Institute of Reproduction and Development
Monash University
Victoria, Australia

CRC Press
Boca Raton   Ann Arbor   London   Tokyo

Library of Congress Cataloging-in-Publication Data

Handbook of in vitro fertilization / editors, Alan O. Trounson, David K. Gardner.
     p.   cm.
    Includes bibliographical references and index.
    ISBN 0-8493-2922-1
    1. Fertilization in vitro, Human.   I. Trounson, Alan.
II. Gardner, David K.
    [DNLM: 1. Fertilization in Vitro—handbooks.   WQ 39 H23558]
RG135.H36   1993
618.1'78059—dc20
DNLM / DLC
for Library of Congress   92-48216
                                                                                                                 CIP

    This book represents information obtained from authentic and highly regarded sources. Reprinted material is quoted with permission, and sources are indicated. A wide variety of references are listed. Every reasonable effort has been made to give reliable data and information, but the author and the publisher cannot assume responsibility for the validity of all materials or for the consequences of their use.

    Neither this book nor any part may be reproduced or transmitted in any form or by any means, electronic or mechanical, including photocopying, microfilming, and recording, or by any information storage and retrieval system, without permission in writing from the publisher.

    All rights reserved. Authorization to photocopy items for internal or personal use, or the personal or internal use of specific clients, is granted by CRC Press, Inc., provided that $.50 per page photocopied is paid directly to Copyright Clearance Center, 27 Congress Street, Salem, MA, 01970 USA. The fee code for users of the Transactional Reporting Service is ISBN 0-8493-2922-1/93/$0.00+$.50. The fee is subject to change without notice. For organizations that have been granted a photocopy license by the CCC, a separate system of payment has been arranged.

    The copyright owner's consent does not extend to copying for general distribution, for promotion, for creating new works, or for resale. Specific permission must be obtained from CRC Press for such copying.

    Direct all inquiries to CRC Press, Inc., 2000 Corporate Blvd., N. W., Boca Raton, Florida, 33431.

© 1993 by CRC Press, Inc.

International Standard Book Number 0-8493-2922-1

Library of Congress Card Number 92-48216
Printed in the United States 1 2 3 4 5 6 7 8 9 0
Printed on acid-free paper

PREFACE

Since the introduction of IVF as a treatment for infertility just over a decade ago, there has been an exponential increase in the amount of research in the area of assisted reproduction. Specific areas which have received a great deal of attention include: ovulation induction, assisted fertilization by microinjection of sperm under the zona pellucida, embryo biopsy and preimplantation diagnosis, embryo metabolism, viability assays, cryopreservation, the ultrastructural analysis of gametes and embryos, and assessment of the female reproductive tract and its receptivity.

It is the aim of this handbook to provide both a theoretical and practical guide to many of the techniques currently used in assisted reproduction, although emphasis has been placed on the practical application of the technologies. Each chapter provides background information and a detailed technical account of the procedures employed. With the rapid development of technologies there has been a concomitant increase in legal and ethical considerations for scientists, clinicians, and society. With scientific advances come social responsibilities. We have therefore included a chapter specifically dealing with the ethical aspects of embryo research.

As with all modern technologies, many of the techniques described are far from optimized, and it is our opinion that some procedures described in this handbook will be superseded in the coming years. The potential areas of rapid development have been highlighted in the final chapter.

This handbook will be of value to scientists, clinicians, IVF technicians and all students of life sciences.

Alan Trounson
David K. Gardner

THE EDITORS

Alan Trounson, Ph.D., is Director, Centre for Early Human Development, and Deputy Director, Monash Institute for Reproduction and Development, Monash University. He is Professor of Obstetrics and Gynecology/Pediatrics, Monash University.

Professor Trounson graduated from the University of New South Wales in 1968 with a B.Sc. in wool and pastoral sciences, and in 1971 with an M.Sc. In 1974 he obtained his Ph.D. degree from Sydney University. From 1974–1976 he was a Research Fellow at Cambridge and in 1976 was a visiting Professor at the University of Calgary. In 1977 he was appointed Senior Research Fellow at Monash University, and by 1984 was a Reader in the Department of Obstetrics and Gynecology. He took up the Directorship of the Centre for Early Human Development in 1985, and in 1991 was awarded a Personal Chair in Obstetrics and Gynecology.

Professor Trounson is a member of the American Fertility Society, the Society for the Study of Reproduction, and the Australian Society of Reproductive Biology, and is an Executive Committee Member of the Australian Fertility Society. He is currently an Editor of the *Journal of Reproduction and Fertility, Human Reproduction, Reproductive Medicine Reviews, Journal of Assisted Reproduction and Genetics, Theriogenology, Reproduction Fertility and Development, Gynaecological Endocrinology,* and *Molecular Reproduction and Development.*

Professor Trounson has held over 40 research grants, published more than 150 research papers, 65 book chapters, and edited 6 books. He has presented over 100 invited lectures at international conferences.

Among other awards, he has received the Wellcome Australia Medal 1991 for contributions to medical research, and the F.C. Donders Chair for Research, University of Utrecht, 1992–1993. His scientific accomplishments include development of human IVF, oocyte donation, cryopreservation of mammalian oocytes and embryos, development of biopsy techniques and the sub-zonal injection of sperm. His current research is focused on nuclear-cytoplasmic relationships during embryo development, sperm-egg interactions, genes in development, oocyte maturation, and embryo developmental competence.

David K. Gardner, D.Phil., is a Research Fellow and Deputy Head of the Embryology and Fertility Research Unit at the Centre for Early Human Development, Monash University.

Dr. Gardner graduated from the University of York with a B.Sc. in biology in 1984, and in 1987 with a D.Phil. degree. After postdoctoral positions in 1988–1989 at Harvard University and the University of York, he took up the position of Research Officer at the Centre for Early Human Development. In 1991 he was appointed Senior Research Officer. He is currently a Research Fellow and Honorary Lecturer in Obstetrics and Gynecology, Monash University, and a Scientific Adviser to Monash IVF and IVF America, Ltd.

Dr. Gardner is a member of the Society for the Study of Reproduction, the Society for the Study of Fertility and the Australian Society for Reproductive Biology.

Dr. Gardner has published more than 30 research papers, book chapters, and abstracts. His research interests include the regulation of energy metabolism in the mammalian preimplantation embryo, optimization of culture systems, the development of viability assays, and *in vitro* fertilization.

CONTRIBUTORS

H. W. G. Baker, M.D., Ph.D.
Department of Obstetrics and
   Gynecology
University of Melbourne
Royal Women's Hospital
Melbourne, Victoria, Australia

Marilyn Bakker
Centre for Early Human
   Development
Monash University
Monash Medical Centre
Clayton, Victoria, Australia

Ilan Calderon
Department of Obstetrics and
   Gynecology
Monash University
Monash Medical Centre
Clayton, Victoria, Australia

Karen Dawson, Ph.D.
Centre of Early Human
   Development
Monash University
Monash Medical Centre
Clayton, Victoria, Australia

Marie Dziadek, D. Phil.
Centre for Early Human
   Development
Monash University
Monash Medical Centre
Clayton, Victoria, Australia

David K. Gardner, D. Phil.
Centre for Early Human
   Development
Monash University
Monash Medical Centre
Clayton, Victoria, Australia

Lyn R. Gras, B.Sc.
Centre for Early Human
   Development
Monash University
Monash Medical Centre
Clayton, Victoria, Australia

David L. Healy, M.D., Ph.D.
Department of Obstetrics and
   Gynecology
Monash University
Monash Medical Centre
Clayton, Victoria, Australia

Ismail Kola, Ph.D.
Centre for Early Human
   Development
Monash University
Monash Medical Centre
Clayton, Victoria, Australia

Michelle Lane, B.Sc.
Centre for Early Human
   Development
Monash University
Monash Medical Centre
Clayton, Victoria, Australia

Henry J. Leese, Ph.D.
Department of Biology
University of York
Heslington, York, U.K.

D.Y. Liu, Ph.D.
Department of Obstetrics and
   Gynecology
University of Melbourne
Royal Women's Hospital
Melbourne, Victoria, Australia

F. L. H. Ng, M. Sc.
Mount Elizabeth IVF Centre
Mount Elizabeth Hospital
Singapore

Apichart Oranratnachai, M. D.
Department of Obstetrics and
  Gynecology
Chiang Mai University
Chiang Mai, Thailand

Jeremy Osborn, Ph.D.
Centre for Early Human
  Development
Monash University
Monash Medical Centre
Clayton, Victoria, Australia

Peter Rogers, Ph.D.
Department of Obstetrics and
  Gynecology
Monash University
Monash Medical Centre
Clayton, Victoria, Australia

A. Henry Sathananthan, Ph.D.
Department of Human Biosciences
LaTrobe University
Carlton, Victoria, Australia

Jillian M. Shaw, Ph.D.
Centre for Early Human
  Development
Monash University
Monash Medical Centre
Clayton, Victoria, Australia

Juan J. Tarín, Ph.D.
Department of Pediatrics,
  Obstetrics and Gynecology
Valencia University
Valencia, Spain

Alan Trounson, Ph.D.
Centre for Early Human
  Development
Monash University
Monash Medical Centre
Clayton, Victoria, Australia

TABLE OF CONTENTS

Chapter 1
Endrocrinology of IVF 1
Ilan Calderon and David Healy

Chapter 2
Oocyte Retrieval and Maturation 17
Jeremy Osborn

Chapter 3
Preparation and Analysis of Semen for IVF/GIFT 33
H.W.G. Baker, F.L.H. Ng, and D.Y. Liu

Chapter 4
In Vitro Fertilization and Embryo Development 57
Alan Trounson and Jeremy Osborn

Chapter 5
Embryo Culture Systems 85
David K. Gardner and Michelle Lane

Chapter 6
Embryo Biopsy for Preimplantation Diagnosis 115
Juan J. Tarín and Alan Trounson

Chapter 7
Fertilization Using Micromanipulation Techniques 131
Alan Trounson and A. Henry Sathananthan

Chapter 8
Genetic Analysis of the Preimplantation Embryo 151
Marie Dziadek and Marilyn Bakker

Chapter 9
Chromosomal Analysis of Preimplantation Mammalian Embryos 173
Ismail Kola, A. Henry Sathananthan, and Lyn Gras

Chapter 10
Assessment of Embryo Metabolism and Viability 195
David K. Gardner and Henry J. Leese

Chapter 11
Cryopreservation of Oocytes and Embryos 213
Jillian Shaw, Apichart Oranratnachai, and Alan Trounson

Chapter 12
Ultrastructure in Fertilization and Embryo Development 237
A. Henry Sathananthan

Chapter 13
Uterine Receptivity 263
Peter Rogers

Chapter 14
Ethical Aspects of IVF and Human Embryo Research 287
Karen Dawson

Chapter 15
Future Prospects 303
Karen Dawson and Alan Trounson

Index 313

Chapter 1

ENDOCRINOLOGY OF IVF

Ilan Calderon and David Healy

TABLE OF CONTENTS

I.	Introduction	2
II.	Folliculogenesis	2
III.	Endocrine Evaluation before IVF Treatment	3
IV.	Stimulation Protocols	4
	A. GnRH Agonist/HMG-Boost Protocol	5
	B. GnRH Agonist/HMG-Down Regulation Protocol	6
	C. Clomiphene Citrate/HMG	7
	1. HMG Doses	8
	D. Natural Cycle.	9
V.	Growth Hormone in Ovulation Induction	9
VI.	Cycle Monitoring	9
	A. Natural Cycle Monitoring	10
VII.	Ovarian Hyperstimulation Syndrome	11
VIII.	Polycystic Ovarian Syndrome (PCOS)	12
IX.	Luteal Phase Support	12
X.	Conclusion	13
References		14

I. INTRODUCTION

The first successful *in vitro* fertilization (IVF) and embryo transfer (ET) treatment described by Edwards and Steptoe[1] in 1978 led to much new clinical and research-oriented work in the field of endocrine infertility. IVF was initially presented as a treatment for severe female mechanical factor infertility but was quickly utilized in other areas in the field of infertility, such as unexplained infertility, male factor infertility, immunological infertility, endometriosis, cervical factor infertility, and even ovarian failure.

Gynecological endocrinology plays an important role in the management of IVF patients. Understanding of the endocrinological basis of normal ovulation and the different induction of ovulation protocols is essential for successful IVF treatment. This chapter will try to give a theoretical and practical guide to the endocrinological management of the IVF patient.

II. FOLLICULOGENESIS

The initiation of follicular growth is a continuous process that does not depend on hormonal stimulation. Most follicles will undergo rapid atresia. However, under the hormonal changes in the beginning of the cycle, a group of follicles will respond to small rises in serum follicle stimulating hormone (FSH) by progressing to the preantral stage2 (Figure 1). At this stage, the follicle is about 200 μm in diameter with multiple granulosa cell layers. Under the influence of FSH, the number of FSH receptors on the granulosa cell increases to about 1500 receptors per cell,3 and at the same time the granulosa cells start to produce estradiol 17B (E_2) by aromatizing androgens that are supplied by the theca cells. E_2 and FSH together cause proliferation of granulosa cells and increase the number of FSH receptors on the granulosa cell plasma membrane. Production of follicular fluid increase its accumulation in the intracellular space eventually connecting to form a cavity — the antrum. The size of the antral follicle is about 500 μm in diameter. By day 5–7, the dominant follicle is selected because of its ability to convert androgens to estrogens. The other follicles will not continue to grow and will undergo atresia. Intra-ovarian growth factors such as insulin-like growth factors, epidermal growth factor, and the inhibin family may be important in regulating the processes of follicle dominance and atresia.[4] The dominant follicle continues to grow and secretes E_2 and inhibin, which exert negative feedback on FSH production causing a decline in serum FSH levels. The high levels of estrogens induce high affinity receptors for LH, and, at the same time, FSH generates the appearance of lutenizing hormone (LH) receptors on granulosa cells. Inhibin and E_2 production gradually increases, and plasma E_2 levels achieve a threshold concentration required for the generation of the LH surge which starts 14 to 24 h after the serum E_2 reaches peak concentration. The LH surge initiates luteinization and the beginning of progesterone production by the granulosa cells of the dominant follicle. It is also responsible for the resumption of

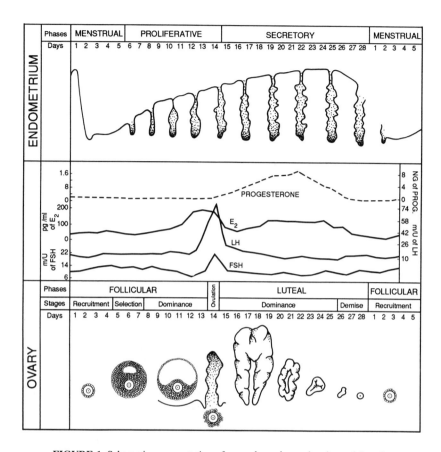

FIGURE 1. Schematic representation of normal ovarian and endometrial cycle.

meiosis in the oocyte and the synthesis of prostaglandins that are essential for follicular rupture. Ovulation occurs 24 to 36 h after the onset of the LH surge, when the follicle, which is about 20 mm, ruptures and the oocyte is released from the ovary.

After ovulation, the dominant follicle becomes the corpus luteum, producing progesterone, estradiol, and inhibin, which suppress the growth of new follicles in the ovary. At the end of the cycle, luteolysis causes decline in both steroids and inhibin, allowing the elevation in serum LH and FSH that is necessary for the initiation of a new cycle.

III. ENDOCRINE EVALUATION BEFORE IVF TREATMENT

IVF is an expensive and relatively invasive technique, and therefore it should be applied only to those patients who have appropriate indications. The current indications at the Monash University Infertility Medical Centre program for IVF treatment and the number of patients treated for each indication

TABLE 1
Frequency of Clinical Indications for Various IVF-ET or GIFT
(Gamete Intra-Fallopian Transfer) Procedures in the Monash
University Infertility Medical Centre, 1990

	Total	Single indication	Multiple indication
1. Male factor infertility	418	258	160
2. Unexplained infertility	346	346	
3. Tubal disease	345	247	98
4. Endometriosis	161	89	72
5. Male or female immune infertility	79	53	26
6. Oocyte donation	72	72	
i. Primary ovarian failure			
ii. Secondary ovarian failure			
iii. Maternal genetic disorder			
iv. Failed IVF			
7. Embryo cryopreservation — prior to chemotherapy or radiotherapy	2	2	
8. Surrogacy — absent uterus	None in 1990		

in 1990 are listed in Table 1. An endocrinological evaluation should be performed on all IVF patients before starting the IVF program. This assessment includes plasma LH, FSH, and prolactin levels in the follicular phase and plasma progesterone (P_4) and E_2 levels in the midluteal phase. This will enable one to confirm ovulation or a clinical diagnosis of polycystic ovary syndrome and to exclude hyperprolactinemia, anovulation, and occult ovarian failure.[5] The diagnosis of polycystic ovarian disease prior to initiation of IVF cycle is especially important since these patients have special difficulties in multiple folliculogenesis (see Section VIII).

IV. STIMULATION PROTOCOLS

The first IVF baby was born as a result of an oocyte picked up in a natural cycle.[1] However, the success rate of this protocol was very low, and the Monash group first reported large numbers of eggs and improved pregnancy rates using a stimulation protocol of clomiphene citrate and human menopausal gonadotropin (HMG) together.[6] Several other regimens using these two medicines were subsequently reported. The common problems with these protocols were that endogenous gonadotropins led to premature luteinization in 30 to 40% of the cases, and, in others, ovulation occurred at an inconvenient time of the day. Several investigators tried to overcome this problem using estrogen and progestagen pills to suppress LH secretion and to prevent the premature luteinization and the untimely ovulation.[7] However, the major step in simplifying IVF induction of ovulation protocols and preventing these unwanted phenomena came with the introduction of GnRH analogues. GnRH analogues were created by a series of modifications in the gonadotropin releasing hormone molecule that led to the availability of new compounds. These compounds initially enhanced gonadotropin release from the pituitary but, with continuing administration, caused down-regulation of the pituitary and reduced LH and FSH secretion for as long as the analogue was given. This effect was a powerful tool with which to control the stimulated IVF cycle.

Initially, the use of GnRH analogue was confined to women with a history of poor response to other stimulation protocols, premature LH surge, and elevated plasma LH and FSH levels,[8-13] but there are now several reports advocating their use in all IVF cycles including those women with normal basal gonadotropins.[14-16] Brzyski and colleagues reported an increased number of mature oocytes retrieved in GnRH analogue treatment compared to treatment cycles without GnRH analogue; this increase in oocyte numbers was not associated with increased E_2 levels.[15] The mechanism by which GnRH analogues improve follicular response is not yet known. Palermo and associates reported improvement in synchronization of follicular development leading to a larger cohort of developing follicles,[13] while others related it to the longer gonadotropin stimulation in the GnRH analogue cycles.[16] According to some authors, pituitary suppression is more effective when the therapy commences in midluteal phase of the previous cycle rather than in the early follicular phase of the treatment cycle.[17]

The current protocols for induction of ovulation in the Monash University/ Infertility Medical Centre IVF program are

1. GnRH agonist/HMG-boost protocol
2. GnRH agonist/HMG-down regulation protocol
3. Clomiphene citrate/HMG
4. Natural cycle

The objective of the first three protocols is to obtain a cohort of co-dominant follicles in both ovaries with adequate E_2 levels suitable for oocyte retrieval on days 11 to 15.

A. GnRH AGONIST/HMG-BOOST PROTOCOL

This protocol (Figure 2) is currently the protocol of choice for first cycle patients and previously normal response subjects in our IVF program. In this protocol, the GnRH agonist (Leuprolide, 1 mg SC, Abbott Pharmaceuticals, Sydney, or Buserelin, 600 μg SC or IM, Hoechst AG, Melbourne) begins on day two of the cycle and continues until the day before the human chorionic gonadotropin (hCG) injection. Human menopausal gonadotropin (HMG, Pergonal, Serono, Australia) starts on day three of the cycle and continues according to individual endocrine and ovarian ultrasonic response until the day before the hCG injection. hCG 5000 IU in single IM injections is given according to E_2 levels and follicular size, and egg pickup follows 36 h later. This protocol "boosts" the exogenous gonadotropin injected into the patient by a rise in serum concentration of her endogenous FSH and LH released in initial response to the GnRH agonist.

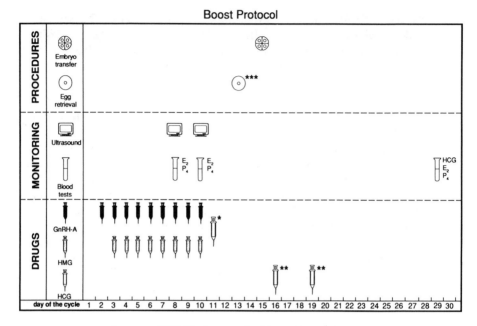

*	5000 IU given preferably on day 11, depending on Ultrasound and blood test results
**	1000 IU boosters given on day 3 and day 6 after oocyte retrieval
***	36 hours after HCG injection

FIGURE 2. Schematic illustration of "Boost" induction of ovulation protocol.

B. GnRH AGONIST/HMG-DOWN REGULATION PROTOCOL

This protocol (Figure 3), which in our unit is reserved only for patients with inadequate (serum E_2 < fifth centile) or abnormal endocrine responses, is used as a primary stimulation protocol in many IVF units around the world with satisfactory results. Disadvantages of this protocol include greater consumption of GnRH agonist and HMG and therefore greater patient cost, as well as the uncertainty of possible pregnancy upon initiation of GnRH agonist treatment. In this protocol, the GnRH analogue starts on day 21 of the previous cycle and continues by daily injections until the day before the hCG injection. HMG commences after achievement of adequate pituitary and ovarian suppression on the same dose and regimen as the boost protocol. The criteria for pituitary and ovarian suppression are E_2 levels <180 pmol/l, LH levels <2 IU/l and P_4 levels <2 nmol/l. hCG administration criteria and dosage are the same as for the boost protocol.

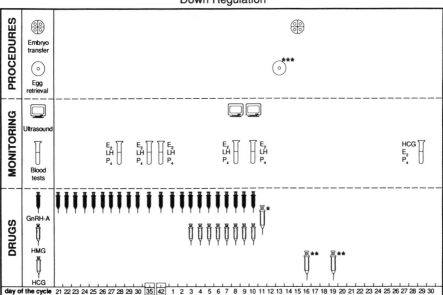

*	5000 IU given preferably on day 11, depending on Ultrasound and blood test results
**	1000 IU boosters given on day 3 and day 6 after oocyte retrieval
***	36 hours after HCG injection

FIGURE 3. Schematic illustration of "Down Regulation" induction of ovulation protocol.

C. CLOMIPHENE CITRATE AND HMG PROTOCOL

This protocol (Figure 4) used to be the preferred protocol in most IVF units prior to development of GnRH analogues; it was abandoned in our program because of the high cancellation rate due to untimely LH surges and some reports of the possible adverse effect of clomiphene citrate on the embryo. In our unit, this protocol is used only for the following patients:

1. Patients who have responded well (≥ five oocytes retrieved) to clomiphene citrate and HMG in the past and who did not respond to the boost protocol;
2. Patients who did not want to use GnRH agonists and who previously responded well (≥ five oocytes) to the combination of clomiphene citrate and HMG.

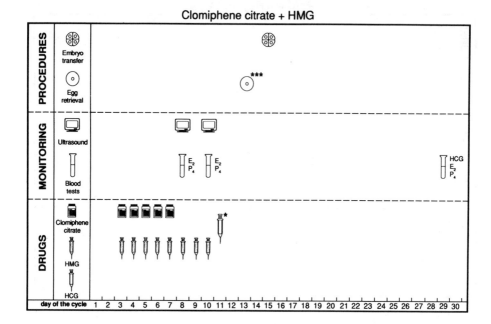

| * | 5000 IU given preferably on day 11, depending on Ultrasound and blood test results |
| *** | 36 hours after HCG injection |

FIGURE 4. Schematic illustration of "Clomiphene Citrate and HMG" induction of ovulation protocol.

In this protocol, clomiphene citrate 100 mg/d commences on day three of the cycle and proceeds for five days. HMG begins on day three and continues, as do the other protocols, until the day of hCG injection minus 1 d. hCG (5000 IU in IM injections) is given when the estimated leading follicle is 18 to 19 mm in diameter with serum E_2 levels >1800 pmol/l.

1. HMG Doses

HMG starting dose is empirically determined according to patient history. HMG starting doses for the different patient groups in our program are listed in Table 2. The duration and daily doses of HMG are adjusted according to individual patient age and response as judged by serum E_2 levels and follicular number and size in an ultrasound scan of the ovary.

Patient age and follicular phase serum FSH values are two useful predictors of gonadotropin dosage.

TABLE 2
HMG Starting Dose in IVF Ovarian Protocols at Monash University

Patient group	HMG Starting dose (IU per day)
1. 1st cycle <37 years old	150
2. 1st cycle with baseline scan suggesting polycystic ovarian syndrome	75
3. 1st cycle patient 37–39 years old	225
4. 1st cycle patient ≥40 years old	300
5. Previous normal response (≥5 oocytes)	150
6. Previous ovarian hyperstimulation syndrome	75
7. Previous poor response (serum E_2 <5th centile)	300

D. NATURAL CYCLE

This protocol does not involve any drug administration and therefore will be addressed later in this chapter.

V. GROWTH HORMONE IN OVULATION INDUCTION

The most common reason for cancellation in an IVF cycle is a low or abnormal (< fifth centile) serum E_2 response to ovarian hyperstimulation. This group of patients usually responds poorly in subsequent cycles with a very low probability of pregnancy.[18] Some of these patients have occult ovarian failure characterized by elevated plasma FSH concentration in the presence of regular menstrual cycle.[5] This condition may represent an early stage of premature ovarian failure.

The optimal ovarian stimulation protocol for this group of patients remains unclear. Check and associates reported their results in 100 cases with hypergonadotrophic amenorrhea. They achieved ovulation in 19% of the cases, with pregnancy rate of 5.2% using gonadal suppression with estrogen or GnRH-analogues and stimulation by HMG.[19]

A new approach to induction of ovulation in these patients is the use of growth hormone in hyperstimulation protocols. Recently, several studies demonstrated a beneficial effect of growth hormone on induction of ovulation. The addition of 12 to 24 IU of growth hormone injections on alternate days in the follicular phase augments the ovarian response to stimulation by gonadotropins.[20,21] This stimulation protocol is, however, still experimental and is used in our program only as a clinical trial.

VI. CYCLE MONITORING

As clinical knowledge about the nature of IVF cycles accumulates, cycle monitoring has become easier and less complicated. In the Monash University/ Infertility Medical Centre, IVF program cycle monitoring initially comprised daily serum E_2, LH, and P_4 estimations and ovarian ultrasound determinations.

Currently cycle monitoring consists of blood sampling for estradiol, LH, and P_4 levels and ultrasound scan of the ovary only on days eight and ten of the cycle.

According to the results on day eight, a decision about HMG dose is made using the following criteria:

1. $1000 > E_2 < 6000$ pmol/l — continue with the same dose
2. $E_2 < 1000$ pmol/l — increase HMG dose
3. $E_2 > 6000$ pmol/l — decrease HMG dose

On the second visit (day ten), if six or more follicles are ≥16 mm and E_2 is >4000 pmol/l, hCG will be given the following day, followed by oocyte retrieval 36 h later. If the criteria for hCG administration has not been met, a third blood sample and ultrasound scan are necessary to determine the right time for hCG injection and egg pickup. About 10% of patients on the IVF program are discharged before egg pickup. Cancellation criteria in our unit are

1. P_4 >8 nmol/l on day nine or ten
2. Less than 3 follicles >16 mm and E_2 less than 3000 pmol/l on day nine or ten
3. LH >30 i.u/l on day nine or ten

It is uncertain why not all women with regular menstrual cycles respond to ovarian hyperstimulation protocols in a satisfactory fashion. O'Shea and associates investigated spontaneous menstrual cycles after failure of multiple IVF folliculogenesis in 131 consecutive cycles. Thirty-six percent of the cycles were endocrinologically normal, while the rest had a range of endocrine abnormalities including low luteal phase progesterone, premature progesterone elevation, occult ovarian failure, LH/FSH ratio >3 in early follicular phase, and hyperprolactinemia.[22]

Repetition of the same superovulation regimen after inadequate stimulation in IVF program results in improved folliculogenesis in only 10% of our patients. A review of patient history and the previous response to IVF folliculogenesis is therefore necessary before a decision is made about the next stimulation cycle protocol.

A. NATURAL CYCLE MONITORING

Unlike other protocols, natural cycle patients do not receive any induction of ovulation drugs and therefore need monitoring only. Information from the patient's previous natural cycles is computed to calculate the expected midpoint of the next cycle.[23] Three days before the calculated midpoint, blood samples for plasma E_2, LH and P_4 levels are taken, and ultrasound scan of the ovary is performed. Blood samples are taken daily after starting, and another ultrasound scan is performed 2 d later if required. Three thousand IU of hCG are given when follicular size is ≥ 17 mm and the serum E_2 levels are ≥ 500 pmol/l.

Oocyte retrieval then follows, 34 h after hCG injection. If there is a sign of LH surge before hCG injection, treatment should be cancelled.

VII. OVARIAN HYPERSTIMULATION SYNDROME

The major serious complication of ovulation induction in IVF-ET is ovarian hyperstimulation syndrome (OHSS). The syndrome is characterized by high serum E_2 levels, ovarian enlargement, abdominal distension, weight gain, and, in severe cases, increased capillary permeability leading to a shift of fluid out of the intravascular space. The etiology and pathogenesis of ovarian hyperstimulation syndrome is not yet known, but its incidence is closely correlated to high serum E_2 levels during the late follicular phase. The incidence of ovarian hyperstimulation syndrome varies between 1 and 30%, as reported in various publications.[24,25] This variety is probably due to the difference in the definition of ovarian hyperstimulation syndrome. Ovarian hyperstimulation syndrome is classically divided into three categories:

1. Mild ovarian hyperstimulation syndrome, with high serum E_2 levels, mild abdominal distension, and large ovaries of about 5 cm due to the presence of multiple follicular and corpus luteal cysts;
2. Moderate ovarian hyperstimulation syndrome, characterized by more abdominal distension, gastrointestinal symptoms such as nausea, vomiting, and less frequently diarrhea, some gain in weight, and ovaries enlarged up to 12 cm;
3. Severe ovarian hyperstimulation syndrome, which can be a life-threatening situation, characterized by pronounced abdominal distension, ascites, pleural effusion, electrolyte imbalance, oliguria, and sometimes hypovolemic shock. The ovaries are enlarged to more than 12 cm in diameter.

The treatment of ovarian hyperstimulation syndrome is conservative. Bed rest and symptomatic relief are usually sufficient for mild and moderate ovarian hyperstimulation syndrome. In mild cases, symptoms subside usually within a few days, while in moderate cases, symptoms can require up to three weeks to subside. When pregnancy occurs, hyperstimulation syndrome will last longer.

Severe hyperstimulation syndrome can be life threatening, and patients therefore should be hospitalized and monitored closely. Patients are put on bed rest; daily body weight and fluid balance monitoring are necessary. Hematocrit, coagulation, kidney function, electrolyte, and albumin/globulin ratio studies are obtained daily. Pelvic examination should be avoided because of the fragility of the enlarged ovaries, and ovarian surgery is contraindicated. When necessary, intravenous plasma expanders are given, but to maintain central venous pressure, diuretics should not be given, since the fluids in the abdominal or thoracic cavity are not responsive to diuretics, and the further intravascular depletion can cause hypotension, shock, and thrombosis. Indomethacin has been shown to have beneficial effects on hyperstimulation syndrome, but its safety in early pregnancy is unknown.[26] The acute clinical manifestation of the severe form of ovarian hyperstimulation syndrome usually disappears within several days if there are no complications. If pregnancy does not occur, the ovarian enlargement subsides usually within 30 to 40 d. If, however, pregnancy occurs, the high serum E_2 levels will continue to the end of the first trimester.

Prevention of OHSS is vital. Low body mass index and polycystic ovary syndrome are two clinical predictors, and HMG dosage should be reduced in such patients. When OHSS is suspected before hCG injection, hCG should be withheld. If, however, OHSS is diagnosed after oocyte retrieval, embryos should be frozen in order to avoid conception and replaced later in a natural cycle.[27] We use hCG at a dose of 5000 IU rather than 10,000 IU for final oocyte maturation before retrieval to help prevent OHSS. Moreover, supplementary injection of l000 IU hCG may be administered 3 and 6 d after oocyte retrieval rather than higher hCG doses in any fixed regimen (see below).

VIII. POLYCYSTIC OVARIAN SYNDROME (PCOS)

A group of patients who need special consideration in induction of ovulation for IVF treatment are patients suffering from polycystic ovarian syndrome. This syndrome that was first described by Stein and Leventhal in 1935 consists of a broad spectrum of abnormalities in women with characteristic endocrine dysfunction. The syndrome consists of amenorrhea or oligomenorrhea, anovulatory infertility, hypergonadism, obesity, and bilateral polycystic ovaries. Induction of ovulation in polycystic ovarian syndrome patients undergoing IVF treatment is associated with high rates of ovarian hyperstimulation syndrome. Identification of these patients before commencing ovarian hyperstimulation protocol is essential to prevent this complication. In our IVF program, baseline ultrasound scan of the ovaries is used to identify these patients, (multiple [10 or more] cysts 2 to 8 mms in diameter and enlarged ovaries), and the ovarian stimulation protocol is modified by reducing HMG starting dose to 75 IU per d and careful follow-up of serum E_2 levels and follicular number and size (Table 2).

IX. LUTEAL PHASE SUPPORT

Luteal phase support in clinical IVF is still a matter of some debate. The hormone profile in the luteal phase of IVF cycles has been blamed for the discrepancy between the high fertilization rate and the relatively low pregnancy rate. A number of theories have been proposed to explain this phenomenon. These include the effect of high serum E_2 levels in the follicular phase on luteal hormone profile,[28] the effect of follicular aspiration during oocyte collection due to aspiration of a large number of granulosa cells in this procedure,[29] and the effect of abnormal early embryo development. Lejeune and colleagues suggested that high serum P_4 concentrations and high P_4/E_2 ratio in early luteal phase have had a favorable influence on implantation in IVF pregnancy.[30] However, reports by Trounson and associates and Leeton and co-workers did not show a significant beneficial effect with the use of progesterone supplementation in the luteal phase.[31,32] Higher progesterone concentrations in the luteal phase can be achieved with hCG treatment compared to progesterone treatment during luteal phase.[33] Casper and colleagues demonstrated a significant improvement in pregnancy rate using exogenous hCG in a double-blind randomized trial.[34] Buvat and associates reported the use of multiple low doses of hCG with increase in luteal phase length, luteal phase progesterone levels, and P_4/E_2 ratio.[35] A meta-analysis of five clinical trials reported by Daya in 1988 found insufficient evidence to recommend the routine use of progesterone as luteal phase support after oocyte retrieval.[36] However, in most of these trials, induction of ovulation protocols consisted of HMG or HMG/CC medicines; it is known that the luteal phase is not shortened in these procedures. The use of GnRH analogues in IVF folliculogenesis protocols causes a shorter luteal phase due to LH suppression, and luteal phase support is therefore necessary. In a recent study, Hutchinson-Williams and co-workers reported the use of a single dose of hCG (10,000 IU) given 5 d after the original hCG dose as luteal phase support in IVF treatment. They found improvement in the luteal phase hormone profile, but no statistical difference in pregnancy rate was found. They advocated the use of such luteal phase support for all IVF cycles.[37] In our IVF program, all IVF patients in whom induction of ovulation protocol includes GnRH analogue receive luteal phase support that consists of 1000 IU of hCG injection on days three and six after oocyte pickup.

X. CONCLUSION

In the last 15 years, IVF and associated procedures have become important components in the treatment of infertile couples. These procedures are performed routinely in hundreds of centers around the world. Stimulation and monitoring of IVF cycles are less complicated today than they were ten years ago. An improved understanding of normal folliculogenesis and the greater availability of superior ovarian stimulation protocols have led to the retrieval of larger numbers of good quality eggs and a subsequent improvment in pregnancy rate.

With the acceptance of IVF and associated procedures as integral parts of the treatment for infertile couples, our objectives for the future should be improvement of the endocrinological control of the cycle, leading to improvement of pregnancy rates and to improvements of the outcomes of IVF pregnancies.

REFERENCES

1. Steptoe, P. C. and Edwards, R. G., Birth after the re-implantation of a human embryo, *Lancet*, II, 366, 1978.
2. Vermesh, M. and Kletzky, O. A., Longitudinal evaluation of the luteal phase and its transition into the follicular phase, *J. Clin. Endocrinol. Metab.*, 65, 653, 1987.
3. Erickson, G. F., An analysis of follicle development and ovum maturation, *Sem. Reprod. Endocrinol.*, 4, 233, 1986.
4. Findlay, A. K., The ovary, in *Growth Factors in Endocrinology*, Robertson, D. M. and Herington, A.C., Eds., in press.
5. Cameron, I. T., O'Shea, F. C., Rolland, J. M., Hughes, E. G., deKretser, D. M., and Healy, D. L., Occult ovarian failure: a syndrome of infertility, regular menses and elevated follicle-stimulating hormone concentrations, *J. Clin. Endocrinol. Metab.*, 67, 1190, 1988.
6. Trounson, A. O., Leeton, J. F., Wood, E. C., Webb, J., and Wood, J., Pregnancies in humans by fertilisation in vitro and embryo transfer in the controlled ovulatory cycle, *Science*, 212, 616, 1981.
7. Patton, P. E., Burry, K. A., Wolf, D. P., Kiessling, A. A., and Craemer, M. J., The use of oral contraceptives to regulate oocyte retrieval, *Fertil. Steril.*, 49, 716, 1988.
8. Edelstein, M. C., Brzyski, R. G., Jones, G. S., Oehninger, S., Sieg, S. M., and Muasher, S. J., Ovarian stimulation for in vitro fertilization using pure follicle-stimulating hormone with and without gonadotropin-releasing hormone agonist in high-responder patients, *JIVET*, 7, 172, 1990.
9. Porter, R. N., Smith, W., Craft, I. L., Abdulwahid, N. A., and Jacobs, S. A., Induction of ovulation for in vitro fertilisation using Buserelin and gonadotropins, *Lancet*, 2, 1284, 1984.
10. Serafini, P., Stone, B., Kerin, J., Batzofin, J., Quinn, P., and Marrs, R. P., An alternate approach to controlled ovarian hyperstimulation in "poor responders": pretreatment with a gonadotropin-releasing hormone analog, *Fertil. Steril.*, 49, 90, 1988.
11. Neveu, S., Hedon, B., Bringer, J., Chinchole, J. M., Arnal, F., Humeau, C., Cristol, P., and Viala, J. L., Ovarian stimulation by a combination of a gonadotropin-releasing hormone agonist and gonadotropins for in vitro fertilization, *Fertil. Steril.*, 47, 639, 1987.
12. Bettendorf, G., Braendle, W., Sprotte, C. H., Poels, W., Lichtenberg, W., and Lindner, C., Pharmacologic hypogonadism — an advantage for HMG-induced follicular maturation and succeeding fertilization, *Horm. Metab. Res.*, 18, 656, 1987.
13. Palermo, R., Amodeo, G., Navot, D., Rosenwaks, Z., and Cittadini, E., Concomitant gonadotropin-releasing hormone agonist and menotropin treatment for the synchronized induction of multiple follicles, *Fertil. Steril.*, 49, 290, 1988.
14. MacLachlan, V., Besanko, M., O'Shea, F., Wade, H., Wood, C., Trounson, A., and Healy, D. L., A controlled study of luteinizing hormone-releasing hormone agonist (Buserelin) for the induction of foliculogenesis before in vitro fertilization, *N. Engl. J. Med.*, 320, 1233, 1989.
15. Brzyski, R. G., Jones, G. S., Oehninger, S., Acosta, A. A., Kruithoff, C. H., and Muasher, S. J., Impact of leuprolide acetate on the response to follicular stimulation for in vitro fertilization in patients with normal basal gonadotropin levels, *JIVET*, 6, 290, 1989.
16. Meldrum, D. R., Wisot, A., Hamilton, F., Gutlay, A. L., Kempton, W., and Huynh, D., Routine pituitary suppression with leuprolide before ovarian stimulation for oocyte retrieval, *Fertil. Steril.*, 51, 455, 1989.

17. **Meldrum, D. R., Wisot, A., Hamilton, F., Gutlay, A. L., Huynh, D., and Kempton, W.**, Timing of initiation and dose schedule of leuprolide influence the time course of ovarian suppression, *Fertil. Steril.*, 50, 400, 1988.
18. **Pellicer, A., Lightman, A., Diamond, M. P., Russell, J. B., and DeCherney, A. H.**, Outcome of in vitro fertilization in women with low response to ovarian stimulation, *Fertil. Steril.*, 47, 812, 1987.
19. **Check, J. H., Nowroozi, K., Chase, J. S., Nazari, A., Shapse, D., and Vaze, M.**, Ovulation induction and pregnancies in 100 consecutive women with hypergonadotropic amenorrhoea, *Fertil. Steril.*, 53, 811, 1990.
20. **Homberg, R., Eshel, A., Abdalla, H. I., and Jacobs, H. S.**, Growth hormone facilitates ovulation induction by gonadotrophins, *Clin. Endocrinol.*, 29, 113, 1988.
21. **Blumenfeld, Z. and Lunenfeld, B.**, The potentiating effect of growth hormone on follicle stimulation with human menopausal gonadotropin in a panhypopituitary patient, *Fertil. Steril.*, 52, 328, 1989.
22. **O'Shea, F. C., Healy, D. L., Besanko, M. D., MacLachlan, V. B., Morrow, L. M., Shukovski, L., Thomas, A., and Okamoto, S. H.**, Unsatisfactory superovulation responses in IVF: classification and endocrine assessment of a subsequent spontaneous menstrual cycle, *Proc. Fertil. Soc. Aust.*, (Abst) A4, 1985.
23. **McIntosh, J. E. A., Matthews, C. D., Crocker, J. M., Broom, T. J., and Cox, L. W.**, Predicting the luteinizing hormone surge: relationship between the duration of the follicular and the luteal phases and the length of the human menstrual cycle, *Fertil. Steril.*, 34, 125, 1980.
24. **Golan, A., Ron-El, R., Herman, A., Weinraub, Z., Soffer, Y., and Caspi, E.**, Ovarian hyperstimulation syndrome following D-Trp-6 luteinizing hormone-releasing hormone microcapsules and menotropin for in vitro fertilization, *Fertil. Steril.*, 50, 912, 1988.
25. **Schenker, J. G. and Weinstein, D.**, Ovarian hyperstimulation syndrome: a current survey, *Fertil. Steril.*, 30, 255, 1978.
26. **Schenker, J. G. and Polishuk, W. Z.**, The role of prostaglandins in ovarian hyperstimulation syndrome, *Eur. J. Obstet. Gynecol. Reprod.*, 6, 47, 1976.
27. **Smitz, J., Camus, M., Devroey, P., Erard, P., Wisanto, A., and Van Steirteghem, A. C.**, Incidence of severe ovarian hyperstimulation syndrome after GnRH/HMG superovulation for in-vitro fertilization, *Hum. Reprod.*, 5, 933, 1990.
28. **DeCherney, A. H., Tarlatzis, B. C., and Laufer, N.**, Follicular development: lessons learned from human in vitro fertilization, *Am. J. Obstet. Gynecol.*, 153, 911, 1985.
29. **Kreitmann, O., Nixon, W. E., and Hodgen, G. D.**, Induced corpus luteum dysfunction after aspiration of the preovulatory follicle in monkeys, *Fertil. Steril.*, 35, 671, 1981.
30. **Lejeune, B., Camus, M., Deschacht, J., and Leroy, F.**, Differences in the luteal phases after failed or successful in vitro fertilization and embryo replacement, *JIVET*, 3, 358, 1986.
31. **Leeton, J., Trounson, A., and Jessup, D.**, Support of the luteal phase in in vitro fertilization programs: results of a controlled trial with intramuscular prolutin, *JIVET*, 2, 166, 1985.
32. **Trounson, A., Howlett, D., Rogers, P., and Hoppen, H. O.**, The effect of progesterone supplementation around the time of oocyte recovery in patients superovulated for in vitro fertilization, *Fertil. Steril.*, 45, 532, 1986.
33. **Nader, S., Berkowitz, A. S., Ochs, D., Held, B., and Winkel, C. A.**, Luteal-phase support in stimulated cycles in an in vitro fertilization/embryo transfer program: progesterone versus human chorionic gonadotropin, *JIVET*, 5, 81, 1988.
34. **Casper, R. F., Wilson, E., Collins, J. A., Brown, S. E., and Parker, J. A.**, Enhancement of human implantation by exogenous chorionic gonadotropin, *Lancet*, 2, 1191, 1983.

35. **Buvat, J., Marcolin, G., Guittard, C., Herbaut, J. C., Louvet, A. L., and Dehaene, J. L.,** Luteal support after luteinizing hormone-releasing hormone agonist for in vitro fertilization: superiority of human chorionic gonadotropin over oral progesterone, *Fertil. Steril.*, 53, 490, 1990.
36. **Daya, S.,** Efficacy of progesterone support in the luteal phase following in-vitro fertilization and embryo transfer: meta-analysis of clinical trials, *Hum. Reprod.*, 3, 731, 1988.
37. **Hutchinson-Williams, K. A., DeCherney, A. H., Lavy, G., Diamond, M. P., Naftolin, F., and Lunenfeld, B.,** Luteal rescue in in vitro fertilization-embryo transfer, *Fertil. Steril.*, 53, 495, 1990.

Chapter 2

OOCYTE RETRIEVAL AND MATURATION

Jeremy Osborn

TABLE OF CONTENTS

I.	Introduction	18
II.	Oocyte Collection	18
III.	Temperature Control	19
IV.	Follicle Flushing	20
V.	Oocyte Identification	20
VI.	Assessment of Oocyte Maturation	21
VII.	Direct Determination of Nuclear Maturity in Oocytes	23
	A. Cumulus Spreading	23
	B. Removal of Cumulus Cells using Hyaluronidase	25
VIII.	Timing of Insemination	27
IX.	Preparation of Oocytes for GIFT	28
X.	Conclusions	29
References		30

I. INTRODUCTION

In the thirteen years that have elapsed since the birth of Louise Brown, the techniques involved in the collection of human oocytes for *in vitro* fertilization (IVF) or gamete intrafallopian transfer (GIFT) have become increasingly more sophisticated and more directly oriented to the patients' needs. Thus, transvaginal ultrasound-directed oocyte recovery performed within a day-surgery setting under mild sedation has replaced the use of laparoscopy under general anesthesia in the hospital operating rooms. In addition, the recognition that oocytes collected and inseminated at the completion of meiotic maturation show higher fertilization rates compared to those exposed to spermatozoa at earlier stages[1] has emphasized the need for accurate assessment of the oocyte and its surrounding cumulus cells.

In this chapter, the procedures currently used at the Infertility Medical Centre, Melbourne, for the collection, identification, and assessment of human oocytes prior to insemination will be discussed. It should be noted, however, that these methods may be changed to varying degrees to suit the needs of other clinics.

II. OOCYTE COLLECTION

Most oocyte collections are now performed vaginally using a fine needle attached to a transvaginal ultrasound probe.[2] At the Infertility Medical Centre, a single lumen 17 gauge needle (William Cook Australia Pty Ltd., Brisbane, Australia), connected by fine Teflon tubing to a Kmar aspiration regulator suction pump controlled by a Kmar-2000 vacuum regulator (William Cook Ltd.), is used. Use of syringes which create variable and uncontrolled suction has largely been discontinued following the unequivocal evidence that the shearing forces which are produced result in a high incidence of fractured zonae and polyspermy.[3]

In our system, flushing of the follicle is accomplished by attaching an 18 gauge cannula to a syringe and inserting the former into the flared end of the vacuum line at the silicone bung. Flushing of the follicles is now rarely performed, and, as a result, the inefficient procedure of disconnecting the silicone bung and injecting medium back into the follicle through the aspiration line has been discontinued. However, where follicle flushing is routinely carried out, a double lumen needle, as supplied by William Cook Ltd. or Casmed, UK, provides the opportunity of applying vacuum and flushing simultaneously or independently without any dead space in the cannula or vacuum system. In all cases, the needles have an ultrasound reflective etched mark at the tip to maximize visualization.

The combination of ultrasound and minimal flushing has greatly reduced both the length of the procedure and the need for extensive anesthesia. As a result, most of our patients now undergo oocyte collection under mild sedation, using Midazolam (Roche, Basle, Switzerland) as a relaxant and Fentanyl

(Jansen-Cilag, Sweden) to relieve pain. Both of these drugs have a short biological half-life, and their effects wear off quickly, allowing the patient to go home within 1 h of the procedure. Alternatives to sedation include the injection of local anesthetic, such as Lignocaine or Zylocaine, around the ovary or the use of epidural analgesia. However, the former is often ineffective, it may blur the ultrasound view, and it may have toxic effects, while the latter is a major procedure for a relatively minor operation, which may result in paralysis for up to 8 h, in occasional urinary retention, and in an overnight stay in the hospital.

III. TEMPERATURE CONTROL

The observation that a 10 min exposure to room temperatures results in spindle disruption and microtubule disassembly, which may lead to an abnormal distribution of chromosomes,[4] emphasizes the need for maintaining temperatures as close as possible to 37°C during the collection and handling of human oocytes. Throughout oocyte recovery, every effort should be made to ensure that the follicular aspirate is collected into prewarmed tubes and that the medium used for flushing the follicles is also kept at 37°C. To this end, we have developed a set of heating blocks, kept at 37°C, which provide spaces for the test tubes during fluid collection as well as for a flask containing flushing medium and a flushing syringe. The temperature of these blocks is always checked prior to the start of each procedure, and such checks should not be compromised for the sake of expedience. It is clearly impossible to prevent all temperature loss from the lines connecting the aspiration needle to the collection tube. Nevertheless, this system minimizes the extent to which the cumulus-oocyte complex is subjected to temperature fluctuations during its transition from the follicle to the test tube.

In most IVF clinics, laboratory manipulations take place in a bench top or free standing laminar flow cabinet, and, at the very least, the stage of the microscope should be covered by a warm plate and the petri dishes preheated in a hot box at 37°C and kept warm on a warming tray. More recently, a Danish company (Henning Knudsen Engineering, Denmark) has designed a laminar flow bench in which part of the table plate is maintained at 37°C. The stereomicroscope is built into the table plate, thus obviating the need for an additional warm stage, and, similarly, the petri dishes can be heated on the table plate. Although this approach goes some way towards improving conditions for the oocytes, they are still suboptimal. By contrast, a humidicrib or isolette enables all procedures to be performed in a humidified, gassed environment maintained at 37°C without the need for additional warm plates or stages. The concept of using a modified baby incubator in this way was first described by Testart et al.,[5] and elegant commercial versions complete with stereomicroscope and 5% CO_2 controller are now available. The advantages of an enclosed, carefully controlled environment for handling oocytes and embryos are immediately apparent. The disadvantages of having to equilibrate the system for 60 min before use and of working in a confined space are soon overcome, and, in our hands, the reliability and mobility of such a unit has enabled both IVF and GIFT to be performed successfully in satellite clinics lacking the normal laboratory facilities.

IV. FOLLICLE FLUSHING

The flushing of follicles during oocyte recovery is no longer a routine procedure and in many units has been abandoned altogether.[6] Where there are many follicles present in the ovary, it is now common practice to aspirate a number of follicles in quick succession and to use the fluid from one follicle to "flush" another. Under these conditions, there is no significant difference in the number of oocytes recovered with or without flushing. However, in natural and in poorly stimulated cycles where follicle numbers are low, it is advisable to aspirate and flush each individual follicle until an oocyte is obtained. The media used for flushing vary from phosphate buffered saline to simple salt solutions (i.e., Earle's solution, Whittingham's T6, Human Tubal Fluid;[7] see Chapter 5) buffered with HEPES. In all cases, the medium should be supplemented with Heparin to prevent clotting and contain penicillin and streptomycin, should have an osmolarity of 280 to 284 mOsmol, and, should have passed through a 0.22 μm filter. The make of syringe used for flushing is also of some importance. To avoid possible toxicity associated with syringes containing rubber plungers and siloxane lubricants, we have routinely used glass syringes washed and sterilized under the same stringent conditions used for tissue culture glassware. These have now been superceded by disposable two-piece syringes (Injekt, Braun Medical Ltd., Germany).

V. OOCYTE IDENTIFICATION

Although there have been significant changes in the clinical techniques used for collecting oocytes, little has changed in the methods used in the laboratory for identifying the oocyte in the aspirate. All aspirates are collected into 16 ml test tubes (Falcon, Becton Dickinson Pty Ltd., Melbourne, Australia) and are kept in a warming block at 37°C prior to examination. The contents of the tubes are poured into 92 × 21 mm petri dishes (Nunclon, Nunc, Denmark) and examined under a stereomicroscope. The size of the expanded cumulus cell-oocyte complex makes it easily identifiable, even in the presence of red blood and granulosa cells. In fact, it is often easier to see the cumulus mass in fluid containing blood than in clear follicular fluid. Occasionally, small pieces of the cumulus mass may be detached from the main oocyte cell complex during recovery, and the latter is found in a different aspirate. Moreover, it is important to realize that in a luteinized follicle the granulosa cells may also be secreting large amounts of mucopolysaccharides and that these form sticky clumps which superficially resemble a cumulus mass. Indeed, during an oocyte collection, many IVF embryologists are often misled by the presence of this material and continually inform the clinician of the recovery of large numbers of cumulus cells. However, these clumps are easily distinguished from the cumulus mass by their transparent appearance and lack of cells.

Once the cumulus-oocyte mass is found, the degree of cumulus expansion and corona dispersal is assessed, and the appearance of the oocyte is noted. It is quite easy at this time to identify oocytes that are grossly misshapen, have a ruptured zona pellucida with oozing cytoplasm, or have a dark, centrally located accumulation of organelles that is so often indicative of meiotic immaturity. However, it is more difficult to visualize the polar body and the perivitelline space in most oocytes after recovery, and, as a result, oocytes are invariably graded for maturity on the basis of the morphological characteristics of the cumulus mass, the corona radiata, the ooplasm, and the detached granulosa cells (see Section VI.). After classification, the cumulus-oocyte complex is washed, either in HEPES-buffered medium or culture medium, and transferred to the incubation medium. It is important that as few red blood cells as possible are transferred with the cumulus mass, and, where necessary, contaminating blood clots and/or large amounts of attached granulosa cells should be removed using fine (25 gauge) needles. Oocytes may be maintained in HEPES-buffered medium throughout the recovery and then transferred to incubation medium. This minimizes pH and temperature shock to the oocytes and prevents the continuous opening and closing of the incubator door, which in itself may have deleterious consequences.[8]

VI. ASSESSMENT OF OOCYTE MATURATION

The distinctive features used to classify the oocyte-cumulus cell complex as either immature (Grade 1), intermediate (Grade 2), mature (Grade 3), postmature (Grade 4), or atretic (Grade 5) are summarized in Table 1 and incorporate the criteria described in previous studies.[9-13]

It is well known that the majority of oocytes derived from complexes with a dense, poorly expanded cumulus and tight corona are immature, with an intact germinal vesicle (GV).[13] Moreover, in unstimulated cycles, there is a good correlation between the degree of cumulus expansion and coronal dispersal and the meiotic status of the oocyte, such that 95% of the oocytes associated with expanded mature complexes are at metaphase II (MII).[14] However, there is a marked asynchrony in follicular development in stimulated cycles[15] which results in different degrees of cumulus cell complex mucification at the time of aspiration.[11,14,16] To add to the confusion, this interfollicular asynchrony in cumulus morphology may also be associated with an intrafollicular asynchrony between the degree of cumulus cell dissociation and oocyte maturation, which then leads to further inaccuracies in the assessment of oocyte maturity. Thus, cumulus-oocyte complexes described as "mature" at aspiration may contain oocytes with an intact GV, or they may have progressed to metaphase I (MI), where germinal vesicle breakdown (GVBD) has occurred, but the first polar body has not been emitted. By

TABLE 1
Morphological Parameters Used for Assessment of Oocyte Maturity

Oocyte status	Grade	Description	In vitro maturation time (h)
Immature	1	Poorly expanded, dense compact cumulus; compact and adherent not radiating corona; aggregated granulosa cells; oocyte obscured; GV observed; cytoplasm may be dark with clumped organelles	24–30
Intermediate	2	Expanded cumulus and slightly compact corona (? partially radiating); well-dispersed granulosa; oocyte may be visible	6–24
Mature	3	Very expanded cumulus and well-dispersed radiating corona, evenly distributed around oocyte; loosely aggregated granulosa; clear zona and ooplasm; polar body visible	4–6
Postmature	4	Expanded cumulus with clumps of cells; radiant corona but often clumped, irregular, and incomplete; visible zona; ooplasm may be granular or dark	4–6
Atretic	5	Absent cumulus or present in small amounts: aggregated; corona, if present, is clumped and irregular; dark, misshapen ooplasm; visible zona	4–6

contrast, oocytes recovered in an intermediate cumulus mass may have completed meiosis and have reached the MII stage with a polar body.[11] Such discrepancies may be partially explained by differences in the dissociation rates of cumulus and corona cells after human chorionic gonadotrophin (hCG) injection and the difficulty of distinguishing, under the stereomicroscope, the subtle change in cumulus cell density associated with the progress of the oocyte from MI to MII. The relationship between cumulus/corona dissociation and the resumption of meiosis after hCG has been described by Bomsel-Helmreich et al.[16] and is summarized in Table 2. At the time of hCG administration (0 h), the oocyte has an intact GV and the densities of the cumulus and corona cells are the same. At 8 h after hCG, the oocyte remains unchanged, even though some dissociation of the cumulus and corona cells has occurred. Dissociation of the cumulus and corona cells continues at a similar rate until 15 h after hCG, when the resumption of meiosis is accompanied by a marked increase in the dissociation rate of the cumulus cells. Thus, by 20 h after hCG, the oocyte has reached MI and the cumulus cell density has fallen to 210 + 15 cells/mm^2. By contrast, the corona has a much higher density than the cumulus (2035 + 128 cells/mm^2). At 35 h, the oocyte is at MII, and the cumulus has dissociated further to 41 + 7 cells/mm^2, although the corona still shows a higher cell density. The difference in density of cumulus cells at 20 h after hCG compared to 35 h (210 vs. 40

TABLE 2
Timing of Cumulus and Corona Cell Dissociation

Hours post hCG	Stage of meiosis	Cell density/mm^2	
		Cumulus	Corona
0	GV	6908 ± 180	6929 ± 262
8	GV	5096 ± 127	5551 ± 143
20	MI	210 ± 15	2035 ± 128
35	MII	41 ± 7	1147 ± 110

From Bomsel-Helmreich, O., Huyen, L. V. N., Durand-Gasselin, I., Salat-Baroux, J., and Antoine, J.-M., *Fertil, Steril,* 48, 586, 1987. With permission.

cells/mm^2) is not detectable by stereomicroscopic observation, and, consequently, a cumulus mass may appear completely dissociated even though the oocyte is still at MI.

VII. DIRECT DETERMINATION OF NUCLEAR MATURITY IN OOCYTES

It is clear from the preceding section that the morphological assessment of the cumulus/corona cell complex provides only an approximation of oocyte maturity. While this approach has proved fairly satisfactory for most IVF clinics, there is no doubt that many oocytes will be inseminated prematurely, particularly when standardized times from recovery to insemination are used. The correct timing of insemination with respect to the completion of maturation has been emphasized in studies where immature (GV and MI) oocytes have been penetrated by sperm but were incapable of supporting normal pronuclear development.[17,18] Moreover, there is some evidence to suggest that premature exposure of immature oocytes to sperm precludes their subsequent fertilization after reinsemination even though meiotic maturation to MII has been completed.[1] This may result from changes in the composition of the zona pellucida brought about by an untimely release of cortical granule contents.[19] The problems associated with premature or even postmature insemination may be partially overcome by staggering the insemination times of immature and intermediate cumulus complexes according to the criteria shown in Table 1. However, this will still result in a number of oocytes being inseminated at the incorrect time. It is obvious, therefore, that only the direct determination of the meiotic status of the oocyte will allow a more accurate timing of insemination. There are two techniques available for performing this examination, (1) "cumulus spreading" and (2) the removal of cumulus cells using hyaluronidase.

A. CUMULUS SPREADING

This technique and the results obtained from it have been described in considerable detail by Veeck.[20] Consequently, only the main points will be summarized here. Essentially, the procedure consists of placing the cumulus cell-oocyte complex in a small droplet of culture medium on the flat surface of a sterile petri dish and, by jarring the dish, spreading the medium and flattening the cumulus mass. The oocyte is then examined under an inverted microscope for evidence of maturity. It is important that good optics, preferably phase contrast or Nomarski interference, are used and that the cumulus cells are well spread. Under these conditions, it is possible to distinguish the presence of the GV, the absence of both the GV and first polar body (MI), or the presence of the first polar body (MII). In addition, other characteristics of the oocyte, such as the size and degree of fragmentation of the polar body and the existence of vacuoles or refractile bodies in the cytoplasm, may be determined. These atypical morphologies are of some considerable interest since they are associated with anomalies at fertilization.[20]

Examination of the oocyte should be performed as rapidly as possible to minimize pH and temperature changes. We have found it more convenient to carry out these procedures in HEPES-buffered medium and have observed that this does not affect the fertilizability of the oocytes (Osborn, unpublished observations). After classification, the complex is resuspended with HEPES-buffered medium, washed with equilibrated culture medium, and returned to an equilibrated culture dish or tube. Invariably, some of the cumulus cells remain attached to the petri dish after spreading. Usually, this is not a problem. However, if desiccation of the complex occurs, through either prolonged observation times or excessive spreading of the cells, the oocyte may be severely damaged.

Insemination schedules and fertilization results for the various types of oocytes identified after flattening are shown in Table 3. It is assumed that a short period of time after extrusion of the first polar body is required by oocytes to gain full cytoplasmic competence before insemination. Consequently, oocytes at MII are inseminated 2 to 5 h after collection. By contrast, immature oocytes are examined every 2 to 3 h after collection and are inseminated 1 to 3 h after expulsion of the first polar body. Oocytes in which the meiotic status is undetermined but which have a highly expanded cumulus mass are inseminated at a fixed interval of 5 to 6 h after collection. The high fertilization rates shown in Table 3 emphasize the merits of staggered insemination. However, it is of interest to note that, even with prolonged culture, oocytes recovered at the GV or early MI stage show significantly lower rates of fertilization (Table 3).[21] Augmented maturation and fertilization of immature oocytes have been accomplished by the addition of gonadotrophins, epidermal growth factor, and granulosa cells to the culture medium[22-24] but without achieving evidence of improved developmental competence. However, a recent report has demonstrated that live births can occur after *in vitro* maturation of oocytes. Cha et al.[25] have shown that 56% of immature follicular oocytes recovered from unstimulated ovaries after ovariectomy and cultured in medium containing 50% preovulatory follicular fluid matured to MII. Of these, 81% fertilized, 64% cleaved normally, and, in one patient with premature ovarian failure, the

TABLE 3
Comparison of Fertilization Outcomes According to Meiotic Stage of Maturation at Oocyte Collection

Meiotic status at collection	Number examined	Interval between collection and insemination (h)	Percent fertilized	Percent triploidy
MII	1811	2–5	92	7
Undetermined	532	5–6	90	9
MI	516	3–7	86	8
MI	468	8–15	84	5
MI	234	>15	69	5
GV	1137	24–30	49	4

From Veeck, L., *Ann. N.Y. Acad. Sci.*, 541, 259, 1988. With permission.

transfer of five embryos from *in vitro* matured oocytes resulted in the birth of triplets. We have repeated this work and have demonstrated similar rates of maturation and fertilization *in vitro* (Osborn and Trounson, unpublished observations). Although it is possible that the developmental potential of immature GV oocytes recovered in stimulated cycles could also be improved by being cultured in mature follicular fluid, there is a clear distinction between these oocytes and those collected in an unstimulated cycle, in that the former have been exposed to hCG *in vivo*.

The cumulus spreading technique allows the identification of the nuclear status of the oocyte without any detrimental effect on fertilization, development, or pregnancy rates.[20,21] Indeed, a more accurate timing of insemination is associated with increased fertilization rates (Table 2). The disadvantage of the technique is that it is very time-consuming, requiring repetition of the procedure every 2 to 3 h, thereby increasing the number of pH and temperature shifts to which the oocyte is exposed.

B. REMOVAL OF CUMULUS CELLS USING HYALURONIDASE

The use of hyaluronidase to free oocytes of their cumulus cells and assess their meiotic maturity was first described by Laufer et al.[11] They observed that, in HMG-stimulated cycles, only 39% of oocytes were at MII immediately after aspiration and that a clear asynchrony existed between the degree of cumulus expansion and the stage of meiotic maturation. However, after 8 h of preincubation, 73% of the oocytes were at MII, and 87% of these fertilized. In a more recent study, Howlett and Rogers[26] used bovine hyaluronidase to determine the relationship between cumulus grading and meiotic status in clomiphene citrate (CC)/HMG cycles. As expected, cumulus-oocyte complexes scored as "good" contained the highest proportion of MII oocytes, while those evaluated as "poor" had mostly immature (GV/MI) oocytes. Again, fertilization rates of MII oocytes after enzymatic removal of cumulus cells were equivalent to those of cumulus-enclosed oocytes. Over the past two years, we have used hyaluronidase to examine the relationship between the meiotic status of the oocyte, the time after oocyte collection, and the ovarian stimulation regimen. We have modified previously described methods to minimize possible erosion of the zona pellucida and to leave most of the corona radiata intact. Our technique involves the following steps:

1. Dissolve 50 IU (1 vial) of leech hyaluronidase (Sigma Chemical Co., St. Louis, MO) in 8 ml of HEPES-buffered medium 7 to give 6.25 IU/ml. Add 2 µl of a stock solution of 40 mg/ml trypsin inhibitor (Sigma Chemical Co., St. Louis, MO) to give a final concentration of 0.01 mg/ml. Dispense 0.5 ml aliquots into 5 ml Falcon tubes and freeze at − 20°C until use.
2. Approximately 1 h before the intended time of cumulus removal, thaw an aliquot of hyaluronidase and dilute 1:2 with HEPES-buffered medium containing 10% heat inactivated serum. The hyaluronidase solution, now at a concentration of ~3 IU/ml is placed in the upper left hand well of a Nunc 4-well dish and HEPES-buffered medium with serum is placed in the remaining three wells. All solutions are warmed to 37°C before use.
3. Cumulus cell-oocyte complexes, either singly or in groups, are placed in the enzyme solution and gently pipetted up and down, using a 9 in. Pasteur pipette, until the cumulus mass begins to disperse (usually 3 to 5 min).
4. Using a hand-drawn pipette with a bore slightly larger than the diameter of the oocyte and corona cells, the oocyte is removed from the dispersed cumulus and washed through the three changes of buffered medium.
5. Oocytes are examined for the presence of the first polar body, using either the stereo or inverted microscope. Where necessary, the number of corona cells can be further reduced using a series of drawn pipettes until the oocyte is clearly visualized. This is often the case for MI oocytes or MII oocytes with small or fragmented polar bodies. Care should always be taken not to disrupt the integrity of the zona pellucida.
6. After assessment, oocytes are washed in and then transferred to incubation medium. Depending on the time of cumulus removal relative to oocyte recovery, MII oocytes are usually inseminated 4 to 6 h after collection.

As in "cumulus spreading," GV and MI oocytes still need constant reassessment for extrusion of the first polar body. However, a distinct advantage of using hyaluronidase is that the oocytes are not subjected to the frequent handling inherent in the "spreading" technique and can be examined while still in incubation medium.

Hyaluronidase is now routinely used in our clinic for the removal of cumulus cells prior to microinjection or insemination with male factor sperm and when cumulus-oocyte complexes are categorized as immature after collection. To date, the technique has not been adopted for determining nuclear maturity

TABLE 4
Distribution of Meiotic Stages in Human Oocytes Examined at Different Times after Recovery

Time after oocyte recovery (h)	Number of oocytes	Meiotic stage (%)		
		GV	MI	MII
0–2	205	16.1	20.5	63.4[a]
2–4	268	14.6	7.1	78.4[b]
4–6	107	10.3	4.7	85.0[bc]
6–8	64	3.1	14.1	82.8[bcd]
Total	644	13.2	11.7	75.2

Note: Different superscripts indicate significant differences ($p < 0.01$) between rows in proportion of mature (MII) oocytes

in all collected oocytes as there remains some anxiety that hyaluronidase may compromise the fertilizability of some oocytes. However, it is clear that there is no significant difference in either the cleavage or pregnancy rates of those oocytes that do fertilize as compared to cumulus-enclosed oocytes (Osborn, unpublished observations).

VIII. TIMING OF INSEMINATION

Despite the clear evidence that the maturity of the oocyte affects the subsequent outcome in terms of both oocyte fertilizability and embryo quality,[11,20,21] there remains some controversy in the literature over the need for a period of culture *in vitro* between oocyte collection and insemination. On the one hand, it has been shown that, irrespective of the stage of oocyte maturation, the fertilization rate is not significantly influenced by the duration of the preinsemination interval.[27,28] Conversely, other authors have observed that a short delay in insemination of between 4 to 6 h minimizes the incidence of polyspermic fertilization and increases the proportion of oocytes that fertilize normally and implant.[29-31] There is no doubt that meiotically immature oocytes are severely compromised by premature exposure to spermaotozoa. Delayed fertilization, cleavage failure, and fragmentation are common sequelae of attempted fertilization of immature oocytes.[32,33] However, it is also apparent that meiotically mature oocytes still benefit from a few hours of preincubation for completion of the events associated with meiotic (Table 4) and cytoplasmic maturation[20,34,35] and that fertilization rates are significantly increased after a delay of 4 h (Table 5). It is of interest to note that increasing the maturation time *in vivo* by extending the hCG/oocyte retrieval interval from 36 h to 39 h does not increase the risk of preoperative ovulation[36] and may obviate the need for preinsemination incubation of the oocytes.[31]

TABLE 5
Fertilization Rates in Relation to Time of Insemination

Time after oocyte recovery (h)	Number of oocytes	Number and % fertilized	Number and % polyspermic
0–1	119	76 (63.9)[a]	5 (4.2)
1–4	227	166 (73.1)[a]	8 (3.5)
>4	781	622 (79.6)[b]	62 (7.9)
Total	1127	864 (76.7)	75 (6.7)

Note: [a] versus [b] ($p < 0.03$)

IX. PREPARATION OF OOCYTES FOR GIFT

Since the first description of the gamete intrafallopian transfer (GIFT) technique by Asch et al.,[37] there have been a great many reports in the literature establishing its efficacy in the alleviation of infertility in couples where the female partner has at least one patent fallopian tube. The variables affecting the probability of pregnancy with GIFT have been analyzed in several studies using large numbers of patients,[38-40] and, as in IVF, the age of the female partner and the number of oocytes transferred are important prognostic factors associated with success rates. However, GIFT differs from IVF in that the oocytes are exposed to and transferred with spermatozoa to the fallopian tube usually within 30 min of recovery. The inability of immature oocytes to fertilize normally after premature insemination has already been discussed and emphasizes the need for meiotically mature oocytes to be selected for GIFT. Indeed, the transfer of mature oocytes is critical, and there is an important association between the number of fully mature oocytes transferred and pregnancy rates.[41] Thus, if only immature oocytes are recovered (i.e., Grades 1 and 2 in Table 1), careful consideration should be given to either abandoning the GIFT attempt and proceeding with *in vitro* maturation followed by IVF with subsequent tubal transfer of zygotes[42] or embryos[43] or placing the oocytes into the tubes without spermatozoa, followed by delayed intrauterine insemination.[44]

The loading of the catheter for gamete transfer is quite straight forward. At the Infertility Medical Centre, we use the Cook Teflon GIFT catheter (William Cook, Melbourne, Australia), which is 5-French in gauge and 45 cm in length and has markings placed at 2 and 4 cm from the tip of the catheter which aid accurate placement of the gametes within the ampullary lumen of the fallopian tube. Prior to loading, the catheter is rinsed with HTF or similar medium and loaded sequentially with (1) a small air space (<5 μl), (2) an aliquot of sperm suspension containing 100 to 150,000 progressively motile sperm, (3) another small air space, (4) oocytes, (5) another air space, and finally (6) a small volume of medium. The total transfer volume varies depending on the sperm concentration (i.e., larger volumes and numbers of sperm may be needed for male factor patients) and the number and size of the cumulus-oocyte masses, but should not exceed 75µl. If necessary, the overall volume can be reduced by either omitting the air spaces and/or loading the oocytes into the catheter in the sperm suspension. In most clinics, oocytes are maintained in bicarbonate-buffered culture medium with 10% heat-inactivated maternal serum during oocyte recovery, and the selection of mature oocytes for transfer is accomplished using the criteria described in Table 1. However, oocytes have also been collected and transferred in HEPES-buffered medium and filtered preovulatory follicular fluid without compromising the outcome.[45,46]

Catheterization of the fallopian tubes is generally performed at laparoscopy under a general anesthetic, and it is important that the gametes are not expelled until the catheter is deep inside the lumen of the tube. Previously, gametes were transferred to both tubes during the GIFT procedure. However, a comparison of unilateral vs. bilateral tubal cannulation has shown no difference in pregnancy rates,[47] and unilateral transfer is now the method of choice in our clinic. The hope for the future is that GIFT will be routinely carried out non-surgically using a transvaginal ultrasound-probe to guide the catheter into the tubal isthmus. Although the advantages of this technique are self-evident and a number of pregnancies have been reported,[48] the results have not so far proved superior to the conventional GIFT procedure.

As an alternative to GIFT, several groups have evaluated the efficacy of directly transferring gametes into the uterus or peritoneal cavity. These procedures, known colloquially as DOST (Direct Oocyte-Sperm Transfer),[49] TOAST (Transcervical Oocyte and Sperm Transfer; Grudzinskas, personal communication), and POST (Peritoneal Oocyte and Sperm Transfer)[50] have all been performed on relatively small groups of patients in uncontrolled studies, and their merits are debatable. Nevertheless, pregnancies have been obtained using these techniques, and some consideration should be given perhaps to comparing them with GIFT in a randomized prospective manner to establish their role relative to the latter. However, the advantages of these procedures as outpatient or office-based alternatives to GIFT are less apparent if the development of ultrasound-GIFT is successful.

X. CONCLUSIONS

The use of ultrasound, day surgeries, and mild anesthesia have all had a major impact, from both the patient's and clinician's perspective, on the procedure of oocyte collection. By contrast, the techniques involved in the identification and assessment of the oocyte have to a great extent remained unchanged in most clinics. It is clear that an unavoidable consequence of the asynchrony in follicle development induced by superovulation is the recovery of oocytes at differing stages of maturation. The use of standardized periods of time from collection to insemination will therefore result in many oocytes being exposed to spermatozoa prematurely, resulting in low or abnormal rates of fertilization. Correct identification of the meiotic status of the oocyte therefore plays a crucial role in maximizing the chances of normal fertilization and embryonic development.

REFERENCES

1. **Tesarik, J., Pilka, L., and Travnik, P.,** Zona pellucida resistance to sperm penetration before the completion of human oocyte maturation, *J. Reprod. Fertil.,* 83, 487, 1988.
2. **Wikland, M., Lennart, E., and Hamberger, L.,** Transvesical and transvaginal approaches for the aspiration of follicles by the use of ultrasound, *Ann. N.Y. Acad. Sci.,* 442, 182, 1985.
3. **Lowe, B., Osborn, J. C., Fothergill, D. J., and Lieberman, B. A.,** Factors associated with accidental fractures of the zona pellucida and multipronuclear human oocytes following in-vitro fertilization, *Hum. Reprod.,* 3, 901, 1988.
4. **Pickering, S.J., Braude, P. R., Johnson, M. H., Cant, A., and Currie, J.,** Transient cooling to room temperature can cause irreversible disruption of the meiotic spindle in the human oocyte, *Fertil. Steril.,* 43, 255, 1990.
5. **Testart, J., Lassalle, B., and Frydman, R.,** Apparatus for the in vitro fertilization and culture of human oocytes, *Fertil. Steril.,* 38, 372, 1982.
6. **Kingsland, C. R., Taylor, C. T., Aziz, N., and Bickerton, N.,** Is follicular flushing necessary for oocyte retrieval? A randomized trial, *Hum. Reprod.,* 6, 382, 1991.
7. **Trounson, A. O.,** Fertilization and embryo culture, in *Clinical in vitro Fertilization*, Wood, C. and Trounson, A. O., Eds., Springer-Verlag, Berlin, 1989, 30.
8. **Gardner, D. K. and Lane, M.,** unpublished data, 1992.
9. **Ben-Rafael, Z., Kopf, G. S., Blasco, L., Flickinger, G. L., Tureck, R. W., Strauss, J. F., and Mastroianni, L.,** Follicular maturation parameters associated with the failure of oocyte retrieval, fertilization and cleavage in vitro, *Fertil. Steril.,* 45, 51, 1986.
10. **Hill, G. A., Freeman, M., Bastias, M. C., Rogers, B. J., Herbert, C. M., Osteen, K. G., and Wentz, A. C.,** The influence of oocyte maturity and embryo quality on pregnancy rate in a program for in vitro fertilization-embryo transfer, *Fertil. Steril.,* 52, 801, 1989.
11. **Laufer, N., Tarlatzis, B. C., DeCherney. A. H., Masters, J. T., Haseltine, FF. P., MacLusky, N., and Naftolin, F.,** Asynchrony between human cumulus-corona cell complex and oocyte maturation after human menopausal gonadotrophin treatment for in vitro fertilization, *Fertil. Steril.,* 42, 366, 1984.
12. **Marrs, R. P., Saito, H., Yee, B., Sato, F., and Brown, J.,** Effect of variation of in vitro culture techniques upon oocyte fertilization and embryo development in human in vitro fertilization procedures, *Fertil. Steril.,* 41, 519, 1984.
13. **Veeck, L. L., Wortham, J. W. E., Jr., Witmyer, J., Sandow, B. A., Acosta, A. A., Garcia, J. E., Jones, G. S., and Jones, H. W., Jr.,** Maturation and fertilization of morphologically immature human oocytes in a program of in vitro fertilization, *Fertil. Steril.,* 39, 594, 1983.
14. **Testart, J., Frydman, R., DeMouzon, J., Lassalle, B., and Belaisch, J. C.,** A study of factors affecting the success of human fertilization in vitro. I. Influence of ovarian stimulation upon the number and condition of oocytes collected, *Biol. Reprod.,* 28, 415, 1983.
15. **Hillier, S. G., Afnan, A. M., Margara, R. A., and Winston, R. M.,** Superovulation strategy before in vitro fertilization, *Clin. Obstet. Gynaecol.,* 12, 687, 1985.
16. **Bomsel-Helmreich, O., Huyen, L. V. N., Durand-Gasselin, I., Salat-Baroux, J., and Antoine, J.-M.,** Timing of nuclear maturation and cumulus dissociation in human oocytes stimulated with clomiphene citrate, human menopausal gonadotrophin and human chorionic gonadotrophin, *Fertil. Steril.,* 48, 586, 1987.
17. **Lopata, A. and Leung, P.C.,** The fertilizability of human oocytes at different stages of meiotic maturation, *Ann. N.Y. Acad. Sci.,* 541, 324, 1988.

18. Tesarik, J. and Kopecny, V., Developmental control of the human male pronucleus by ooplasmic factors, *Hum. Reprod.*, 4, 962, 1989.
19. Shabanowitz, R. B. and O'Rand, M. G., Characterization of the human zona pellucida from fertilized and unfertilized eggs, *J. Reprod. Fertil.*, 82, 151, 1988.
20. Veeck, L., Oocyte assessment and biological performance, *Ann. N.Y. Acad. Sci.*, 541, 259, 1988.
21. Flood, J. T., Chillik, C. F., van Uem, J. F. H. M., Iritani, A., and Hodgen, G. D., Ooplasmic transfusion: prophase germinal vesicle oocytes made developmentally competent by microinjection of metaphase II egg cytoplasm, *Fertil. Steril.*, 53, 1049, 1990.
22. Prins, G. S., Wager, C., Weigal, L., Gianfortoni, J., Marut, E. L., and Scommegna, A., Gonadotrophins augment maturation and fertilization of human immature oocytes cultured *in vitro*, *Fertil. Steril.*, 47, 1035, 1987.
23. Das, K., Stout, L. E., Hensleigh, H. C., Tagatz, G. E., Phipps, W. R., and Leung, B. S., Direct positive effect of epidermal growth factor on the cytoplasmic maturation of mouse and human oocytes, *Fertil. Steril.*, 55, 1000, 1991.
24. Dandekar, P. V., Martin, M. C., and Glass, R. H., Maturation of immature oocytes by coculture with granulosa cells, *Fertil. Steril.*, 55, 95, 1991.
25. Cha, K. Y., Koo, J. J., Ko, J. J., Choi, D. H., Han, S. Y., and Yoon, T. K., Pregnancy after in vitro fertilization of human follicular oocytes collected from non-stimulated cycles, their culture in vitro and their transfer in a donor oocyte program, *Fertil. Steril.*, 55, 109, 1991.
26. Howlett, D. and Rogers, P. A. W., The use of hyaluronidase to assess oocyte maturity in an in vitro programme, *JIVET*, 3, 135, 1986.
27. Harrison. K. L., Wilson, L. M., Breen, T. M., Pope, A. K., Cummins, J. M., and Hennessey, J. F., Fertilization of human oocytes in relation to varying delay before insemination, *Fertil. Steril.*, 50, 294, 1988.
28. Fisch, B., Kaplan-Kraicer, R., Amit, S., Ovadia J., and Tadir, Y., The effect of preinsemination interval upon fertilization of human oocytes in vitro, *Hum. Reprod.*, 4, 954, 1989.
29. Trounson, A. O., Mohr, L. R., Wood, C., and Leeton, J. F., Effect of delayed insemination on in vitro fertilization, culture and transfer of human embryos, *J. Reprod. Fertil.*, 64, 285, 1982.
30. Khan, I., Staessen, C., Van den Abbeel, E., Camus, M., Wisanto, A., Smitz, J., Devroey, P., and Van Steirteghe, A. C., Time of insemination and its effect on in-vitro fertilization, cleavage and pregnancy rates in GnRH agonist/HMG-stimulated cycles, *Hum. Reprod.*, 4, 921, 1989.
31. Jamieson, M. E., Fleming, R., Kader, S., Ross, K. S., Yates, R. W. S., and Coutts, J. R. T., In vivo and in vitro maturation of human oocytes: effects on embryo development and polyspermic fertilization, *Fertil. Steril.*, 56, 93, 1991.
32. Trounson, A. O., Willadsen, S. M., and Rowson, L. E. A., Fertilization and developmental capability of bovine follicular oocytes matured in vitro and in vivo and transferred to oviducts of the rabbit and cow, *J. Reprod. Fertil.*, 51, 321, 1977.
33. Zenzes, M. T., Belkien, L., Bordt, J., Kan, I., Schneider, H. P. G., and Nieschlag, E., Cytologic investigation of human in vitro fertilization failures, *Fertil. Steril.*, 43, 883, 1985.
34. Sathananthan, A. H. and Trounson, A. O., Ultrastructure of cortical granule release and zona interaction in monospermic and polyspermic human ova fertilized in vitro, *Gamete Res.*, 6, 225, 1982.
35. Sundstrom, P. and Nilsson, B. O., Meiotic and cytoplasmic maturation of oocytes collected in stimulated cycles is asynchronous, *Hum. Reprod.*, 3, 613, 1988.

36. **Gudmundsson, J., Fleming, R., Jamieson, M. E., McQueen, D., and Coutts, J. R. T.,** Luteinization to oocyte retrieval delay in women in whom multiple follicular growth was induced as part of an in vitro fertilization/gamete intrafallopian transfer program, *Fertil. Steril.*, 53, 735, 1990.
37. **Asch, R. H., Ellsworth, L. R., Balmaceda, J. P., and Wong, P. C.,** Pregnancy after translaparoscopic gamete intrafallopian transfer, *Lancet*, II, 1034, 1984.
38. **Asch, R. H., Balmaceda, J. P., Cittadini, E., Casas, P. F., Gomel, V., Hohl, M. K., Johnston, I., Leeton, J., Escudero, F. J. R., Noss, U., and Wong, P. C.,** Gamete intrafallopian transfer. International cooperative study of the first 800 cases, *Ann. N.Y. Acad. Sci.*, 541, 723, 1988.
39. **Craft, I. and Brinsden, P.,** Alternatives to IVF: the outcome of 1071 first GIFT procedures, *Hum. Reprod.*, 4 (Suppl.), 29, 1989.
40. **Jansen, R. P. S., Anderson, J. C., Birrell, W. S. R., Lyneham, R. C., Sutherland, P. D., Turner, M., Flowers, D., and Ciancaglini, E.,** Outpatient gamete intrafallopian transfer: a clinical analysis of 710 cases, *Med. J. Aust.*, 153, 182, 1990.
41. **Guzick, D. S., Balmaceda, J. P., Ord, T., and Asch, R. H.,** The importance of egg and sperm factors in predicting the likelihood of pregnancy from gamete intrafallopian transfer, *Fertil. Steril.*, 52, 795, 1989.
42. **Yovich, J. L., Blackledge, D. G., Richardson, P. A., Matson, P. L., Turner, S. R., and Draper, R.,** Pregnancies following pronuclear stage tubal transfer, *Fertil. Steril.*, 48, 851, 1987.
43. **Balmaceda, J. P., Gastaldi, C., Remohi, J., Borrero, C., Ord, T., and Asch, R. H.,** Tubal embryo transfer as a treatment for infertility due to male factor, *Fertil. Steril.*, 50, 476, 1988.
44. **Leung, C. K. M., Leong, M. K. H., Chan, Y. M., Wong, C. J. Y., Chan, H. H. Y., and Tucker, M. J.,** Fallopian replacement of eggs with delayed intrauterine insemination (FREDI): an alternative to gamete intrafallopian transfer (GIFT), *JIVET*, 6, 129, 1989.
45. **Yee, B., Rosen, G. F., Chacon, R. R., Soubra, S., and Stone, S. C.,** Gamete intrafallopian transfer: the effect of the number of eggs used and the depth of gamete placement on pregnancy initiation, *Fertil. Steril.*, 52, 639, 1989.
46. **Tucker, M. J., Chan, Y. M., Chan, S. Y. W., Wong, C. J. Y., Mao, K. R., Leong, M. K. H., and Leung, C. K. M.,** The use of human follicular fluid in gamete intrafallopian transfer, *Hum. Reprod.*, 4, 931, 1989.
47. **Haines, C. J. and O'Shea, R. T.,** The effect of unilateral versus bilateral tubal cannulation and the number of oocytes transferred on the outcome of gamete intrafallopian transfer, *Fertil. Steril.*, 55, 423, 1991.
48. **Risquez, F., Mathieson, J., and Zorn, J.-R.,** Tubal cannulation via the cervix: a passing fancy — or here to stay? *JIVET*, 7, 301, 1990.
49. **Sterzik, K., Rosenbusch, B., Grab, D., and Lauritzen, C.,** Pregnancies following direct oocyte-sperm transfer (DOST): a simple alternative to conventional in vitro fertilization (IVF), *JIVET*, 8, 241, 1991.
50. **Sharma, V., Pampiglione, J. S., Mason, B. A., Campbell, S., and, Riddle, A.,** Experience with peritoneal oocyte and sperm transfer as an outpatient-based treatment for infertility, *Fertil. Steril.*, 55, 579, 1991.

Chapter 3

PREPARATION AND ANALYSIS OF SEMEN FOR IVF/GIFT

H. W. G. Baker, F. L. H. Ng, and D. Y. Liu

TABLE OF CONTENTS

I.	Introduction	34
II.	Pre-IVF Evaluation	34
	A. Clinical Examination of the Man	34
	1. Male Sterility	34
	2. Treatable Conditions	35
	3. Male Subfertility	36
	B. Analysis of Semen	37
	1. Evidence of Infection in the Semen	37
	C. New Sperm Function Tests	38
	1. Sperm Morphology	38
	2. Sperm Motility and Movement Characteristics	39
	3. Acrosomal Status	40
	4. Sperm-Zona Pellucida Binding	42
	5. Relationship Between Sperm Function Tests and IVF Rates	42
III.	Sperm Preparation for IVF	44
	A. IVF Procedures and Modifications	44
	B. Special Collection Problems	45
	C. Principles of Sperm Preparation	45
	D. Preparation Procedures	46
	1. Collection of Semen for IVF	48
	2. Swim-Up Preparation	48
	3. Percoll and Mini-Percoll Gradients	49
	4. Combination of Mini-Percoll and Swim-Up	50
	E. Use of Motility Stimulants	50
IV.	Future Advances	50
	References	51

I. INTRODUCTION

Over the last ten years, *in vitro* fertilization (IVF) has become an established method for management of infertility of diverse causes, ranging from obstruction of the fallopian tubes to idiopathic or poorly explained infertility and male infertility of mild to moderate severity. Methods are being developed for use of sperm aspirated from the testis or epididymis and for micromanipulation of oocytes to inseminate them with a single or small number of spermatozoa. A large amount of information is becoming available on the relationship between sperm function tests and the results of IVF. Also many variations on methods of sperm preparation have been described. Despite these advances, there has been no major improvement in the fertilization rate. Causes of failure of fertilization remain poorly understood. Few controlled trials have been undertaken, so that sperm preparation for IVF remains more of an art than a science. In this chapter we provide details for the practical evaluation and management of the male partner and some popular methods of sperm preparation. We also review selected aspects of tests of sperm function for the prediction of results of IVF and potential improvements in IVF procedures for male factor infertility.

II. PRE-IVF EVALUATION

A detailed fertility evaluation of both partners is necessary to determine the optimal method of treatment, to give some guide to the prognosis, and to ensure that no other treatment should be instituted before the IVF procedure. The male partner needs to be aware that he must provide semen of good quality on the day of oocyte collection, preferably by masturbation in a special room close to the IVF laboratory. Preliminary semen analyses provide an opportunity to identify problems with collection as well as to determine the quality of the semen and to perform trial preparations if necessary. Because of the variability of semen quality in men, several tests may be required if the semen is known to be abnormal or if the cause of the couple's infertility is not obvious. Occasionally, fertilization fails because of an unexpectedly poor semen sample on the day of IVF.

A. CLINICAL EXAMINATION OF THE MAN
The main purpose of the investigation of the male is to determine the potential fertility of his sperm; however, inquiry about the possibility of transmitting serious hereditary disorders or infection such as hepatitis or human immunodeficiency viruses should be considered. If there is a disorder in the male, this requires detailed investigation.[1,2] The types of male infertility are summarized in Table 1.

1. Male Sterility
Patients with primary seminiferous tubule failure of whatever cause are usually irreversibly sterile, with azoospermia and often testicular atrophy and

TABLE 1
Types of Male Infertility

Untreatable sterility	13%
Primary seminiferous tubule failure	12%
Total teratospermia and immotile sperm	1%
Treatable conditions	12%
Gonadotrophin deficiency	0.5%
Obstructive azoospermia	5%
Sperm autoimmunity	6%
Disorders of sexual function	0.5%
Reversible toxic effect	0.02%
Untreatable subfertility	75%
Oligospermia	38%
Asthenospermia and mixed teratospermia	37%

elevated serum FSH levels. The histological picture of the testis may include hyalinized tubules, Sertoli cell only syndrome, germ cell arrest, or severe hypospermatogenesis. Clinically significant androgen deficiency may also be present. For such men, parenting is only possible through the use of donor insemination or adoption. While artificial insemination with donor semen has reasonably good results, with pregnancy rates in the region of 10 to 15% per cycle, many clinics would now use IVF with donor sperm if pregnancy had not been achieved within 6 to 12 inseminations. This is to conserve precious donor semen, since usually the results of IVF are excellent, with high fertilization rates and pregnancy rates.[3]

2. Treatable Conditions

Gonadotropin deficiency, coital disorders, and reversible toxin effects (e.g., from treatment with Salazopyrin) are individually uncommon causes of male infertility, and rarely would IVF be needed in such situations. Obstructive azoospermia and sperm autoimmunity are more common and less successfully treated. Vasectomy reversals produce moderately successful results, although perhaps only 50% of couples have a pregnancy within 12 months of the operation. Often the failures are related to sperm autoimmunity, restenosis, unsuspected epididymal blockages, spermatogenic disorders, or female factors such as advanced age. Results of vasoepididymostomies for epididymal obstruction depend very much on the level of the obstruction. Those in the tail have reasonably good results, with approximately 50% of couples achieving a pregnancy within 12 to 24 months. Those obstructions in the head have poor results with perhaps only 30% having sperm in the semen and less than 10% producing a pregnancy within two years. Patients with unsuccessful vasovasostomies or vasoepididymostomies, obstructions in the head of the epididymis, or congenital absence of the vasa may be treated by epididymal sperm aspiration and IVF. Although good results have been achieved by one group with patients with congenital absence of the vasa, the general experience is that the fertilization (<35%) and pregnancy (2 to 5%) rates are low.[4,5] The addition of oocyte micromanipulation procedures may improve the results of IVF with epididymal sperm.

Men with sperm autoimmunity, with high levels of antisperm antibodies in their serum and coating their sperm, with inability of the sperm to penetrate normal mid-cycle cervical mucus usually have complete failure of fertilization *in vitro*. Treatment with glucocorticoids in high dose will reduce the antibody level and improve the semen quality in approximately 50% of men, and pregnancies occur during the therapy in about 25% of the wives.[6] If the semen quality improves and a pregnancy does not occur, then IVF may be worthwhile, especially if the level of antibodies on the surface of the sperm has been reduced. If the IgA immunobead test shows less than 80% of sperm with beads bound to the heads, normal fertilization rates are obtained.[7] Techniques for treating sperm *in vitro* to reduce the density of sperm antibodies on their surface have been unsuccessful in our hands. Oocyte micromanipulation procedures may be useful. There are a number of patients who have low level sperm antibodies that do not completely inhibit sperm mucus penetration. In these, normal fertilization rates can usually be obtained without glucocorticoid treatment. It is probably inappropriate to regard these patients as having immunological infertility. They are equivalent to the fertile men who have sperm antibodies present in their serum and on their sperm.

Possibly reversible factors contributing to poor semen analysis results should be detected: incorrect semen collection techniques, too short or too long an interval since previous ejaculation, previous illness, heavy alcohol consumption, obesity, frequent hot spa baths or saunas, and treatment with certain drugs such as Salazopyrin, some antibiotics, narcotics, and steroid hormones.

3. Male Subfertility

Other patients with poor semen quality can be divided into one of two groups. Those with too few sperm for standard IVF (less than two million motile sperm per ejaculate) may be treated in the future by microinjection procedures, but currently the results are very poor. In the remaining patients with more sperm, IVF can be attempted, but the results depend on the semen quality, and a number of groups have now found that sperm morphology is an important predictor of the success rate (see Section II.B).

It is important that both the man and the woman are psychologically prepared for the IVF procedure. As failure of fertilization is almost always caused by sperm defects, it is important that this possibility be broached with the couple, particularly if the semen tests are not absolutely normal. If the man has difficulty collecting semen, then he should practice or have other alternatives offered for collection of semen on the day.

Defects of sperm production of mild to moderate degree are treated reasonably successfully by IVF, but as the fertilization rates are often reduced, the number of pre-embryos for transfer or cryopreservation is reduced, and the overall expectation of pregnancy is lower than when normal semen is used. In general nothing can be done to improve semen quality in this group of patients. Many treatments have been used in the past, including operations for varicoceles, antibiotic treatment for low grade infections, and administration of anti-inflammatory agents, hormones, and nutritional supplements. None of these have been proven to improve semen quality.[8] Patients with obvious inflammation in the semen should be treated. Those with very variable semen quality might be able to have semen stored frozen as backup in case the semen quality is particularly poor on the day of IVF.

B. ANALYSIS OF SEMEN

Because of the variability of semen analysis results from day to day for the one man, it is recommended that at least two samples are analyzed, and these should be collected at least two weeks apart.[9] The duration of abstinence from ejaculation prior to the test should be between 48 h and 1 week. In some instances, shorter durations of abstinence may be valuable, e.g., with necrospermia or where there are sperm antibodies. Samples are collected in a special collection room near the laboratory. If the samples are collected at home or outside the hospital, it is important that they are delivered to the laboratory within 1 h and that the temperature of the sample is not allowed to fluctuate greatly. On cold days, it is preferable to carry the sample inside the clothing. Special sterile disposable plastic jars should be provided for the semen samples. The room for collection should be comfortable and should contain a toilet and hand washing facilities. It may be useful to provide a bed or couch, so that the wife could help with collections, or erotic pictures or video tapes.

1. Evidence of Infection in the Semen

In the past, much care was taken to ensure that there were no pathogenic organisms in the semen, and many samples were cultured for gonococci and other micro-organisms.[10] The usefulness of this approach is now suspect. It is probably reasonable to restrict detailed bacteriological evaluation to those patients in whom there are high white cell numbers in the semen, e.g., >2 million/ml polymorphs. Alternatively, those men with high white cell numbers could be treated with broad spectrum antibacterial agents prior to the IVF attempt. These agents must be chosen carefully, as a number of antibacterial agents do not get into the prostate and semen, and others may have antispermatogenic activity. Commonly used antibacterial agents are Erythromycin, 500 mg, three times a day for 1 week, followed by 250 mg, three times a day for 3 weeks, Doxycycline, 100 mg daily for 1 month, or Noroxin, 200 mg, twice daily for 1 month. Nitrofurantoin and some sulphonamides should not be used because of their antispermatogenic effects. Despite the concern that the infection in the semen might be transmitted to the recipient or might result in problems with the insemination or embryo cultures, IVF procedures have been remarkably free of problems with infection.

C. NEW SPERM FUNCTION TESTS

The standard semen analysis, including sperm concentration, motility, and morphology has been widely used as a fundamental indicator of male fertility. Although the results do not provide precise diagnostic or prognostic information for human fertility *in vivo* or *in vitro*, preliminary semen analysis for IVF is very important.[11-17] Because the results of semen analysis between ejaculates in the same man will vary widely[9] it is necessary to have several recent semen analyses conducted to determine the current quality of the semen before patients commence treatment.

Because of the limitations of standard semen analysis for predicting fertility, many other tests of human sperm function have been introduced to improve assessment. For example, improved sperm morphology assessment, objective measurement of motility, examination of acrosome status, and human sperm-zona binding tests have been reported to provide additional information for prediction of fertility *in vitro*.[18-24] It is important to realize that no single test of sperm function will predict fertility accurately, except where there is an absolute disorder affecting all sperm such as azoospermia or totally absent acrosomes. In other situations, groups of tests will be required to evaluate male fertility.

1. Sperm Morphology

The proportion of sperm with normal morphology has been considered to be the most significant factor related to fertilization rates *in vitro*.[18-24] However, the subjective microscopic method for assessing sperm morphology has led to large variations within and among technicians.[25] Although characteristics of morphologically normal and various abnormal forms have been defined,[26] the technician's experience and skill are extremely important for producing consistent and reliable results. The quality of preparation of the sperm smear and staining of the slides are also important factors influencing assessment of morphology. The errors may be reduced by improving the methods for preparation of the slides and for staining to produce high quality images. In our studies, the sperm were washed with normal saline to remove seminal plasma, the sperm concentration was adjusted to about 80 million/ml, the smear was checked to ensure an even spread of sperm on the slide, and the smear was fixed in 90% ethanol after air drying. Then the slide was stained with the Shorr method.[19,27] We believe it is important to remove the seminal plasma so that there is no stained protein background on the slide; it is also important to adjust the concentration of washed sperm to about 80 million/ml by using a different volume of semen for washing or dilution, according to the sperm concentration of individual semen samples. This method provides a very clear image for the technician to count normal and abnormal morphological sperm and avoids bias related to sperm density. Sperm morphology is considered normal on the following criteria: the head has an oval shape, the acrosomal region (light staining) is greater than half of the sperm head, and there are no abnormalities of tail and midpiece. This improved morphology assessment is similar to the strict scoring method of Kruger et al.[23] Thus, as well as the outline of the head, the density of nuclear stain and the appearance of the acrosomal region are important features of normal sperm morphology.[18,23,27] With our morphology assessment, men with ≥30% of sperm with normal morphology are considered normal; this is now the same as the WHO standard.[26] In general, subgrouping abnormal morphology is not necessary during routine semen analysis because this is of no clinical value and very time consuming. Although subjective methods for assessment of sperm morphology can result in large errors between different technicians and laboratories, these can be minimized by using standards for normal sperm morphology and quality control samples. Each laboratory must have its own standards, and a good technician must have consistent readings; the variation between different readings of the same slide should be less than 15%. Morphology assessment should improve with further development of objective methods for this assessment.[28,29]

Makler[30] has suggested that it may be more valuable clinically if sperm morphology were assessed in the motile subpopulation. In the standard procedure, morphology is determined on a preparation of fixed (immobilized) sperm, and one cannot tell whether morphologically abnormal sperm were previously motile or immotile. It is reported that sperm with abnormal morphology are twice as frequent in the immotile subpopulation as in the motile subpopulation.[30] This is consistent with reports that motile sperm selected by swim-up or Percoll gradient centrifugation techniques have significantly better morphology compared with sperm in the original semen.[31-33] Despite this, our studies showed that percentage normal morphology of sperm in semen had better predictive value for IVF rate than percentage normal morphology of motile sperm in the swim-up suspension. Katz and Overstreet[34] reported that morphologically normal sperm swim faster, straighter, and with higher tail beat frequencies than do morphologically abnormal sperm in semen. Furthermore, the velocity of morphologically normal sperm swimming in human cervical mucus was higher than that of abnormal sperm.[35]

Studies with the zona-free hamster oocyte penetration assay suggest that morphologically abnormal sperm have low fertilizing ability compared with those with normal morphology.[36-38] There is a negative correlation between the proportion of sperm with abnormal morphology and the results of the zona-free hamster oocyte penetration.[37,39] Similarly, we have found that the human zona is highly selective for binding of sperm with normal morphology.[40] Measurement of the head dimension of human sperm bound on the ZP showed that width and area (width × length) were significantly larger for sperm on the ZP than for sperm in the insemination medium. Assessment of the range of characteristics of sperm bound to the ZP should provide useful standards for the assessment of morphology of sperm in semen.[40]

2. Sperm Motility and Movement Characteristics

Sperm motility is also important for fertilizing ability. Sperm must be motile enough to penetrate through cervical mucus and to migrate through the female genital tract to the site of fertilization. Furthermore, sperm need to be motile enough to penetrate the cumulus and the ZP of the oocyte. Men with absolutely immotile sperm, for example those with Kartagener's syndrome, are sterile.[41] Although it has been known for a long time that fertile men have better sperm motility than infertile men,[42] motility was poorly correlated with fertility *in vivo* in a large survey using life table methods and in a study comparing subfertile men who produced a pregnancy with those who remained persistently infertile.[13,43] Motility had some predictive value only in men with sperm concentrations $<5 \times 10^6$/ml.[13] In our IVF program, percentage sperm motility was also poorly correlated with IVF rates when other sperm tests such as morphology were considered.[19,22] However, it is recognized that the microscopic method for assessing motility is subject to large errors. Also, detailed movement characteristics are not measured. Therefore, a number of objective techniques have been developed for assessing the kinetics of human sperm motility. These techniques include cinemicrography, videomicrography, and time-exposure photomicrography.[11,12,34,44,45] However, these methods are time consuming and difficult for routine assessment of sperm motility. Computer systems such as Cellsoft and Hamilton-Thron for computer assisted motility analysis provide objective measurements of sperm movement characteristics, such as average sperm velocities — curvilinear velocity (VCL), straight line velocity (VSL), and average path velocity (VAP), amplitude of lateral head (ALH) displacement, and tail beat cross frequency.[46]

With the older techniques, such as time-exposure photomicrography, it was reported that sperm velocity (VSL), linearity of progression (LIN), and ALH were useful predictors for male infertility.[11,12] Similarly, Holt et al.[47] reported that the swimming speed (VCL) of ejaculated sperm assessed by a semiautomatic image analysis system was highly correlated with fertilization rate *in vitro*. Jeulin et al.[27] showed that the ALH of motile sperm selected by the swim-up technique correlated with the results of IVF. Chan et al.[48] reported that curvilinear velocity (VCL) of swim-up sperm assessed with the Cellsoft system was a useful predictor of fertilization rate *in vitro*. We have studied the relationship between objective motility of sperm in semen assessed with Hamilton-Thron Motility Analyzer (HTM-2030) and IVF rates in a large number of patients, and the results have shown that LIN (VSL/VCL) and VSL were most significantly correlated with IVF rate in logistic regression analysis.[49] Many other characteristics, such as ALH, were not significantly related to IVF rates. Overall, the commercial computer systems provide a practical method for objective assessment of sperm velocity and movement characteristics in a clinical semen laboratory. However, it is still not clear which characteristics of sperm movement will be most useful for predicting fertility. The accuracy and precision of these automatic systems are currently less than optimal.

3. Acrosomal Status

It is known that the human acrosome and acrosome reaction are important for sperm fertilizing ability, both *in vivo* and *in vitro*. A normal acrosome reaction is essential for sperm penetration through the zona pellucida and for fusion with the oolemma.[50-53] Round headed sperm without an acrosome will not bind to and penetrate through the human ZP.[54] These sperm will also not bind to and penetrate the vitellus of ZP-free hamster oocytes.[54-56] Thus, acrosomeless human sperm are sterile.[57,58] Although the condition is an uncommon cause of male infertility, high proportions of round-headed sperm without an acrosome are observed in the ejaculates of some infertile patients.[59]

For a long time there was no simple technique for routine assessment of human acrosome. The human acrosome is too small to be examined by light microscopy. Although the electron microscope is the most effective method for assessing acrosome, it is impractical for routine assessment. There are now some simple and reliable techniques, such as fluorescein isothocyanate labelled lectins, pisum sativum agglutinin, or peanut agglutinin.[60,61] These methods can be performed easily in the clinical laboratory.

In normal fertile men, over 85% of sperm in a fresh ejaculate have a normal intact acrosome.[62] Spontaneous acrosome reactions occur in about 5 to 20% of sperm from fertile men after incubation for 24 h *in vitro*.[63,64] The absence of acrosome reactions in polyzoospermia has been reported.[65] It has been suggested that study of the kinetics of the acrosome reaction may be useful for predicting sperm fertilizing ability.[66] Unfortunately, this idea is not supported by other studies which failed to show a correlation between the ability of human sperm to undergo acrosome reactions and to fertilize oocytes *in vitro*.[67,68]

In the mouse, sperm bind to the ZP of mouse oocytes with an intact acrosome, and the acrosome reaction is subsequently induced by one of the zona proteins, ZP3.[69,70] The situation in humans is unclear since both acrosome intact and reacted sperm are observed on the ZP. Morales et al.[71] have reported that both acrosome intact and reacted sperm can initiate binding to the human ZP. However, no attempts were made to differentiate between adherence and real binding, since the ZP was not washed to remove loosely attached sperm after incubation with a highly concentrated sperm suspension for 1 min. In contrast, when we washed the oocytes to remove loosely adhered sperm after incubation, we showed decreased sperm-ZP binding and increased sperm-oolemma binding of human sperm incubated with the calcium ionophore A23187 to induce the acrosome reaction.[72] Therefore, human sperm may be similar to those of mice in that, for sperm to bind to the ZP, they must be acrosome intact.[73-75]

We have determined the proportion of sperm with a normal intact acrosome and acrosin activity of sperm in semen in over 100 IVF patients; there was a weak correlation between the normal intact acrosome percentage and acrosin activity, but acrosin activity was not significantly correlated with IVF rates. The proportion of sperm with a normal intact acrosome was highly related to IVF rates only in patients with less than 30% of sperm with normal morphology.[20,21] Thus assessment of acrosome status of sperm in semen or insemination medium gives additional information for predicting fertility, particularly in patients with poor sperm morphology.

4. Sperm-Zona Pellucida Binding

Assessment of sperm-oocyte interaction should be a most powerful approach to evaluating human sperm fertilizing ability, since only a small number of sperm can bind to the ZP, and one or few can penetrate the ZP even when large numbers of sperm surround the oocyte *in vitro*. Therefore, a biological test for assessing the ability of human sperm to bind to the ZP may have substantial prognostic and diagnostic value in male fertility. However, the use of mature human oocytes for diagnostic tests of human sperm function is almost impossible, both for ethical reasons and because of limited availability of material. Overstreet et al.[76] reported that the ZP of non-viable or immature human oocytes can support sperm binding and penetration. Failure of sperm-ZP binding may be associated with certain cases of male infertility.[76] In a clinical IVF program, it has been shown that fertilized human oocytes have more sperm bound to the ZP than do unfertilized oocytes.[77] In mouse IVF, the number of sperm bound to the ZP is directly related to sperm-ZP penetration and fertilization rates.[78] We have recently developed a sperm-zona binding ratio test.[79,80] Oocytes which had failed to be fertilized in the clinical IVF program are stored in ammonium sulphate. Patient (test) and fertile donor (control) sperm are labelled with different fluorochromes. An equal number of progressively motile test and control sperm are mixed and incubated with four to six salt-stored ZP. Then the ratio of test and control sperm bound to the ZP are calculated and used as an indicator of the ability of sperm to bind to the ZP. The sperm-ZP binding ratio is highly significant in its relationship to fertilization rate *in vitro*. This test is simple and easy to perform in a clinical laboratory. Because 20 to 40% of oocytes fail to be fertilized *in vitro*, there is a continuous supply of material for such tests. Because these oocytes have been exposed to sperm in IVF, their quality and state of cortical granule and zona reaction are uncertain; it is therefore necessary to use donor sperm to control for oocyte variability.

Burkman et al.[81] established a test called the hemizona assay (HZA). The ZP of immature oocytes from ovarian surgery or IVF are cut into halves using a micromanipulator, normal fertile donor sperm are incubated with one half of the ZP, and patient's sperm are incubated with the other half. The sperm-ZP binding index obtained by HZA is significantly correlated with fertilization rate *in vitro*.[81,82] Therefore, it is suggested that the HZA is useful for assessing male fertility. However, immature human oocytes are in limited supply. Also, it is difficult to cut the hemizonae into equal sizes. Furthermore, it is unclear if there is a difference between sperm binding to the inside or to the outside of the ZP.

5. Relationship Between Sperm Function Tests and IVF Rates

The results of a clinical IVF program provide several advantages for evaluating tests of human sperm function.[19] Since the fertilization rate in IVF ranges up to 60 to 80%, there is a high frequency end point. Thus, in contrast to studies involving pregnancy rates *in vivo*, relatively small numbers of subjects are

TABLE 2
The Most Significant Sperm Factors Related to Fertilization Rates *In Vitro*

Tests	IVF relationship	References
Normal morphology (%)	+++	18–24
Normal intact acrosomes (%)	++	20,21
Linearity (LIN)	++	40
Straight line velocity (VSL)	++	40,47
Sperm-ZP binding	+++	79–83

Note: +++, most significant; ++, highly significant.

required. Because sperm from the same ejaculate used for insemination of oocytes can be tested in the laboratory, the results of IVF and the sperm tests are directly related. It is also possible that oocyte quality and maturity could be assessed to determine if failure of fertilization is due to oocyte defects. As the pregnancy outcome is not different from embryo transfers resulting from IVF with normal or abnormal semen, it is likely that the rate of fertilization *in vitro* is a good measure of sperm fertility.[77,83-86] However, this assumes that once sperm fertilize oocytes, there is not a high rate of subsequent disordered embryo development caused by abnormalities in the sperm associated with male infertility. Although this assumption needs further investigation, at the moment it appears that using the results of IVF can contribute to very powerful studies of the sperm factors which are most important in human fertility.

Because the results of sperm tests such as concentration, motility, and morphology are correlated, and defects in these usually occur in combination, it is necessary to determine which groups of sperm tests give the most information about fertility. Maximum likelihood logistic regression analysis is the most suitable statistical method for determining which sperm factors are independently related to IVF rates.

We have studied sperm factors influencing IVF rates in over 1000 treatment cycles. Sperm samples remaining after preparation of motile sperm for insemination of oocytes were examined for various sperm function tests. These included tests for sperm concentration, motility, morphology, movement characteristics (Hamilton-Thron HTM-2030), membrane integrity — hypoosmotic swelling (HOS), nuclear maturity, acrosome status, acrosin activity, and the ability of sperm to bind to the ZP and oolemma of ZP-free oocytes.[19-22,49,79,80,87] The significant factors related to IVF rates were evaluated in over 100 patients for each study, and then all the data were analyzed by logistic regression analysis. The most significant sperm factors related to IVF rates are summarized in Table 2. Sperm morphology is the most significant standard semen analysis measurement correlating with IVF rates (Figure 1). This has also been found by others.[23,24] Although the sperm-ZP binding ratio test is, so far, the best single predictor of IVF rates, this test is not practical for routine assessment because it is time consuming and limited by oocyte availability. However, this

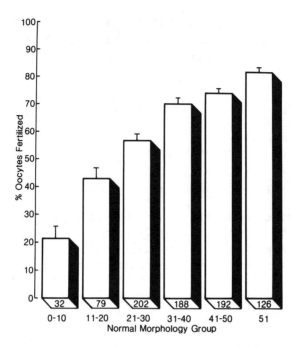

FIGURE 1. The relationship between the percentage of sperm with normal morphology (10% groups to 50% or greater than 50%) in the semen sample used to prepare sperm for insemination and fertilization rates *in vitro*. (Error bars are SEM; number of treatments is indicated on the base of each column; total number of IVF treatments = 819).

test should be useful in patients with poor sperm morphology. Acrosome status also provides additional information for predicting fertility in men with poor sperm morphology.

Many other tests, such as hypoosmotic swelling and tests for nuclear maturity, were not significantly correlated with IVF rates in our studies. Others also showed that the HOS was not of prognostic value for fertilization rate *in vitro*.[88-90] Although we showed that there was a significant difference between HOS test results for patients with IVF rates greater or less than 50%, HOS was not significantly related to IVF rates when other sperm tests such as morphology were included in the logistic regression analysis. As mentioned above, we are skeptical that any single test of sperm function will be found to be of value for predicting fertility in the majority of men.

III. SPERM PREPARATION FOR IVF

A. IVF PROCEDURES AND MODIFICATIONS

The various types of IVF and related procedures are covered in detail in other chapters, but it is important to recognize that some require special modifications of the sperm preparation. For example, if suspensions of spermatozoa are to be introduced into the fallopian tubes, then it is important that the preparation procedure remove debris and bacteria effectively and that it not add particulate material to the sperm suspension which might damage the female genital tract.

If cryopreserved donor sperm are to be used, then special matching and preparation of the sample are usually required. Cryopreserved husband's sperm can also be used if he cannot be present at the time of oocyte collection. Also sperm may have been stored prior to a sterilization procedure (e.g., vasectomy), prior to treatment with an agent which would result in spermatogenic suppression (e.g., chemotherapy with cytotoxic drugs or radiotherapy), during effective treatment (e.g., for sperm autoimmunity), or during a spontaneous improvement if semen quality is variable.

If the semen is abnormal, then some modification of the preparation procedure may be warranted to improve the yield of normal motile sperm. If the semen is severely abnormal, then other procedures such as oocyte micromanipulation may be considered.

B. SPECIAL COLLECTION PROBLEMS

Nontoxic condoms made of Teflon® or other material are available for men unable to collect semen by masturbation for religious or other reasons. It is important that ordinary contraceptive condoms are not used, as most of these are toxic to the sperm, even those without spermicides.[91] Unless the couple are particularly skillful, collections by coitus interruptus are often unsatisfactory because of incomplete recovery of the ejaculate.

If the semen sample on the day of IVF is unexpectedly poor, then a second sample could be collected some hours later, as this might provide sufficient sperm for successful fertilization.

Semen may be collected by use of a vibrator or with electroejaculation from men who are unable to ejaculate normally because of spinal cord injury or other problems.[92] Sperm may also be recovered from the urine of patients with retrograde ejaculation.[93]

Occasional patients are seen in whom the sperm motility declines rapidly with time. These may be managed by collecting the semen close to the time of oocyte insemination and preparing the insemination suspension quickly. Also, there are rare patients in whom delayed fertilization occurs, and in these it may be worth attempting to collect the semen and prepare the spermatozoa 12 to 16 h before insemination. At this stage there is insufficient information to know whether these particular modifications are effective.

C. PRINCIPLES OF SPERM PREPARATION

The goal is to provide the maximum number of normally fertilized oocytes for transfer to the uterus or cryopreservation. With normal semen it is not difficult to obtain sufficient numbers of normal motile sperm for fertilization, and many techniques are successful. On the other hand, with abnormal semen it is often difficult to obtain good sperm by any method. The current practice of many laboratories of having a variety of sperm preparation procedures for choice by the technician is probably satisfactory although somewhat unscientific. As it has been shown above that the proportions of sperm with normal morphology, normal intact acrosomes, greatest VSL and LIN, and best ability to bind to the zona pellucida are associated with higher fertilization rates, the aim of sperm preparation procedures should be to maximize the yield of sperm with these characteristics from poor sperm samples.

The number of sperm for insemination is still poorly defined, but several reviews of results of IVF suggest that there is an increase in fertilization rate with insemination of sperm between 2,000 and 500,000/ml.[94] There may be some increase in risks of polyspermy with the higher sperm concentrations; thus most people aim to inseminate approximately 100,000 sperm/ml. It is now clear that this is grossly in excess of what might be expected to surround the oocyte *in vivo*. Thus, perhaps if better selection of high quality sperm could be achieved, then insemination with lower numbers would be equally successful. In general, most units would attempt to inseminate increased numbers of sperm up to 500,000/ml if there were previous poor fertilization or abnormalities of the sperm such as poor sperm morphology.

In principle, the sperm preparation procedure must be such that damage of the sperm is minimized.[95] Therefore, dilution, temperature change, centrifugation, and exposure to potentially toxic material must be considered. Dilution should be performed slowly, especially with cryopreserved sperm.[10] The media should contain moderate to high concentrations of protein; serum protein appears to be better for this purpose than purified albumin preparations.[96] Perhaps the former contains other materials which support sperm survival, for example by acting as antioxidants. Temperature changes should be gradual. All the preparation of the insemination suspension could be performed at 37°C. Centrifugation should be kept to a minimum within reason, and the force used as low as possible although sufficient to bring down the most motile sperm.

Recently, much interest has been generated in the possibility of oxidants such as free oxygen species being released from leukocytes or abnormal sperm affecting other more normal sperm in sperm pellets.[97,98] This should be avoided or reduced by the antioxidants naturally present in serum, by minimizing centrifugation, and by separating the sperm from the dead sperm and debris early in the preparation procedure. Centrifugation up to 500 g for 5 to 10 min appears to be innocuous.

Capacitation of human sperm by removal of seminal plasma and exposure to protein-containing buffers is another aim of the sperm preparation procedure. Although capacitation is clearly demonstrated in a number of domestic and laboratory animals, it seems to be less obvious in humans. Fertilization can occur as early as 2 or 3 h after insemination.[99]

D. PREPARATION PROCEDURES

The first semen treatment in IVF involved "washing" the spermatozoa by dilution of the semen with culture medium, centrifugation, and resuspension of the pellet in further aliquots of culture medium supplemented with protein.

Usually three washes were performed. Although this technique produced the earlier successes, recently it has been criticized, particularly when used for abnormal semen samples, in that it might damage the sperm by the repeated centrifugation. It has been theorized that centrifugation might result in peroxidation damage of the sperm by free oxygen species.[95] Occasionally, a semen sample is so poor that washing is all that can be done to prepare sperm for insemination, and while fertilization often fails, surprisingly good results sometimes occur.

The swim-up procedure was used from the early 1980s and is probably the most commonly used technique today.[10] A number of modifications of the procedure have been introduced, including swim-down, in which the semen or sperm pellet is layered on top of the culture medium.[100] The swim-over technique involves special concentric tubes, in which the sperm that swim over a barrier then fall or swim down into a central well. Some groups prefer to introduce the sperm suspension beneath the overlay medium, as this may produce a cleaner interface.[100]

Various gradient separation procedures have been introduced. The advantage is that the gradient separation techniques are rapid, requiring 20 min centrifugation compared with an average of 1 h incubation for swim-up; they are also relatively simple to prepare and easy to carry out under sterile conditions. The most popular of these is Percoll density gradient centrifugation, but albumin, Nycodenz, a radiographic contrast medium, and Ficoll, a sucrose polymer, have also been used.[100] Percoll consists of colloidal silica particles coated with polyvinylpyrollidone. The discontinuous Percoll gradient method has been recommended as a technique for rapid and efficient isolation of motile human sperm, free from contamination with other seminal constituents.[101] Sperm form distinct bands at the interfaces between the different Percoll concentrations, and optimal sperm yields are usually in the 85 to 100% Percoll fractions. It has been claimed that since abnormal sperm as well as immotile sperm and debris are largely eliminated by Percoll gradients, fertilization rates and pregnancy rates are increased. While some excellent results have been reported there have been no controlled trials.[102,103] A special small volume Percoll gradient (mini-Percoll) has been introduced by Ord et al.[104] for treatment of severely abnormal semen samples.

In a comparative study of Percoll, mini-Percoll, and swim-up techniques for preparing sperm from abnormal semen samples, we have been unable to show any difference between Percoll and mini-Percoll, but both Percoll techniques produced a substantial increase in the yield of motile sperm (approximately threefold). However, the quality of the sperm recovered was less than with the swim-up technique, which produced consistently better sperm suspensions with higher sperm velocity, and higher proportions of sperm with normal intact acrosomes and normal morphology.[105] Combining mini-Percoll and swim-up produced a significant increase in yield of motile sperm over swim-up alone.[105] Controlled trials of the use of these techniques in IVF are underway.

1. Collection of Semen for IVF

In a room adjacent to the IVF laboratory, the man should collect semen into a sterile disposable plastic jar. The sperm should be prepared soon after liquefaction of the seminal plasma. If liquefaction is delayed or the specimen is particularly viscous, then syringing the sample through a 21 gauge needle may help break up viscous globules.

2. Swim-Up Preparation

All plastic, glassware, and media should be checked for toxicity to sperm or pre-embryos. Sperm should not be allowed to come into contact with rubber as this may immobilize them. A variety of media are suitable for sperm preparation for IVF (see Chapter 7). The medium chosen should be equilibrated with the gas mixture, and the temperature should be maintained constant, usually 37°C. The protein source for the medium needs to be checked for sperm antibodies, and if pools are used, the donors must be tested for viral illnesses including HIV and hepatitis. Heat inactivation of the serum should not be relied upon to obviate the risk of transmitting infections.

The timing of semen collection and preparation does not appear to be critical, especially with good semen samples. In general, the oocytes are inseminated 4 to 6 h after collection, and the sperm can be prepared during this time. With patients with previous delayed fertilization, there may be some benefit from delaying the insemination and storing the prepared sperm for a longer time. Preparing the sperm quickly and inseminating the oocytes within an hour of collection may be worthwhile for those sperm samples which appear to have a rapid decline in motility. The semen should be placed in a sterile area of the laboratory or in a laminar flow hood. The sample must be mixed thoroughly because ejaculation does not result in a homogeneous suspension of sperm in the seminal plasma. Following mixing, a small portion (10 µl) of the sample is taken to check the sperm concentration and motility. With normal semen samples, usually 1 ml of sample is sufficient for preparation of adequate numbers of motile sperm. If the semen sample is poor, then the whole semen volume should be distributed to several tubes for preparation of as many sperm as possible.

Several variations of the swim-up procedure are possible. The seminal plasma can be overlayed directly with culture medium and the sperm allowed to swim from the seminal plasma into the culture medium. Following this, the sperm suspension should be washed to ensure adequate removal of seminal plasma constituents. Alternatively, the semen sample may be diluted and centrifuged and the pellet loosened and overlayed, or the semen sample may be centrifuged without prior dilution of the seminal plasma and the pellet loosened and overlayed with medium for the swim-up procedure. The latter technique may be particularly useful for oligospermic semen samples, as the sperm in some of these appear to be damaged by the dilution procedure.

The semen sample is examined, any particulate material is allowed to settle, and the supernatant is transferred to another tube. If dilution is to be performed, then culture medium is added, the semen sample is centrifuged, the supernatant is aspirated off the pellet, and the pellet is gently resuspended in a small volume of liquid. The overlay medium is then gently pipetted onto the surface of the pellet, and the tube is incubated for 30 to 60 min. Some recommend that the tubes be placed in the incubator on an angle to increase the surface area of the interface. Following the incubation, the upper half to two-thirds of the overlay is aspirated and mixed, and the sperm concentration is counted. Sufficient volume of the sperm suspension is added to each culture well enough to have a final concentration between 5 and 15×10^4 motile sperm/ml. As mentioned above, higher sperm numbers may be used where there has been previous failure of fertilization or where it is known that the sperm have poor morphology. If insufficient sperm are obtained, then the whole sperm preparation may be added to a well, and several oocytes may be placed in this well.

If cryopreserved semen is to be used, then dilution of the semen sample should be slow, with dropwise addition of culture medium to the thawed sample. Pellets formed should be gently resuspended.

3. Percoll and Mini-Percoll Gradients

The stock solution of Percoll (designated 100% Percoll) is prepared by diluting 9 parts of Percoll (obtained from Pharmacia, Uppsala, Sweden) in 1 part of 10-times concentrated culture medium, e.g., Ham's F10. Solutions with different percentages of Percoll are prepared by combining the 100% Percoll with culture medium supplemented with protein. Each Percoll concentration should be allowed to equilibrate in the incubator for 1 to 2 h. Discontinuous three-step Percoll gradients can be formed by carefully pipetting 1 ml of each of 95, 70, and 50% Percoll concentrations into a 10 ml centrifuge tube so that the interfaces are visible between the layers. The semen samples are then gently loaded onto the top of the gradients, usually 1 ml onto the top of each of several gradients. Gradients are then centrifuged in a swinging bucket rotor for 20 min at 450 g at either 37°C or room temperature.

For mini-Percoll gradients, 0.3 ml of each of the 95, 70, and 50% Percoll concentrations are used. The semen sample is washed by diluting in two volumes of culture medium and centrifuged at 500 g for 8 to 10 min. The sperm pellet is then resuspended in a small volume of medium, and equal volumes (~0.3 ml) are loaded onto two or three Percoll gradients, which are then centrifuged at 300 g for 20 min.[104] Following centrifugation of the Percoll gradients, the seminal plasma and upper two layers of 50% and 70% Percoll are aspirated off until the 95% Percoll interface is reached. Alternatively, the 95% layer may be aspirated in and out of a pipette passed through the upper layers to resuspend the sperm before removing it to another tube without disturbing the interface. The recovered 95% Percoll layer is diluted with 2 ml of medium and the sample centrifuged at 500 g for 8 to 10 min. The supernatant is removed, and the sperm pellet is resuspended in culture medium for insemination.

4. Combination of Mini-Percoll and Swim-Up

Aliquots of semen samples are washed by dilution with two volumes of medium and centrifuged at 500 g for 8 to 10 min. The pellets are resuspended in 0.3 ml of medium, layered on mini-Percoll gradients, and centrifuged at 300 g for 20 min. After centrifugation, the seminal plasma and upper two layers of the gradient are aspirated off. The 95% layers are transferred to new tubes, mixed by pipetting, and overlaid with medium for swim-up. Following swim-up, the upper layer is centrifuged at 500 g for 5 to 10 min. The upper layer is centrifuged and the pellet resuspended in 200 µl of medium for insemination. This method appears to improve the yield of motile sperm in up to half the abnormal semen samples treated.[105] This may be because the preliminary mini-Percoll gradient centrifugation separates the cellular debris from the sperm and permits the motile sperm to migrate more readily into the overlay during the subsequent swim-up procedure. There is also a significant increase in sperm motility of the recovered sperm after this procedure, probably because of the additional selection step.

E. USE OF MOTILITY STIMULANTS

A variety of agents have been reported to enhance sperm motility — relaxin, kallikrein, cysteine, taurine, prolactin, pentoxifylline, caffeine, adenosine, and deoxyadenosine.[106,107] A number of groups have used pentoxifylline and 2-deoxyadenosine for IVF.[5,108] At the moment it is not certain that these agents improve the results, but increased yields of motile sperm can be obtained with pentoxifylline.[107,108] The use of pentoxifylline has been reported for both abnormal semen and for sperm retrieved from the epididymis for congenital absence of the vas or epididymal obstruction.[5] The maximally effective dose of pentoxifylline appears to be between 0.3 and 0.6 mmol/l, and many groups use 3.6 mmol (1 mg/ml). The addition of pentoxifylline to the medium used for washing the sperm and for swim-up or Percoll gradient centrifugation will result in increased yields. Pentoxifylline has been reported to provide greater stimulation of motility and velocity than caffeine or 2-deoxyadenosine.[107] There have been reports that some stimulants such as caffeine and 2-deoxyadenosine are associated with reduced sperm penetration assay results.[107,109] Other sperm preparation techniques for special purposes such as micromanipulation are covered in other chapters (see Chapters 6 and 7).

IV. FUTURE ADVANCES

The main problems to be solved in the future are the accurate identification of patients who are likely to have problems with fertilization, effective treatment of defective sperm production or function, and improved sperm preparation for IVF, the aim being to increase fertilization rates with normal and abnormal semen. At this stage it does not appear that the sperm contribute significantly to the other major problem with IVF, namely the low implantation rate.

Improved prediction of the results of IVF will come from the development of new methods of sperm assessment, particularly automated methods for determining sperm morphology and biochemical methods for assessing the ability of sperm to interact with eggs, focused on both sperm-zona binding sites and sperm-oolemma binding sites. Further studies should resolve questions about the involvement of free oxygen species in the pathogenesis of sperm defects, about chemotactic signals between oocytes and sperm, and about the realistic results of micromanipulation procedures for severe sperm defects. New technology may improve these procedures with the development of laser manipulation of sperm and direct injection of a sperm into the ooplasm.

REFERENCES

1. **Baker, H. W. G., Burger, H. G., de Kretser, D. M., and Hudson, B.,** Relative incidence of etiologic disorders in male infertility, in *Male Reproductive Dysfunction: Diagnosis and Management of Hypogonadism, Infertility and Impotence,* Santen, R.J. and Swerdloff, R.S., Eds., Marcel Dekker, New York, 1986, 341.
2. **Baker, H. W. G.,** Male infertility of undetermined etiology, in *Current Therapy in Endocrinology and Metabolism,* Kreiger, D. T. and Bardin, C. W., Eds., B.C. Decker, Philadelphia, 1985, 165.
3. **Kovacs, G. T., King, C., Rogers, P., Wood, C., Baker, H. W. G., and Yates, C.,** In vitro fertilisation, a practical option after failed artificial insemination with donor semen, *Reprod. Fertil. Dev.,* 1, 383, 1989.
4. **Silber, S., Ord, T., Balmaceda, J. P., Patrizio, P., and Asch, R. H.,** Congenital absence of the vas deferens: studies on the fertilising capacity of human epididymal sperm, *N. Engl. J. Med.,* 323, 1788, 1990.
5. **Yates, C. and Temple-Smith, P. D.,** Treatment of obstructive azoospermia by sperm microaspiration retrieval technique for IVF: SMART-IVF, *46th Annual Meeting of the American Fertility Society,* 141(Abstr.), S61, 1990.
6. **Hendry, W. F.,** Detection and treatment of antispermatozoal antibodies in men, *Reprod. Fertil. Dev.,* 1, 205, 1989.
7. **Clarke, G. N., Lopata, A., McBain, J. C., Baker, H. W. G., and Johnston, W. I. H.,** Effect of sperm antibodies in males on human in vitro fertilisation (IVF), *Am. J. Reprod. Immunol. Microbiol.,* 8, 62, 1985.
8. **Baker, H. W. G., Burger, H. G., de Kretser, D. M., Hudson, B., Rennie, G.C., and Straffon, W. G. E.,** Testicular vein ligation and fertility in men with varicoceles, *Brit. Med. J.,* 291, 1678, 1985.
9. **Mallidis, C., Howard, E. J., and Baker, H. W. G.,** Variation of semen quality in normal men, *Int. J. Androl.,* 14, 99, 1991.
10. **Mahadevan, M. M. and Baker, H.W.G.,** Assessment and preparation of semen for in vitro fertilisation, in *Clinical In Vitro Fertilization,* Wood, C. and Trounson, A., Eds., Springer-Verlag, New York, 1984, 83.
11. **Aitken, R. J., Best, F. S. M., Richardson, D. W., Djahanbakhch O., Mortimer, D., Templeton, A. A., and Lees, M.M.,** An analysis of sperm function in case of unexplained infertility: conventional criteria movement characteristics and fertilising capacity, *Fertil. Steril.,* 38, 211, 1982.
12. **Aitken, R. J., Best, F. S. M., Richardson, D. W., Djahanbakhch, O., Templeton, A. A., and Lees, M. M.,** An analysis of semen quality and sperm function in case of oligospermia, *Fertil. Steril.,* 38, 705, 1982.

13. **Zaini, A., Jennings, M. G., and Baker, H. W. G.,** Are conventional sperm morphology and motility assessments of predictive value in subfertile men?, *Int. J. Androl.,* 8, 427, 1985.
14. **Silber, S. J.,** The relationship of abnormal semen parameters to male fertility, *Human Reprod.,* 4, 947, 1989.
15. **Cohen, J., Edwards, R., Fehilly, C., Fischel, S., Hewitt, J., Purdy, J., Rowland, G., Steptoe, P., and Webster, J.,** In vitro fertilisation: a treatment for male infertility, *Fertil. Steril.,* 43, 422, 1985.
16. **Yates C. A. and de Kretser, D. M.,** Male-factor infertility and in vitro fertilisation, *J. In Vitro Fertil. Embryo Transfer,* 4, 141, 1987.
17. **Dunphy, B., Neal, L. M., and Cooke, I. D.,** The clinical value of conventional semen analysis, *Fertil. Steril.,* 51, 324, 1989.
18. **Baker, H. W. G., Liu, D. Y., and Speirs, A.,** Prediction of fertilisation rates in IVF from semen analysis results and diagnostic category, Proc. 9th Ann. Scientific Meet., Fertil. Soc. Aust., Perth, Australia, 26 to 29 September, 1990, Abst. 51.
19. **Liu, D. Y., du Plessis, Y. P., Nayudu, P. L., Johnston, W. I. H., and Baker, H. W. G.,** The use of in vitro fertilisation to evaluate putative tests of human sperm function, *Fertil. Steril.,* 49, 272, 1988.
20. **Liu, D. Y. and Baker, H. W. G.,** The proportion of sperm with poor morphology but normal intact acrosomes detected with pisum sativum agglutinin correlates with fertilisation in vitro, *Fertil. Steril.,* 50, 288, 1988.
21. **Liu, D. Y. and Baker, H. W. G.,** Relationships between human sperm acrosin, acrosomes, morphology and in vitro fertilisation, *Hum. Reprod.,* 5, 298, 1990.
22. **Liu, D. Y., Elton, R. A., Johnston, W. I. H., and Baker, H. W. G.,** Spermatozoal nuclear chromatin decondensation in vitro: a test for sperm immaturity. Comparison with results of human in vitro fertilisation, *Clin. Reprod. Fertil.,* 5, 191, 1987.
23. **Kruger, T. F., Menkveld, R., Stander, F. S. H., Lombard, C. J., Van den Merwe, J. P., Van Zyl, J. A., and Smith, K.,** Sperm morphological features as a prognostic factor in in vitro fertilisation, *Fertil. Steril.,* 46, 1118, 1986.
24. **Kruger, T. F., Acosta, A. A., Simmons, K. F., Swanson, R. J., Matta, J. F., and Oehninger, S.,** Predictive value of abnormal sperm morphology in vitro fertilisation, *Fertil. Steril.,* 49, 112, 1988.
25. **Baker, H. W. G. and Clarke, G. N.,** Sperm morphology: consistency of assessment of the same sperm by different observers, *Clin. Reprod. Fertil.,* 5, 37, 1987.
26. **World Health Organisation,** *WHO Laboratory Manual for Examination of Human Semen and Semen-Cervical Mucus Interaction,* 3rd ed., Cambridge University Press, Cambridge, 1992, 1.
27. **Jeulin, C., Feneux, D., Serres, C., Jouannet, P., Guillet-Rosso, F., Belaisch-Allart, J., Frydman, R., and Testart, J.,** Sperm factors related to failure of human in vitro fertilisation, *J. Reprod. Fertil.,* 76, 1, 1986.
28. **Katz, D. F., Overstreet, J. W., Samuels, S. J., Niswander, P. W., Blood, T. D., and Lewis, E.,** Morphometric analysis of spermatozoa in the assessment of human male fertility, *J. Androl.,* 7, 203, 1986.
29. **Moruzzi, J. F., Wyrobek, A. J., Mayall, B. H., and Gledhill, B. L.,** Quantification and classification of human sperm morphology by computer-assisted image analysis, *Fertil. Steril.,* 50, 142, 1988.
30. **Makler, A.,** Modern methods in semen analysis evaluation, in *Progress in Infertility,* Behrman, S. J., Kistner, R.W., Patton, G. W., Jr., Eds., Little, Brown, Boston, 1988, 633.
31. **Pousette, A., Akerlof, E., Rosenborg, L., and Fredricsson, B.,** Increase in progressive motility and improved morphology of human spermatozoa following their migration through Percoll gradients, *Int. J. Androl.,* 9, 1, 1986.
32. **Andolz, P., Bielsa, M. A., Genesca, A., Benet, J., and Egozcue, J.,** Improvement of sperm quality in abnormal semen samples using a modified swim-up procedure, *Hum. Reprod.,* 2, 99, 1987.

33. **Le Lannou, D. and Blanchard, Y.**, Nuclear maturity and morphology of human spermatozoa selected by Percoll density gradient centrifugation or swim-up procedure, *Fertil. Steril.*, 84, 551, 1988.
34. **Katz, D. F. and Overstreet, J. W.**, Sperm motility assessment by videomicrography, *Fertil. Steril.*, 35, 188, 1980.
35. **Katz, D. F., Morales, P., Samuels, S. J., and Overstreet, J. W.**, Mechanisms of filtration of morphologically abnormal human sperm by cervical mucus, *Fertil. Steril.*, 54, 513, 1990.
36. **Rogers, B. J., Bentwood, B. J., Van Campden, H., Helmbrecht, G., Soderdahl, D., and Hale, R. W.**, Sperm morphology assessment as an indicator of human fertilising capacity, *J. Androl.*, 4, 119, 1983.
37. **Shalgi, R., Dor, J., Rudak, E., Lusky, A., Goldman, B., Mashiach, S., and Nebel, L.**, Penetration of sperm from teratospermic men into zona-free hamster eggs, *Int. J. Androl.*, 8, 285, 1985.
38. **Marsh, S. K., Bolton, V. N., and Braude, P. R.**, The effect of morphology on the ability of human spermatozoa to penetrate zona-free hamster oocytes, *Hum. Reprod.*, 2, 499, 1987.
39. **Kruger, T. F., Swanson, R. J., Hamilton, M., Simmoms, K., Acosta, A. A., Matta, J. F., Oehninger, S., and Morshedi, M.**, Abnormal sperm morphology and other semen parameters related to the outcome of the hamster oocyte human sperm penetration assay, *Int. J. Androl.*, 11, 107, 1988.
40. **Liu, D. Y. and Baker, H. W. G.**, Morphology of human sperm bound to the zona pellucida of oocytes which failed to be fertilised in vitro, *J. Reprod. Fert.*, 94, 71, 1992.
41. **Aitken, R. J., Ross, A., and Lees, M. M.**, Analysis of sperm function in Kartagener's syndrome, *Fertil. Steril.*, 40, 696, 1983.
42. **MacLeod, J. and Gold, R. Z.**, The male factor in fertility and infertility, ICI An analysis of motile activity in the spermatozoa of 1000 fertile men and 1000 men in infertile marriage, *Fertil. Steril.*, 2, 187, 1985.
43. **Baker, H. W. G. and Burger, H. G.**, Male infertility, in *Reproductive Medicine, Serono Symposia Publications,* Steinberger, E., Frajese, G., and Steinberger, A., Eds., Raven Press, New York, 1985, 187.
44. **David, G., Severs, C., and Jouannet, P.**, Kinematics of human spermatozoa, *Gamete Res.*, 4, 83, 1981.
45. **Overstreet, J. W., Katz, D. F., Hanson, F. W., and Fonseca, J. R.**, A simple inexpensive method for objective assessment of human sperm movement characteristics, *Fertil. Steril.*, 31, 162, 1979.
46. **Mortimer, D.**, Objective analysis of sperm motility and kinematics, in *The Handbook of the Laboratory Diagnosis and Treatment of Infertility*, CRC Press, Boca Raton, FL, 1989, 97.
47. **Holt, W. V., Moore, H. D. M., and Hillier, S. G.**, Computer-assisted measurement of sperm swimming speed in human semen: correlation of results with in vitro fertilisation assays, *Fertil., Steril.*, 44, 112–119, 1985.
48. **Chan, S. Y. W., Wang, C., Chan, S. T. H., Ho, P. C., So, W. W. K., Chan, Y. F., and Ma, H. K.**, Predictive value of sperm morphology and movement characteristics in the outcome of in vitro fertilisation of human oocytes, *J. In Vitro Fertil. Embryo Transfer*, 6, 142, 1989.
49. **Liu, D. Y., Clarke, G. N., and Baker, H. W. G.**, Relationship between sperm motility assessed with the Hamilton-Thron Motility Analyzer and fertilisation rates in vitro, *J. Androl.*, 12, 231, 1991.
50. **Sathananthan, A. H., Trounson, A. O., Wood, C., and Leeton, J. F.**, Ultrastructural observation on the penetration of human sperm into the zona pellucida of the human egg in vitro, *J. Androl.*, 3, 356, 1982.
51. **Yanagimachi, R.**, Mechanisms of fertilisation in mammals, in *Fertilisation And Embryonic Development In Vitro*, Mastroianni, L. and Biggers, J. D., Jr., Eds., Plenum Press, New York, 1981, 81.

52. Moore, H. D. M. and Bedford, J. M., The interaction of mammalian gametes in the female, in *Mechanism and Control of Animal Fertilisation*, Hartman, J. F., Ed., Academic Press, New York, 1983, 435.
53. Overstreet, J. W. and Hembree, W. C., Penetration of the zona pellucida of nonliving human oocytes by human spermatozoa *in vitro, Fertil. Steril.*, 27, 815, 1976.
54. von Bernhardi, R., de Ioannes, A. E., Blanco, L. P., Herrera Bustos-Obregon, E., and Vigil, P., Round-headed spermatozoa: a model to study the role of the acrosome in early events of gamete interaction, *Andrologia*, 22, 12, 1990.
55. Lalonde, L., Langlais, J., Antaki, P., Chapdelaine, A., Roberts, K.D., and Bleau, G., Male infertility associated with round-headed acrosomeless spermatozoa, *Fertil. Steril.*, 49, 316, 1988.
56. Weissenberg, R., Eshkol, A., Rudak, E., and Lunenfeld, B., Inability of round acrosomeless human spermatozoa to penetrate zona free hamster ova, *Arch. Androl.*, 11, 167, 1983.
57. Anton-Lamprecht, I., Kotzur, B., and Schopf, E., Round-headed human spermatozoa, *Fertil. Steril.*, 27, 685, 1976.
58. Nistal, M. and Paniagua, R., Morphogenesis of round-head human spermatozoa lacking acrosomes in case of severe teratozoospermia, *Andrologia*, 10, 49, 1978.
59. Florke-Gerloff, S., Topfer-Petersen, E., Muller-Esterl, W., Mansouri, A., Schatz, R., Schirren, C., Schill, E. B., and Engel, W., Biochemical and genetic investigation of round-headed spermatozoa in infertile men including two brothers and their father, *Andrologia*, 16, 187, 1984.
60. Cross, N. L., Morales, P., Overstreet, J. W., and Hanson, F. W., Two simple methods for detecting acrosome-reacted human sperm, *Gamete Res.*, 15, 213, 1986.
61. Mortimer, D., Curtis, E. F., and Miller, R. G., Specific labelling by peanut agglutinin of the outer acrosome membrane of the human spermatozoa, *J. Reprod. Fertil.*, 81, 127, 1987.
62. Wolf, D. P., Bold, J., Byrd, W., and Bechtol, K. B., Acrosome status evaluation in human ejaculated sperm with monoclonal antibodies, *Biol. Reprod.*, 32, 1157, 1985.
63. Byrd, W. and Wolf, D. P., Acrosomal status in fresh and capacitated human ejaculated sperm, *Biol. Reprod.*, 34, 859, 1986.
64. Stock, C. E. and Fraser, L. R., The acrosome reaction in human sperm of proven fertility, *Hum. Reprod.*, 2, 109, 1987.
65. Topfer-Petersen, E., Volcker, C. H., Heissler, E., and Schill, W. B., Absence of the acrosome reaction in polyzoospermia, *Andrologia*, 19, 225, 1987.
66. Topfer-Petersen, E., Heissler, E., and Schill, W. B., The kinetics of the acrosome reaction, an additional sperm parameter? *Andrologia*, 17, 224, 1985.
67. Plachot, M., Mandelbaum, J., and Junca, M. A., Acrosome reaction of human sperm used for in vitro fertilisation, *Fertil. Steril.*, 42, 418, 1984.
68. De Jonge, C. J., Rawlins, R. G., and Zaneveld, L. J. D., Induction of the human sperm acrosome reaction by human oocytes, *Fertil. Steril.*, 50, 949, 1988.
69. Wassarman, P. M., Early events in mammalian fertilisation, *Annu. Rev. Cell. Biol.*, 3, 109, 1987.
70. Wassarman, P. M., The biology and chemistry of fertilisation, *Science*, 235, 553, 1987.
71. Morales, P., Cross, N. L., Overstreet, J. W., and Hanson, F. W., Acrosome intact and acrosome-reacted human sperm can initiate binding to the zona pellucida, *Dev. Biol.*, 133, 385, 1989.
72. Liu, D.Y. and Baker, H. W. G., Inducing the human acrosome reaction with a calcium ionophore A23187 decreases sperm-zona pellucida binding with oocytes that failed to fertilise in vitro, *J. Reprod. Fertil.*, 89, 127, 1990.
73. O'Rand, M. G., Matthews, J. E., Welch, J. E., and Fisher, S. J., Identification of zona binding proteins of rabbit, pig, human and mouse spermatozoa on nitrocellulose blots, *J. Exp. Zool.*, 235, 423, 1985.

74. **Tesarik, J.,** Appropriate time of the acrosome reaction is a major requirement for the fertilising spermatozoa, *Hum. Reprod.,* 4, 957, 1989.
75. **Tesarik, J. and Testart, J.,** Human sperm-egg interaction and their disorders: implications in the management of infertility, *Hum. Reprod.,* 4, 729, 1989.
76. **Overstreet, J. W., Yanagimachi, R., Katz, F., and Hanson, F. W.,** Penetration of human spermatozoa into the human zona pellucida and zona-free hamster egg: a study of fertile donor and infertile patients, *Fertil. Steril.,* 33, 534, 1980.
77. **Mahadevan, M. M., Trounson, A. O., Wood. C., and Leeton, J. F.,** Effect of oocyte quality and sperm characteristics on the number of spermatozoa bound to the zona pellucida of human oocytes inseminated in vitro, *J. In Vitro Fertil. Embryo Transfer,* 4, 223, 1987.
78. **Wolf, D. P. and Inoue, M.,** Sperm concentration dependency in the fertilisation and zonal sperm binding properties of mouse egg inseminated in vitro, *J. Exp. Zool.,* 196, 27, 1976.
79. **Liu, D. Y., Lopata, A., Johnston, W. I. H., and Baker, H. W. G.,** A human sperm-zona pellucida binding test using oocytes that failed to fertilise in vitro, *Fertil. Steril.,* 50, 782, 1988.
80. **Liu, D. Y., Clarke, G. N., Lopata, A., Johnston, W. I. H., and Baker, H. W. G.,** A sperm-zona pellucida binding test and in vitro fertilisation, *Fertil. Steril.,* 52, 281, 1989.
81. **Burkman, L. J., Coddington, C. C., Franken, D. R., Kruger, T. F., Rosenwaks, Z., and Hodgen, G. D.,** The hemizona assay (HZA): development of a diagnostic test for the binding of human spermatozoa to the human hemizona pellucida to predict fertilisation potential, *Fertil. Steril.,* 49, 688, 1988.
82. **Oehninger, S., Coddington, C. C., Scott, R., Franken, D. A., Burkman, L. J., Acosta, A. A., and Hodgen, G. D.,** Hemizona assay: assessment of sperm dysfunction and prediction of in vitro fertilisation outcome, *Fertil. Steril.,* 51, 665, 1989.
83. **Acosta, A. A., Chillik, C. F., Brugo, S., Ackerman, S., Swanson, R. J., Pleban, P., Yuan, J., and Haque, D.,** In vitro fertilisation and the male factor, *Urology,* 28, 1, 1986.
84. **Cohen, J., Edwards, R., Fehilly, C., Fischel, S., Hewitt, J., Rowland, G., Steptoe, P., and Webster, J.,** Treatment of male infertility by in vitro fertilisation: factors affecting fertilisation and pregnancy, *Acta Eur. Fertil.,* 15, 455, 1984.
85. **Cohen, J., Fehilly, C. B., Fishel, S. B., Edwards, R. G., Hewitt, J., Rowland, G. F., Steptoe, P. C., and Webster, J.,** Male infertility successfully treated by in vitro fertilisation, *Lancet,* 1, 1239, 1984.
86. **National Perinatal Statistics Unit & Fertility Society of Australia,** IVF and GIFT Pregnancies Australia and New Zealand 1988, National Perinatal Statistics Unit, Sydney, 1990, 1.
87. **Liu, D. Y., Lopata, A., Johnston, W. I. H., and Baker, H. W. G.,** Human sperm-zona binding, sperm characteristics and in-vitro fertilisation, *Hum. Reprod.,* 4, 696, 1989.
88. **Barratt, C. L. R., Osborn, J. C., Harrison, P. E., Monks, N., Dunphy, B. C., Lenton, E. A., and Cooke, I.,** The hypo-osmotic swelling test and the sperm mucus penetration test in determining fertilisation of human oocyte, *Hum. Reprod.,* 4, 430, 1989.
89. **Chan, S. Y. W., Wang, C., Ng, M., and Ho, P. C.,** Multivariate discriminant analysis on the relationship between the human sperm hypoosmotic swelling test and the human sperm in vitro fertilising capacity, *Int. J. Androl.,* 11, 367, 1988.
90. **Chan, S. Y. W., Wang, C., Chan, S. T. H., and Ho, P.C.,** Differential evaluation of human sperm hypoosmotic swelling test and its relationship with the outcome of in vitro fertilisation of human oocytes, *Hum. Reprod.,* 5, 84, 1990.
91. **Jones, D. M., Kovacs, G. T., Harrison, L., Jennings, M. G., and Baker, H. W. G.,** Immobilization of sperm by condoms and their components, *Clin. Reprod. Fertil.,* 4, 367, 1986.

92. **Bennett, C. J., Seager, S .W., Vasher, E. A., and McGuire, E. J.**, Sexual dysfunction and electroejaculation in men with spinal cord injury: review, *J. Urol.*, 139, 453, 1988.
93. **Mahadevan, M., Leeton, J. F., and Trounson, A. O.**, Noninvasive method of semen collection for successful artificial insemination in a case of retrograde ejaculation, *Fertil. Steril*, 36, 243, 1981.
94. **Wolf, D. P., Byrd, W., Dandekar, P., and Quigley, M. M.**, Sperm concentration and the fertilisation of human eggs in vitro, *Biol. Reprod.*, 31, 837, 1984.
95. **Mortimer, D.**, Sperm preparation techniques and iatrogenic failure of in-vitro fertilisation, *Hum. Reprod.*, 6, 173, 1991.
96. **Liu, D. Y., Clarke, G. N., and Baker, H. W. G.**, The effect of serum on motility of human spermatozoa in culture, *Int. J. Androl.*, 9, 109, 1986.
97. **Aitken, R. J. and Clarkson, J. S.**, Significance of reactive oxygen species and antioxidants in defining the efficacy of sperm preparation techniques, *J. Androl.*, 9, 367, 1988.
98. **Aitken, R. J., Clarkson, J. S., Hargreave, T. B., Irvine, D. S.. and Wu, F. C. W.**, Analysis of the relationship between defective sperm function and the generation of reactive oxygen species in case of oligospermia, *J. Androl.*, 10, 214, 1989.
99. **Lopata, A., McMaster, R., McBain, J. C., and Johnston, W. I. H.**, In-vitro fertilisation of preovulatory human eggs, *J. Reprod. Fertil.*, 52, 339, 1978.
100. **Mortimer, D.**, Semen analysis and sperm washing techniques, in *Control of Sperm Motility*, Gagnon, C., Ed., CRC Press, Boca, Raton, FL, in press.
101. **Gorus, F. K. and Pipeleers, D. G.**, A rapid method for the fractionation of human spermatozoa according to their progressive motility, *Fertil. Steril.*, 35, 662, 1981.
102. **Hyne, R. V., Stojanoff, A., Clarke, G. N., Lopata, A., and Johnston, W. I. H.**, Pregnancy from in vitro fertilisation of human eggs after separation of motile sperm by density gradient centrifugation, *Fertil. Steril.*, 45, 93, 1986.
103. **Guerin, J. F., Mathieu, C., Lornage, J., Pinatel, M. C., and Boulieu, D.**, Improvement of survival and fertilizing capacity of human spermatozoa in an IVF program by selection on discontinuous Percoll gradients, *Hum. Reprod.*, 4, 798, 1989.
104. **Ord, T., Patrizio, P., Marello, E., Balmaceda, J. P., and Asch, R. H.**, Mini-Percoll: a new method of semen preparation for IVF in severe male factor infertility, *Hum. Reprod.*, 5, 987, 1990.
105. **Ng, F. L. H., Liu, D. Y., and Baker, H. W. G.**, Comparison of Percoll, mini-Percoll and swim-up for sperm preparation from abnormal semen samples, *Hum. Reprod.*, 7, 261, 1992.
106. **Lindemann, C. B. and Kanous, K. S.**, Regulation of mammalian sperm motility, *Arch. Androl.*, 23, 1, 1989.
107. **Hammitt, D. G., Bedia, E., Rogers, P. R., Syrop, C. H., Donovan, J. F., and Williamson, R. A.**, Comparison of motility stimulants for cryopreserved human semen, *Fertil. Steril.*, 52, 495, 1989.
108. **Yovich, J. M., Edirisingher, W. R., Cummins, J. M., and Yovich, J. L.**, Influence of pentoxifylline in severe male factor infertility, *Fertil. Steril.*, 53, 715, 1990.
109. **Aitken, R. J., Mattei, A., and Irvine, S.**, Paradoxical stimulation of human sperm motility by 2-deoxyadenosine, *J. Reprod. Fertil.*, 78, 515, 1986.

Chapter 4

IN VITRO FERTILIZATION AND EMBRYO DEVELOPMENT

Alan Trounson and Jeremy Osborn

TABLE OF CONTENTS

I. Introduction 58

II. Insemination of Oocytes *In Vitro* 58
    A. Insemination in Capillary Tubes and Straws 59
    B. Insemination in Microdrops 60
    C. Insemination in Coculture Systems 63

III. Fertilization *In Vitro* 63
    A. Checking for Fertilization 63
    B. Abnormalities of Fertilization 64
    C. Reinsemination 66
    D. Timing of Fertilization Events 67
    E. Transfer of Pronuclear Embryos 68

IV. Embryo Development *In Vitro* 69
    A. Timing of Early Cleavage Events (2- to 8-cells) 69
    B. Morphology of Early Cleavage Stage Human Embryos 71
    C. Cytological and Nuclear Characteristics of Human Embryos Developing *In Vitro* 74
    D. Morphology of Late Preimplantation Human Embryos Grown *In Vitro* 76
    E. Embryo Development and Culture System Used 76
    F. Perforation of the Zona for Assisted Hatching 78
    G. The Transfer of Human Embryos 79

References 80

I. INTRODUCTION

Human oocytes can be fertilized readily *in vitro*, and the fertilized ovum will develop through the preimplantation stages *in vitro*. It is essential that the oocyte has extruded the first polar body before the oocyte is inseminated (Figure 1). Human spermatozoa capacitate *in vitro* after removal of seminal plasma and resuspension in culture medium. Sperm acrosomes must react before they can penetrate the zona pellucida, but there are few human sperm which are acrosome-reacted at any time during incubation in culture medium. It is likely that the fertilizing spermatozoon acrosome reacts when in contact with the zona pellucida. Penetration of the zona requires hyperactive motility of the acrosome-reacted spermatozoon, and the sperm must retain motility until they fuse with the oocyte plasma membrane. Sperm fusion with the oocyte plasma membrane initiates the cortical granule reaction and expulsion of the second polar body from the oocyte. The cortical granule contents released into the perivitelline space cause the zona reaction which prevents supernumary sperm entering or completing penetration of the zona. Microvilli on the oocyte plasma membrane, which initiate fusion with the equatorial segment of the sperm head, draw the whole spermatozoon into the oocyte cytoplasm, and decondensation of the sperm head begins (Figure 1) through factors present in the ooplasm (Male Pronucleus Growth Factor). Pronuclear membranes are formed around the male and female chromosomes, and the pronuclei move to the center of the oocyte and remain there until the pronuclear membranes dissolve (20 to 26 h after insemination). This allows combination of the maternal and paternal chromatids on the metaphase plate of the first cleavage division (syngamy), establishing the embryonic genome (Figure 2). Cleavage occurs within a few hours of syngamy, completing the fertilization process. In this chapter, we explore the practical details of insemination, fertilization, and preimplantation embryo development *in vitro*.

II. INSEMINATION OF OOCYTES *IN VITRO*

Various culture systems have been used successfully for *in vitro* fertilization (IVF), including test tubes, petri dishes, multi-well dishes, and the central well of plastic organ culture dishes. In most cases, the oocytes are cultured in relatively large volumes of medium (0.5 to 1.0 ml) and, for normozoospermic men, are inseminated with 50 to 100,000 normal motile sperm. We have found no difference in either the normal or abnormal rates of fertilization when the numbers of sperm are reduced from 100,000 to 50,000/ml (51.8% vs. 59.8% and 5.2% vs. 4.1%, respectively), and we routinely add 50,000 sperm to each oocyte. For male factor patients, however, fertilization rates are significantly lower than for female factor etiologies, and, as a result, larger numbers of sperm are added to smaller volumes of media to enhance the rates of fertilization. In many cases, though, the treatment of severe male factor infertility with high concentrations of motile sperm is limited by the low numbers of motile sperm present in the ejaculate. For oligoasthenozoospermic patients, it may be

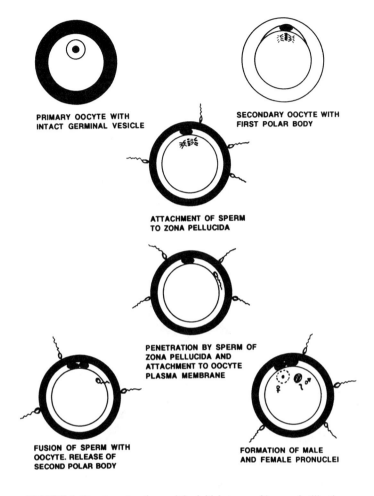

FIGURE 1. Oocyte maturation and the initial stages of human fertilization.

necessary to concentrate the sperm into a small volume following washing to obtain a high concentration and to add the oocytes directly to the concentrated specimen for fertilization.

A. INSEMINATION IN CAPILLARY TUBES AND STRAWS

Successful fertilization of human oocytes in microcapillary tubes and embryo cryopreservation straws using 5 to 10 µl volumes containing 2000 to 4000 normal sperm has been reported [1,2] with fertilization rates comparable to those achieved under standard insemination conditions. More recently, Hammitt et al.[3] have also achieved high fertilization rates with male factor sperm using cryopreservation straws and volumes of 10 to 150 µl. The technique of microinsemination in capillary tubes and cryopreservation straws is described in detail in the papers referred to above. Essentially, both methods use a

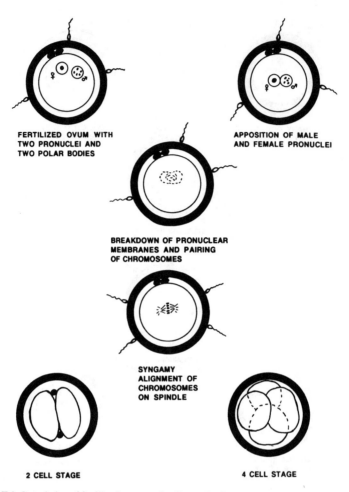

FIGURE 2. Completion of fertilization events leading to the first two cleavage events. All of these stages are dependent on maternal messages produced during oogenesis.

tuberculin syringe with an adaptor to aspirate the sperm-oocyte suspension into the tube or straw. In the former, the sperm-oocyte solution is surrounded by a small amount of sterile, equilibrated liquid paraffin, whereas, in the latter, it is protected by culture medium separated by small columns of air. In each case, the straws are cultured horizontally at 37°C in 5% CO_2 with saturated humidity. After culture overnight, the contents of the tubes or straws are allowed to drain into the center well of an organ culture dish containing culture medium, and then the tubes or straws are rinsed twice to ensure that all of the oocytes are recovered.

B. INSEMINATION IN MICRODROPS

Prior to the introduction of microinsemination using capillary tubes and straws, Cohen et al.[4] showed that successful fertilization could be achieved

TABLE 1
Male Factor Microdrop Results

Male factor category	Number of cycles	Number of oocytes inseminated	% fertilized 2PN	Number of >2PN	Number and % of transfers preg.	
Single defect	5	51	19.6	0.0	0	0
Double defect	33	274	36.4	2.9	20	4 (20.0%)
Triple defect	13	113	25.7	8.8	7	1 (14.3%)
Antibodies	5	46	43.5	2.2	3	0
Failed Fert.	3	28	17.9	3.6	2	0
Bad on the day	8	69	58.0	5.8	7	2 (28.6%)
Total	**67**	**581**	**35.1**	**4.1**	**39**	**7 (18.0%)**

using small numbers of sperm in 0.2 ml microdroplets under oil. We have evaluated the combined methods of insemination in microdrops under oil and use of high concentrations of motile sperm in the treatment of male-factor infertility. Patients were categorized as being male factor if the average concentration was $<20 \times 10^6$ sperm/ml, if motility <40%, if abnormal morphology >50%, and if immunobeads showed the presence of autosperm antibodies, as defined by >50% binding of IgG and/or IgA. These patients were further divided into five major groups: severe single defect, double defect, triple defect, antibodies, and previous failed fertilization as described by Yates et al.[5] In the majority of patients, the decision to use microdrop insemination was made prior to the day of oocyte retrieval and was based on the patient's semen analysis or results of previous IVF cycles. In a number of cycles, however, the decision to use microdrops was made on the day of oocyte recovery.

The technique of microdrop insemination is relatively simple. Motile spermatozoa are prepared using discontinuous two-step (45%/90%) Percoll gradients[5] and concentrated by centrifugation after washing. Twenty to thirty µl drops of the concentrated sperm suspension, containing 4 to 18×10^6 sperm/ml are placed under pre-equilibrated liquid paraffin oil in Nunc four-well dishes (Roskilde, Denmark). After a further period of equilibration, oocytes are transferred to the drops in as small a volume of insemination medium as possible to avoid diluting the sperm solution. The cumulus-oocyte complex can be reduced in size either by cutting mechanically with 26-gauge needles or by incubation in hyaluronidase. The former is preferable, as we have found that hyaluronidazed oocytes tend to float to the top of the microdrop and remain there throughout the insemination period. These oocytes invariably degenerate. Sperm and oocytes are incubated at 37°C in 5% CO_2 for 16 to 20 h prior to evaluation for fertilization. Normally fertilized oocytes are then cultured for a further 24 to 48 h before transfer to the uterus or fallopian tubes.

The results of 67 cycles in which oocytes were inseminated with male factor sperm in microdrops are shown in Table 1. The overall rates for normal and polyspermic fertilization were 35.1% (204/581) and 4.1% (24/581), respectively. The normal fertilization rates in the double defect, antibody, and "bad semen quality on the day" groups were all significantly higher than those

TABLE 2
Fertilization Rates in Oocytes Inseminated in Microdrops with and without Cumulus Cells

Cumulus status	Number of cycles	No. of oocytes inseminated	% Fertilized 2PN	No. of >2PN	No. & % transfer preg.
With	52	467	37.9[a]	4.1	32 7 (21.9)
Without	15	114	23.7[b]	4.4	7 0 (0.0)

Note: [a] versus [b]: $p < 0.00046$.

TABLE 3
Microdrop Fertilization Rates in Male Factor Patients after a Conventional Insemination Cycle

Insemination conditions	No. of cycles	No. of oocytes inseminated	No. & % of oocytes fertilized	No. & % of transfer cycles
Conventional	24	206	29 (14%)	11 (46%)
Microdrops	24	254	139 (55%)	19 (79%)

observed in the severe single defect, triple defect, and failed fertilization groups (p values ranging from 0.0001 to 0.05) but were not significantly different in the polyspermic fertilization rate in the triple defect group compared to the single and double defect groups ($p < 0.0266$ and 0.0114, respectively). There was, however, no significant difference between the six groups in pregnancy rates of patients who were transferred embryos.

A comparison of fertilization rates in oocytes inseminated in microdrops with and without cumulus cells (Table 2) shows a highly significant difference ($p < 0.0046$) between the two groups and emphasizes the problems encountered with hyaluronidazed oocytes or when cumulus cells are absent.

The efficacy of inseminating oocytes for individual couples is demonstrated in Table 3, where the fertilization rates in microdrops are compared with those resulting from conventional techniques in the preceding IVF cycle. These results show that there is a highly significant difference in the fertilization rate obtained with microdrop insemination (55% vs. 14%; $p < 0.0001$), resulting in significantly more treatment cycles proceeding to embryo transfer ($p < 0.016$).

It is clear that the treatment of male factor infertility can be successfully achieved by inseminating oocytes in microdrops containing high concentrations of motile spermatozoa. The use of high sperm concentrations does not appear to increase the incidence of polyspermy or reduce the capacity of the resulting embryos to implant and produce pregnancies. The relative merits of microdrops compared to capillary tubes or embryo cryopreservation straws are yet to be determined. Definite proof of the comparative value of these microinsemination techniques will not only require insemination of oocytes from the same cohort in either tubes, straws, or drops but will also necessitate comparisons with oocytes inseminated under standard conditions with normal numbers of sperm.

C. INSEMINATION IN COCULTURE SYSTEMS

In a recent study, Bongso et al.[6] have compared the fertilization rates between oocytes inseminated in medium alone and oocytes inseminated in the presence of medium conditioned by human tubal ampullary cells. They found that significantly more oocytes fertilized in ampullary coculture than in the controls (85% vs. 67%; $p < 0.01$) and that this occurred for sperm samples with normal and reduced sperm motility. They observed that insemination of oocytes should be carried out in the presence of freshly detached cells from passaged monolayers, as the sperm bound to monolayer cells, and their motility was impeded. Although these results were obtained with a small number of patients (32), they are of some interest and clearly warrant further investigation. If it appears that human ampullary coculture cells release certain factors into the culture medium that increase the fertilizability of sperm, then the combination of conditioned medium and microinsemination techniques may further improve the chances of fertilization with male factor sperm.

III. FERTILIZATION *IN VITRO*

A. CHECKING FOR FERTILIZATION

In most cases, fertilization checks are carried out on the morning of the day after egg recovery, some 12 to 20 h after insemination. By this time, the cumulus mass has become completely dispersed and forms a monolayer of cells upon which the oocyte, still surrounded by the corona cells, rests. Unlike the cumulus cells, the corona cells remain attached to the oocyte by the vestiges of their transzonal processes and completely obscure the ooplasm and perivitelline space. Two methods are available for removing these cells, both of which involve some manipulation of the oocyte.

In the first, cells are dissected away using fine (26 gauge) needles attached to 1 ml tuberculin syringes. Using this method, one needle is used to "pin down" the oocyte, while the other strips off as many cells as necessary for evaluation. In the second and most commonly used method, a finely drawn pipette is used to denude the oocyte of cells.

Both techniques have advantages and disadvantages. The diameter of the pipette must not be smaller than that of the oocyte, otherwise excessive compression may result in the rupture of the zona pellucida. Similarly, it is possible to pierce the zona with the needle. Conversely, if the bore of the pipette is too large, then insufficient numbers of cells will be removed. There is no doubt that, by using a micropipette of the correct diameter, a large number of oocytes can be checked in a short time, minimizing temperature and pH changes. However, on some occasions, the corona cells are very difficult to remove using pipettes, and needles should be used to avoid damage to the oocyte. In some clinics, sets of graded pipettes are prepared for denuding oocytes. This is probably unnecessary, as, with experience, pipettes of the correct bore can be drawn as required. However, it is useful to have two pipettes of slightly different diameter, first to strip most of the outer corona cells and second to remove the inner cells adhering to the zona.

There are a number of important guidelines to observe when performing fertilization checks. First, always use separate needles or pipettes for each patient. Second, speed is of the essence, particularly if the oocytes are cultured in large volumes of media in four-well or organ culture dishes. Every effort should be made to reduce temperature and pH change. If necessary, the corona-enclosed oocytes can be transferred to HEPES-buffered culture medium during the time needed to assess the oocytes prior to their return to fresh culture medium. Third, although it is advisable to perform the fertilization checks as quickly as possible, it is also essential that they are done efficiently and that each oocyte is examined carefully. As will be shown in the following section, it is important that any anomalies in fertilization checks should be performed between 16 to 20 h after insemination and ideally at 18 h. After 20 h, there is an increasing possibility that pronuclear dissolution will have occurred, and the oocyte can be classified as unfertilized. By contrast, if the checks are performed too early, pronuclear formation may not have occurred, and again, the oocyte may be assessed as being unfertilized. In both cases, the oocytes will have divided by the following day and may be classified as showing delayed fertilization.[7]

B. ABNORMALITIES OF FERTILIZATION

The criteria for normal fertilization are the presence of two pronuclei in the cytoplasm and two polar bodies in the perivitelline space. However, the combination of problems that arise from the use of low powered microscopes, from insufficient denuding of the egg, and from fragmentation of the first polar body often makes accurate visualization of the polar bodies difficult; as a result, only the pronuclei are used as a guide to the status of fertilization. Where two pronuclei are observed, the eggs are usually classified as having fertilized normally. By contrast, where more than two pronuclei (usually three but possibly four or five) are visible in the ooplasm, the oocytes are assumed to be polyspermic and to have been penetrated by more than one sperm (see Figure 3). Invariably, these eggs are discarded without further observation, even though it is known that the additional pronuclei are in some cases cytoplasmic vacuoles and can be distinguished by their lack of nucleoli under phase contrast optics on an inverted microscope.[8]

The reported incidence of polypronuclear embryos in IVF cycles varies, but generally ranges between 5% and 10%.[9] The majority results from penetration of the oocyte by two or more sperm. An increased risk of polyspermy is associated with early or late inseminations,[10] rupture of the zona pellucida,[11] and insemination with high numbers of motile sperm.[12] In most clinics, transfer of embryos containing three or more pronuclei is avoided because they could

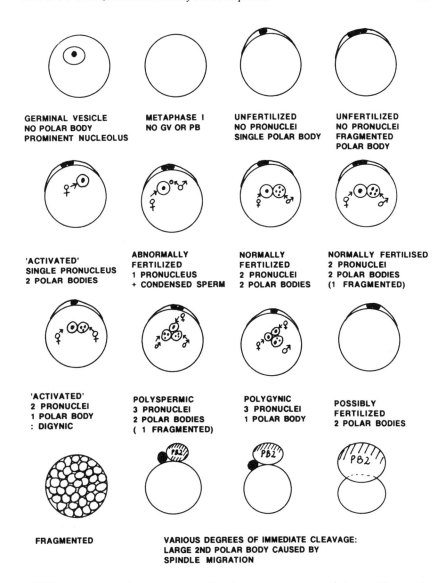

FIGURE 3. The normal appearance of fertilization stages and range of abnormalities seen in human oocytes during the process of fertilization *in vitro*.

result in genetic abortions, the formation of hydatidiform moles, or even triploid infants. Vigilance is required to identify these embryos at the pronuclear stage because they often cleave normally and are morphologically indistinguishable from normally fertilized embryos. Recently, several groups have attempted correction of polyspermy through microsurgical removal of a single pronucleus.[13,14] However, Wiker et al.[15] have concluded that the parental origin of human pronuclei cannot be determined morphologically using standard optics and advise caution when contemplating the microsurgical removal

TABLE 4
Fertilization Outcome of 1364 Oocytes

Number of oocytes inseminated:	1364	
Number fertilized normally:	738	(54.1%)
Number polypronuclear:	56	(4.1%)
Number unfertilized:	486	(35.6%)
Number with delayed fertilization:	54	(4.0%)
Number with ruptured zonae:	39	(2.9%)
Number degenerated/vacuolated:	12	(0.9%)
Number immature (germinal vesicles):	10	(0.8%)
Number with immediate cleavage:	8	(0.6%)
Number activated:	8	(0.6%)

of paternal pronuclei. Indeed, the relevance of such procedures is questionable, since only 24% of tripronuclear oocytes develop into triploid embryos after the first cleavage division[16] and since there is a clear correlation between the pattern of the first cleavage division and the subsequent karyotype of these embryos.

The nature and incidence of other anomalies commonly observed at the fertilization check are shown in Figure 3 and Table 4. In this series of 1364 inseminated oocytes, 54.1% fertilized normally and 4.1% were polypronuclear. Additional abnormalities included ruptured zonae, activation, degenerated and vacuolated oocytes, delayed fertilization, immediate cleavage, and immature oocytes with intact germinal vesicles. The second largest category (35.6%) consisted of unfertilized oocytes. It is usually assumed that most IVF failures are due to the functional incompetence of the sperm. This is invariably the case in male-factor infertility. However, failure of fertilization also occurs in cycles where semen parameters appear normal, and it is likely that oocytes abnormalities may play a larger role in the cause of human IVF failure than has been estimated previously.

C. REINSEMINATION

In the event that oocytes fail to fertilize upon the initial insemination, reinsemination provides a potential means by which fertilization can be achieved. Fertilization rates of 25 to 74% have been reported after reinsemination,[17-19] and pregnancies have been achieved following the transfer of reinseminated embryos. However, implantation and pregnancy rates are low and in the fullest study to date,[20] only two pregnancies were obtained from 76 embryo transfers (2.6%) with only 1.3% (2/158) of the embryos transferred implanting. More recently, Pool et al.[19] have used donor sperm to reinseminate oocytes first exposed to husband's sperm without fertilization. In four cases of male infertility, reinsemination with donor sperm gave an average fertilization rate of 70% and in two cases clinical pregnancy resulted. Although these results are only preliminary, Pool et al.[19] concluded that the reinsemination of oocytes with donor sperm when fertilization by husband fails, a procedure they refer to as "Donor Rescue," may be used to treat male factor infertility.

D. TIMING OF FERTILIZATION EVENTS

The process of fertilization in the human can be divided into three main stages: (1) the attachment to and subsequent penetration of the zona pellucida by the spermatozoon; (2) gamete fusion, sperm incorporation and activation of the oocytes; (3) decondensation of the sperm nucleus and formation of the male and female pronuclei. Using living gametes, zona penetration and sperm-oocyte fusion cannot be detected easily with the microscope, and, as a result, there is relatively little information available regarding the timing of these early fertilization events. (See Figures 1 and 2.) Moreover, spermatozoa are usually left in contact with the oocytes overnight, and fertilization is not assessed until 16 to 20 h after insemination. However, studies on fixed, zona-enclosed oocytes have shown the presence of decondensed spermatozoa in the ooplasm within 45 min after insemination,[21] suggesting that zona attachment, penetration, and sperm-oocyte fusion can occur very rapidly. More recently, we have found that approximately 30% of oocytes inseminated with normal sperm exhibit a clear second polar body by 4 h after insemination and that evidence of oocyte activation can be observed as early as 2.5 h after insemination.[22]

The mechanics of gamete fusion in the human and the time course of sperm nuclear decondensation and male pronuclear formation have been analyzed using polyspermic zona-free oocytes. In an elegant ultrastructural study, Sathananthan et al.[23] described the early stages of sperm fusion and incorporation. As in most eutherian mammals, in humans the plasma membrane overlying the midsegment of the sperm has special fusogenic properties which are only acquired after the acrosome reaction. Once initial membrane fusion occurs, the rest of the sperm head is incorporated into the ooplasm horizontally by a process similar to phagocytosis. Following its penetration into the ooplasm, the sperm head undergoes a series of complex ultrastructural changes resulting in its transformation into a fully developed male pronucleus. Using human zona-free eggs prepared from oocytes that failed to fertilize *in vitro*, Tesarik and Kopecny[24] and Lassalle and Testart[25] have described the main morphological changes and the time course of human sperm nucleus transformation. This continuous process can be divided into four stages. Briefly, stage 1 is characterized by the disappearance of the sperm nuclear envelope, a medium degree of chromatin condensation, and enlargement of the sperm head. Sperm nuclear decondensation is completed in about 1 h and is followed by a partial recondensation within 1 h after the end of the nuclear decondensation phase. In stage 2, the sperm chromatin re-expands, and, between 2 to 3 h after the onset of sperm head decondensation, a dense outline appears around the sperm nucleus consisting of aggregations of small cytoplasmic vesicles. This is considered to be the beginning of pronuclear formation. The main events occurring in stage 3 are the completion of nuclear envelope reformation, the restructuring of chromatin, the assembly of nucleolar precursors, and the linear growth of the pronucleus. Nuclei may persist for a long period at stage 3 before progressing to stage 4 when nucleolar precursor development and changes in chromatin distribution are completed.

Newly formed pronuclei, completely surrounded by a primitive nuclear envelope, appear in zona-free oocytes as early as 2 h after insemination,[25] but in our own studies on zona-intact oocytes, we have not detected any pronuclei microscopically in living oocytes before 5 h.[22] Fully developed stage 4 male pronuclei are first observed approximately 12 h after insemination,[24] and, together with the female pronucleus, they migrate towards the central region of the oocyte where they become closely associated and flatten where they meet. Simultaneously, the nucleoli appear to cluster, aligning themselves equatorially on adjacent sides of the closely associated area between the pronuclei.[26] Details on the timing of pronuclear dissolution prior to syngamy are sparse. However, in a recent study, Osborn[27] has shown that only 7.5% of normally fertilized eggs showed dismantling of the pronuclear envelopes within 20 to 22 h after insemination. This figure increased to 18% and 23.5% at 22 to 24 h and 24 to 26 h, respectively. Concomitantly, the proportion of fertilized eggs undergoing the first cleavage division increased from 1.1% at 20 to 22 h to 3.5% and 16% at 22 to 24 h and 24 to 26 h, respectively. However, even at 26 to 30 h after insemination, 33% of the zygotes still had two clear pronuclei.

E. TRANSFER OF PRONUCLEAR EMBRYOS

In the majority of IVF clinics, normally fertilized oocytes are cultured for a further 24 to 48 h *in vitro* before replacement in the uterus. Nevertheless, successful pregnancies have resulted from the intrauterine transfer of pronucleate embryos.[28] In a prospective, controlled clinical trial, Warnes et al.[29] showed that there was no difference in pregnancy rate between transfers performed the day after oocyte recovery (pronuclear) or the following day (cleaved). The practice of transferring embryos into the uterus on day 1 has not been universally adopted, largely because it is felt that once embryos have undergone at least one cleavage division, it is easier to determine which embryos should be transferred, cryopreserved, or discarded. It is recognized, however, that *in vitro* culture conditions are suboptimal, and it can be argued that increased pregnancy rates should result after the replacement of pronucleate embryos. Indeed, the improved pregnancy rate of GIFT over IVF, which allows fertilization *in vivo* and minimizes the duration of culture *in vitro*, supports this view. There is no doubt that GIFT is an effective form of therapy for those infertile couples in which the female partner has at least one patent fallopian tube. However, in certain cases of non-tubal infertility, the combination of fertilization *in vitro* and the subsequent transfer of pronuclear embryos into the fallopian tubes enhances the chances of pregnancy. The advantage of this technique, usually known as pronuclear stage tubal transfer (PROST)[30] or zygote intrafallopian transfer (ZIFT),[31,32] is that it allows the selection of normally fertilized oocytes for transfer as well as the use of techniques such as microinsemination and microinjection to enhance fertilization. To date, PROST/ZIFT has been applied successfully to couples with either unexplained infertility, or repeated failures in the GIFT program and to severe male factor infertility. The disadvantage of the procedure is that conventionally it has been an invasive, two-step procedure: ultrasound-guided retrieval and laparoscopic replacement. More recently, however, pregnancies have been obtained by retrograde catheterization of the fallopian tubes and ZIFT; it is likely that transcervical tubal cannulation will become the appropriate alternative to laparoscopic embryo transfer.

IV. EMBRYO DEVELOPMENT *IN VITRO*

Human embryos develop in simple culture medium to the hatched blastocyst stage.[10] During the first two cleavage divisions, the embryo is reliant on maternal mRNA produced during oogenesis, and the new embryonic transcripts are thought to be activated during the 4-cell stage of development.[33] Because human embryos are normally transferred before the 8-cell stage, the initial cleavage divisions are likely to reflect the adequacies of oocyte maturation rather than the developmental competence of the embryo. Human oocytes can also be parthenogenetically activated[34] and readily undergo apparently normal or abnormal cleavage. Under these circumstances, it is rather difficult to develop morphological and cleavage rate criteria which correlate closely with embryo viability.

A. TIMING OF EARLY CLEAVAGE EVENTS (2- TO 8-CELLS)

The mean time for the first three cleavage divisions reported by Trounson et al.[10] were 35.6, 45.7, and 54.3 h after insemination. In a detailed analysis of the early cleavage rate of human embryos, Cummins et al.[35] plotted the expected cleavage rate of embryos as a regression of logarithmically corrected embryo cell number against time after insemination (Figure 4). The mean expected times for the 2-, 4-, and 8-cell stages were 33.6, 45.5, and 56.4 h, respectively. These authors devised an embryo development rating (EDR) based on the formula

$$EDR = (TO/TE)\ 100$$

where TO is the observed time of the cleavage stage and TE is the expected time for that cleavage stage (derived from Figure 4). An EDR of 100 corresponds to an embryo at the cleavage stage expected. They were able to show a significant association of pregnancy with EDR in multiple and single embryo transfers, with increasing pregnancy rates with increasing EDR. Embryos with an EDR of 110 to 130 were more likely to result in pregnancy than slower cleaving embryos, but, interestingly, those embryos cleaving very rapidly (EDR > 130) produced pregnancies at rates similar to those of embryos with average cleavage rates (EDR 90 to 109). These rapidly dividing embryos probably include abnormal embryos, such as those derived from tripronuclear oocytes which cleave from 1 to 3-cells, then to 6-cells, etc.[16] Prediction of pregnancy was further improved by adding an embryo quality rating based on the regularity or symmetry of the embryos' blastomeres, the proportion of fragmented cells, and the clarity of the blastomere cytoplasm. Essentially,

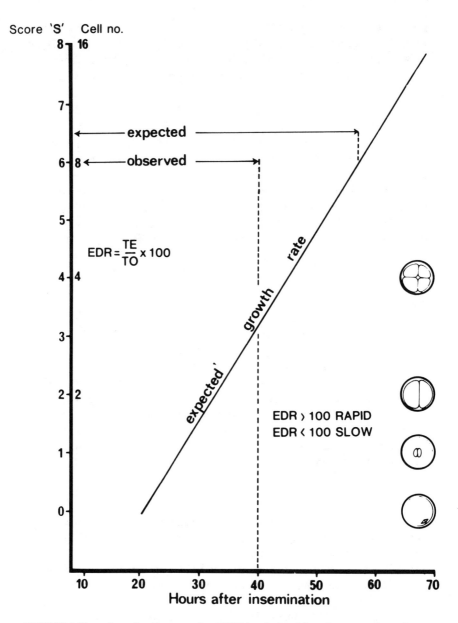

FIGURE 4. The embryo development rating (EDR) is calculated from the expected growth rate regression which has been plotted from cleavage rate data in an IVF program. An example is given for an eight-cell embryo, expected to be at this stage at 58 h but observed at 40 h. The EDR in this case is $(58/40) \times 100 = 145$. (Reproduced with permission from Cummins et al.[35]).

those embryos with abnormalities in these morphological characteristics had low viability irrespective of their cleavage rate.[35]

This information is very useful to assess the performance of IVF laboratory procedures. The aim is to maximize the number of normal embryos with EDR of 90 to 130. Changes to procedures such as the introduction of new culture media should also be assessed against the quality and cleavage rate of embryos, since a combination of embryo quality and the number of embryos transferred will be the primary determinant of IVF pregnancy rate and the proportion of multiple births. Steer et al.[36] combined the score for embryo quality with the number of embryos transferred to establish the cumulative embryo score (CES). This was derived from the formula

$$CES = \Sigma_n((EG \times CN)_a + (EG \times CN)_b + (EG \times CN)_c + \ldots\ldots)$$

where EG is the embryo grade, and CN is the cell number of each of the embryos (a,b,c.....) transferred. Four grades of embryos were defined: grade 4, equal sized symmetrical blastomeres; grade 3, uneven blastomeres with <10% fragmentation; grade 2, 10 to 50% blastomeric fragmentation; and grade 1, >50% blastomeric fragmentation or pronucleate single cell embryos.

The CES for 390 women less than 36 years of age and the mean number of embryos transferred are shown in Figure 5. Pregnancy rate increased significantly with the CES to a value of 42 but showed no further increase. All of the quadruplet and the majority of triplet pregnancies (14/18) occurred when the CES was higher than 42. These interesting data provide some quantitative indication of the number of embryos to transfer in relation to the grade and cleavage stage of the embryos involved. Put simply, it is sensible to transfer larger numbers of low quality embryos and to restrict the number of good quality embryos transferred.

The relationship between embryo quality and multiple pregnancy has also been demonstrated by Staessen et al.[37] who transferred three grades of embryos, those with regular cells and no fragments (A), those with some irregular cells and less than 20% of the embryo's volume containing anucleate fragments (B), and those with 20 to 50% of their volume containing anucleate fragments (C). Pregnancy rate for embryos with 3-cells or more was 24% (A), 12% (B), and 0 (C). When A and B embryos graded 0, 1, or 2 were transferred, twin pregnancies increased from 0 to 8% to 39%, respectively. These data again strongly support the need to monitor closely the quality and number of embryos replaced and to advise some patients about both pregnancy and multiple pregnancy expectations.

B. MORPHOLOGY OF EARLY CLEAVAGE STAGE HUMAN EMBRYOS

There have been many reports of the association between the morphological appearance and pregnancy success rates in IVF,[38-41] but the association with the usual criteria of size and regularity of blastomeres and the presence or absence of cytoplasmic fragments with capacity for continued development after transfer is weak and not particularly useful. In a report by Erenus et al.,[42] a simple grading system of three categories based on the three criteria of regularity of blastomere size, granularity of blastomere cytoplasm, and fragmentation showed a highly significant relationship to pregnancy rate. This was shown also to be related to

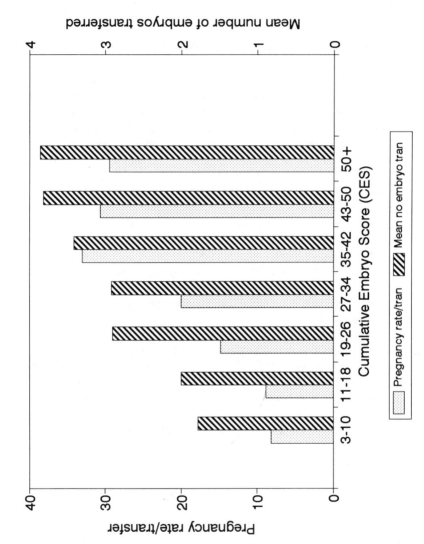

FIGURE 5. The relationship between the cumulative embryo score (CES) and the mean number of embryos transferred and pregnancy rate per transfer. (Data derived from Steer et al.[36])

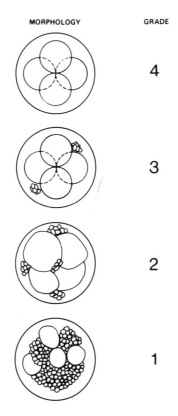

FIGURE 6. Embryo grading system for four-cell embryos: Grade 4: regular, spherical blastomeres with no extracellular fragmentation; Grade 3: regular, spherical blastomeres with some extracellular fragmentation; Grade 2: blastomeres slightly irregular in size and shape with considerable extracellular fragmentation; Grade 1: barely defined blastomeres with considerable extracellular fragmentation. (Reproduced with permission from Bolton et al.[43])

both cleavage rate and the number of embryos transferred. These criteria are more sensibly incorporated into the EDR or CES systems.

A well-defined grading system was reported by Bolton et al.[43] and is shown in Figure 6. They examined the developmental capacity of human embryos *in vitro* and showed that the better quality embryos (Grades 3 and 4) developed to blastocysts at a very much higher rate (23 and 18%, respectively) than poor quality embryos (Grades 1 and 2; 5 and 6%, respectively). While they found an association between cleavage rate and capacity to develop to blastocysts *in vitro*, those embryos which were up to a cleavage division retarded still had the capacity to develop to blastocysts (2- and 3-cells by the time of transfer, 17 and 21% developed to blastocysts vs. 26% for 4-cell embryos). However, the predictive value of both embryo quality and cleavage rate was only 34%. It is apparent that morphology and cleavage rate are only some of the criteria necessary to predict the capacity for development to blastocysts *in vitro*. Noninvasive tests of embryo viability are therefore highly desirable (see Chapter 10).

In their study of 317 pronucleate oocytes, the majority developed to 2-cells (98%) and 4-cells (85%), but thereafter there was a dramatic decline in the proportion developing through subsequent divisions (Figure 7), and only 17% of the original oocytes developed into fully expanded blastocysts. The high loss of developmental capacity probably includes intrinsic factors, such as developmental and genetic errors, and extrinsic factors, such as sub-optimal culture conditions.

C. CYTOLOGICAL AND NUCLEAR CHARACTERISTICS OF HUMAN EMBRYOS DEVELOPING *IN VITRO*

The cell number, nuclear number, and nuclear integrity of human embryos on days 2, 3, and 5 after insemination have been examined in some detail by Winston et al.[44] Their study of embryos derived from apparently normal oocytes with two pronuclei showed that embryos graded as normal, with even blastomeres and no fragmentation, were most likely to have single nuclei in each cell at days 2 and 3. Embryos of decreasing quality (increasing lack of cell symmetry and fragmentation) had increasing proportions of anucleate and polynucleate cells. Multinucleate blastomeres and cytoplasmic fragments have been frequently reported in early cleavage stage embryos.[45,46]

The high frequency of disturbance to normal cytokinesis and nucleokinesis during early cleavage divisions is likely a major contribution to the relatively low viability of human embryos. In the study by Winston et al.,[44] 62 (39%) of 159 normally fertilized oocytes developed to cavitated blastocysts during five d in culture. However, only 39% of these blastocysts had more than 29 nuclei, and all had multinucleated cells. When calculated as the percentage of fertilized oocytes, it is apparent that only about 13% are capable of developing to blastocysts with sufficient nucleated cells to form both inner cell mass and trophectoderm, and the subsequent lineages for normal development. Winston et al.[44] believe they may have overestimated the number of cells with single nuclei, but it is interesting that their estimate approaches the expected implantation rate of human embryos transferred to patients. While the quality grade of the embryos at 42 to 46 h after insemination was related to the cell numbers in blastocysts, only 46% of the blastocysts formed from the best quality embryos had more than 29 nuclei. Even fewer (20%) of second grade and none of third or fourth grade embryos formed blastocysts with 30 or more nuclei. On day 5 after insemination, it could be expected that embryos should have made at least six cleavage divisions, with 60 or more cells, but few (18%) of even the best quality embryos had this many nuclei.

It is possible that the cleavage retardation and the nuclear abnormalities observed in human embryos may be related to sub-optimal culture conditions. It is also likely they derive from abnormalities of oocyte maturation and the events of fertilization *in vitro* because a large number of nuclear and cytoplasmic abnormalities are also observed in unfertilized and fertilized human oocytes examined after insemination *in vitro*.[47,48]

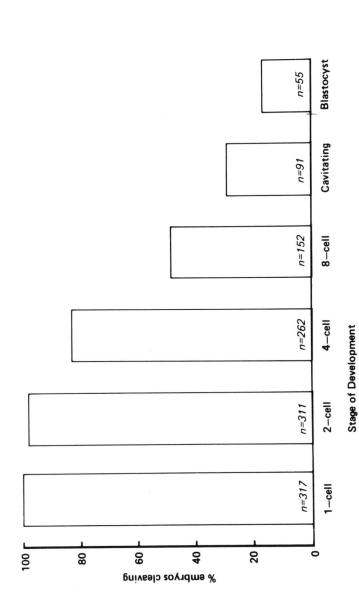

FIGURE 7. Percentage of 317 spare human preimplantation embryos surviving each cleavage division through to blastocyst formation *in vitro*. (Reproduced with permission from Bolton et al.[43])

D. MORPHOLOGY OF LATE PREIMPLANTATION HUMAN EMBRYOS GROWN *IN VITRO*

A large percentage (45%) of human blastocysts grown *in vitro* have visible morphological abnormalities, including more than one cavity, necrotic areas, no visible inner cell mass, irregular trophoblast cells, severe contraction,[49] and variable cell numbers (24 to 90 cells).[50] It is also apparent that there is no increase in implantation rate when embryos are cultured to the blastocyst stage prior to transfer to patients.[51] In studies where supernumary embryos were cultured to the blastocyst stage after transfer of early cleavage stage embryos to patients 2 to 3 d after insemination, there have been variable correlations between pregnancy and the capacity of a patient's embryos to blastulate. Bolton et al.[43] reported similar rates of embryos developing to blastocysts in pregnant (31%) and non-pregnant patients (28%), whereas Sjögren et al.[52] reported high rates in pregnant patients (100%) compared to non-pregnant patients (53%). In the latter report, 34% of spare embryos developed to blastocysts compared with 63% of spare embryos of pregnant patients. Despite these correlations, the predictive value of blastocyst formation for pregnancy was rather low.[52]

Dorkras et al.[53] report that cavitation, as distinct from blastulation, occurred in 31% of embryos developing from 1-cell fertilized oocytes (bipronucleate and multipronucleate oocytes). However, many of these embryos are vacolated morulae attempting unsuccessful or incomplete blastulation and are not typical blastocysts (Figure 8). Only 19% of fertilized oocytes developed to typical blastocysts, involving a single layer of trophectoderm and an inner cell mass. When all abnormal oocytes were excluded, the percentage of blastocysts increased to 27%.

The abnormal cavitating morulae do not produce human Chorionic Gonadotrophin (hCG). The earliest detection of hCG secretion from a human blastocyst was day 6 after insemination, which was one day after the earliest time of blastocyst formation (49% blastulated on day 5).[53] However, as shown in Figure 9, the first significant rise in mean hCG for 26 human blastocysts was day 8, peaking on day 10, and decreasing to baseline levels by day 14. Blastocyst escape from the zona pellucida (hatching) usually occurs days 7 to 9.[53] Interestingly, blastocysts derived from oocytes with single pronuclei (possibly parthenogenetic) also produced hCG in quantities similar to bipronucleate oocytes.[53]

E. EMBRYO DEVELOPMENT AND CULTURE SYSTEM USED

It has been proposed that improved embryo quality and viability can be achieved by coculture of human embryos with somatic cells, in particular with human tubal ampullary epithelial cells.[54] While some improvement in cleavage to blastocysts was evident in coculture (69% of pronucleate oocytes cavitated) when compared with simple T6 medium with 15% serum (33% of pronucleate oocytes cavitated), there was no improvement in the percentage of properly expanding and hatched blastocysts.[54] Similar improvements in the percentage

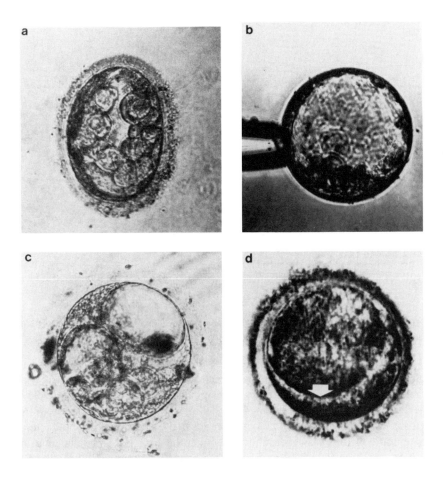

FIGURE 8. Blastocysts and cavitating morulae. (a) Cavitating morula, (b) typical blastocyst, (c) day 5 embryo with multiple cavities, (d) day 5 embryo with a single large cavity; the arrow denotes the sharp borders (magnification × 40). (Reproduced with permission from Dorkras et al.[53])

of human embryos developing to blastocysts have been reported in CZB medium designed to improve mouse embryo development in culture (56% development to blastocysts in CZB compared to 20% in Earle's balanced salt solution), although there was no improvement in implantation rates of embryos cultured in CZB.[55] The CZB medium has an increased lactate to pyruvate ratio, EDTA, and glutamine, and it lacks glucose for initial stages of culture. A beneficial effect on the rate of development of human embryos to expanded blastocysts was reported in coculture with Vero cells (African monkey kidney cells).[56] However, there is a need to examine more closely the morphology of embryos grown in these new culture conditions and to conduct adequate prospective controlled trials to assess their benefit for embryo development *in vitro*. The role of culture medium components in embryo developments is discussed extensively in Chapter 5.

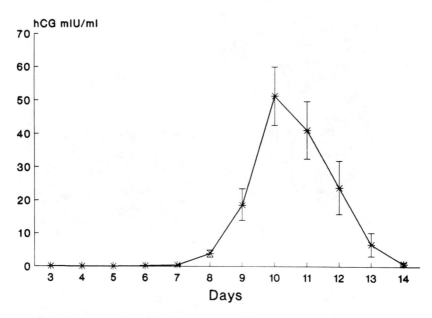

FIGURE 9. Mean (+ SEM) daily hCG secretion by 26 human blastocysts from days 3 to 14 of culture. (Reproduced with permission from Dorkras et al.[53])

There is interest developing in the production and sequence of expression of cytokines in early human embryo development,[57] the production of growth factors in culture medium from human embryos (for example, platelet-derived growth factor is detected in medium in which human blastocysts grow),[58] and the response of human embryos to the addition of growth factors to culture media. However, there is rather little convincing evidence at present that significant improvements can be made to human embryo development and viability by addition of cytokines and growth factors to culture media. This is an important area of current research.

F. PERFORATION OF THE ZONA FOR ASSISTED HATCHING

It has been reported[59] that the mechanical perforation of the zona pellucida in 4-cell human embryos will improve the implantation of embryos transferred to patients. The small slit made in the zona aided embryos in hatching from the zona pellucida. A zona drilling procedure, where the zona was digested by squirting acidified Tyrode's medium (pH 2.35) at the zona to form a gap of 10–36 μm, was used by Cohen et al.[60] to show that implantation rate could be increased in embryos with thick zonae (>15 μm). In embryos with thin zonae (<13 μm), implantation was reduced. By selecting embryos for zona drilling, they increased implantation rates from 18% to 25%. These observations suggest that embryos with thick zonae (>15 μm), or those with a poor prognosis because of retarded cleavage and fragmentation may benefit from zona drilling to aid their hatching and implantation.

G. THE TRANSFER OF HUMAN EMBRYOS

Preimplantation embryos are usually transferred to the uterus using a variety of transfer catheters. Embryos may also be transferred to the fallopian tubes by laparoscopy or ultrasound guidance,[61,62] hysteroscopy,[63] or nonhysteroscopic falloposcopy[64] through the cervix, uterine cavity, and utero-tubal junction. However, there is little evidence that the replacement of cleavage stage embryos in the fallopian tube improves their survival and implantation over that achieved by transfer to the uterine cavity. In fact, in a prospective randomized trial, Balmaceda et al.[65] showed that implantation rates were the same for embryos replaced in the uterus (17.4%) and in the fallopian tubes (21.5%) in patients transferred embryos during hormonal replacement cycles in an oocyte donation program. Embryos were replaced 44 to 48 h after insemination at the 2- to 4-cell stage. Our own clinical experience is that there is no difference in implantation or pregnancy rate between laparoscopic and ultrasound guided tubal embryo transfer (TEST) and uterine replacement of embryos.

The use of ultrasound to guide the replacement of human embryos in the uterine cavity has shown no significant improvement in pregnancy rate over that obtained without any ultrasound guidance.[66] Other studies examining the retention of radiopaque dye in the uterus after "mock" embryo transfer showed that the dye remained in the uterine cavity in only 68% of patients in the optimum embryo transfer position (knee-chest for anteverted and supine for retroverted or axial uterus) and in 48% for the non-optimum position (supine for anteverted uterus).[67] Dye moved into the fallopian tubes in 38%, into the cervix in 9%, and into the vagina in 12% of cases. It was recommended that a mock transfer be performed to determine the correct position for embryo transfer for each patient.

The type of embryo transfer catheter may influence pregnancy rate. For example, it has been reported that the fine, relatively rigid Tom Cat catheter resulted in higher pregnancy rates than the Frydman catheter, which has a soft distal end with an end opening (28% compared with 16% pregnancy rates, respectively).[68] In some cases a cervical introducer[69] may be needed to avoid difficult transfers in patients with tortuous cervical canals, and when using in soft side opening catheters. Other modifications[70] improve their ease of use and transfer success rates.

It was reported that the transfer of embryos in 100% human serum improved pregnancy rates when compared to culture medium without serum.[71] However, a prospective randomized trial comparing transfer of embryos in medium containing 75% human serum, 8% human serum, and 2.25% human serum albumin showed no significant difference in pregnancy rates between the three media (43%, 27%, and 36% pregnancy rates, respectively).[72]

Choices regarding the procedures of IVF, GIFT, and ZIFT will depend on the patency of a patient's fallopian tubes, access to laparoscopy, and the policy of the clinic involved. Bollen et al.[73] reported implantation rates of 14%, 8%, and 18% for IVF, GIFT, and ZIFT, respectively, when three embryos or oocytes were transferred. However, others have reported consistently higher implantation and pregnancy rates for GIFT than for IVF. It is recommended that patients with at least one patent fallopian tube be treated by GIFT or ZIFT, and those with blocked fallopian tubes be treated by IVF and embryo transfer to the uterus. Under optimal conditions, the maximum number of oocytes or embryos transferred should be restricted to two or three depending on the quality of embryos available. Under these conditions 20 to 30% of IVF patients and 30 to 40% of GIFT patients will have clinical pregnancies with a minimum of multiple fetuses.

REFERENCES

1. **Van der Ven, H. H., Hoebbel, K., Al-Hasani, S., Diedrich, K., and Kerbs, D.,** Fertilization of human oocytes in capillary tubes with very small numbers of spermatozoa, *Hum. Reprod.,* 4, 72, 1989.
2. **Ranoux, C. and Seibel, M. M.,** New techniques in fertilization: intravaginal culture and microvolume straw, *J. In Vitro Fertil. Embryo Transfer,* 7, 6, 1990.
3. **Hammitt, D. G., Walker, D. L., Syrop, C. H., Miller, T. M., and Bennett, M. R.,** Treatment of severe male-factor infertility with high concentrations of motile sperm by microinsemination in embryo cryopreservation straws, *J. In Vitro Fertil. Embryo Transfer,* 8, 101, 1991.
4. **Cohen, J., Edwards, R., Fehilly, C., Fishel, S., Hewitt, J., Purdy, J., Rowland, G., Steptoe, P., and Webster, J.,** *In Vitro* Fertilization: a treatment for male infertility, *Fertil. Steril.,* 43, 422, 1985.
5. **Yates, C. A., Thomas, C., Kovacs, G. T., and de Kretser, D. M.,** Andrology, male factor infertility and IVF, in *Clinical in vitro Fertilization,* Wood, C. and Trounson, A.O., Eds.,. Springer-Verlag, Berlin, 1989, 95.
6. **Bongso, A., Ng, S.-C., Fong, C.-Y., and Ratnam, S.,** Improved fertilization rates of human oocytes in coculture, *J. In Vitro Fertil. Embryo Transfer,* 8, 216, 1991.
7. **Ron-El, R., Nachum, H., Herman, A., Golan, A., Caspi, E., and Soffer, Y.,** Delayed fertilization and poor embryonic development associated with impaired semen quality, *Fertil. Steril.,* 55, 338, 1991.
8. **Van Blerkom, J., Bell, H., and Henry, G.,** The occurrence, recognition and developmental fate of pseudo-multipronuclear eggs after *in vitro* fertilization of human oocytes, *Hum. Reprod.,* 2, 217, 1987.
9. **Dandekar, P. V., Martin, M. C., and Glass, R. H.,** Polypronuclear embryos after *in vitro* fertilization, *Fertil. Steril.,* 53, 510, 1990.
10. **Trounson, A. O., Mohr, L. R., Wood, C., and Leeton, J. F.,** Effect of delayed insemination on *in vitro* fertilization, culture and transfer of human embryos, *J. Reprod. Fertil.,* 64, 285, 1982.
11. **Lowe, B., Osborn, J. C., Fothergill, D., and Lieberman, B. A.,** Factors associated with accidental fractures of the zona pellucida and multipronuclear human oocytes following *in vitro* fertilization, *Hum. Reprod.,* 3, 901, 1988.
12. **Englert, Y., Puissant, F., Camus, M., Degueldre, M., and Leroy, F.,** Factors leading to tripronuclear eggs during human *in vitro* fertilization, *Hum. Reprod.,* 1, 117, 1986.
13. **Gordon, J. W., Grunfield, L., Garrisi, G. J., Navot, D., and Laufer, N.,** Successful microsurgical removal of a pronucleus from tripronuclear human zygotes, *Fertil. Steril.,* 52, 367, 1989.

14. **Malter, H. and Cohen, J.**, Embryonic development after microsurgical repair of polyspermic human zygotes, *Fertil. Steril.*, 52, 373, 1989.
15. **Wiker, S., Malter, H., Wright, G., and Cohen, J.**, Recognition of paternal pronuclei in human zygotes, *J. In Vitro Fertil. Embryo Transfer*, 7, 33 1990.
16. **Kola, I., Trounson, A., Dawson, G., and Rogers, P.**, Tripronuclear human oocytes: altered cleavage patterns and subsequent karyotypic analysis of embryos, *Biol. Reprod.*, 37, 395, 1987.
17. **Trounson, A. and Webb, J.**, Fertilization of human oocytes following reinsemination *in vitro*, *Fertil. Steril.*, 41, 816, 1984.
18. **Ben-Rafael, Z., Kopf, G. S., Blasco, L., Tureck, R. W., and Mastroianni, L.**, Fertilization and cleavage after reinsemination of human oocytes, *Fertil. Steril.*, 45, 58, 1986.
19. **Pool, T. B., Martin, J. E., Ellsworth, L. R., Perez, J. B., and Atiee, S. H.**, Zygote intrafallopian transfer with "donor rescue": a new option for severe male factor infertility, *Fertil. Steril.*, 54, 166, 1990.
20. **Pampiglione, J. S., Mills, C., Campbell, S., Steer, C., Kingsland, C., and Mason, B. A.**, The clinical outcome of reinsemination of human oocytes fertilized *in vitro*, *Fertil. Steril.*, 53, 306, 1990.
21. **Plachot, M., Junca, A. M., Mandelbaum, J., Cohen, J., Salat-Baroux, J., and Lage, C. D.**, Timing of *in vitro* fertilization of cumulus-free and cumulus-enclosed human oocytes, *Hum. Reprod.*, 4, 237, 1986.
22. **Osborn, J. C.**, Unpublished observations.
23. **Sathananthan, A. H., Ng, S. C., Edirisinghe, R., Ratnam, S. S., and Wong, P. C.**, Human sperm-egg interaction *in vitro*, *Gamete Res.*, 15, 317, 1986.
24. **Tesarik, J. and Kopecny, V.**, Development of human male pronucleus: ultrastructure and timing, *Gamete Res.*, 24, 135, 1989.
25. **Lassalle, B. and Testart, J.**, Sequential transformations of human sperm nucleus in human egg, *J. Reprod. Fertil.*, 91, 393, 1991.
26. **Wright, G., Wiker, S., Elsner, C., Kort, H., Massey, J., Mitchell, D., Toledo, A., and Cohen, J.**, Observations on the morphology of pronuclei and nucleoli in human zygotes and implications for cryopreservation, *Hum. Reprod.*, 5, 109, 1990.
27. **Osborn, J. C.**, Asynchronous pronuclear development in human embryos fertilized *in vitro*, Proc. Xth Annu. Sci. Meet. Fertil. Soc. Aust., 1991, 94.
28. **Ahuja, K. K., Smith, W., Tucker, M., and Craft, I.**, Successful pregnancies from the transfer of pronucleate embryos in an outpatient *in vitro* fertilization program, *Fertil. Steril.*, 44, 181, 1985.
29. **Warnes, G. M., Quinn, P., Kirby, C. A., Broom, T. J., and Kerin, J. F.**, The effect of transferring pronuclear embryos on pregnancy outcome after *in vitro* fertilization, *Ann. N. Y. Acad. Sci.*, 541, 465, 1988.
30. **Yovich, J. L., Blackledge, P. A., Richardson, P. A., Matson, P. L., Turner, S. R., and Draper, R.**, Pregnancies following pronuclear stage tubal transfer, *Fertil. Steril.*, 48, 851, 1987.
31. **Hamori, M., Stuckensen, J. A., Rumpf, D., Kniewald, T., Kniewald, A., and Marquez, M. A.**, Zygote intrafallopian transfer (ZIFT): evaluation of 42 cases, *Fertil. Steril.*, 50, 519, 1988.
32. **Devroey, P., Staeesen, C., Camus, M., De Grauwe, E., Wisanto, A., and Van Steirteghem, A. C.**, Zygote intrafallopian transfer as a successful treatment for unexplained infertility, *Fertil. Steril.*, 52, 246, 1989.
33. **Braude, P.R., Bolton, V.N., and Moore, S.**, Human gene expression first occurs between the four- and eight-cell stages of preimplantation development, *Nature*, 332, 459, 1988.
34. **Winston, N.J., Johnson, M.H., Pickering, S.J., and Braude, P.R.**, Parthenogenetic activation and development of fresh and aged human oocytes, *Fertil. Steril.*, 56, 904, 1991.

35. **Cummins, J.M., Breen, T.M., Harrison, K.L., Shaw, J.M., Wilson, L.M., and Hennessey, J.F.,** A formula for scoring human embryo growth rates in in vitro fertilization: its value in predicting pregnancy and in comparison with visual estimates of embryo quality, *J. In Vitro Fertil. Embryo Transfer,* 3, 284, 1986.
36. **Steer, C.V., Mills, C.L., Tan, S.L., Campbell, S., and Edwards, R.G.,** The cumulative embryo score: a predictive embryo scoring technique to select the optimal number of embryos to transfer in an in vitro fertilization and embryo transfer programme, *Hum. Reprod.,* 7, 117, 1992.
37. **Staessen, C., Camus, M., Bollen, N., Devroey, P., and Van Steirteghem, A.,** The relationship between embryo quality and the occurrence of multiple pregnancies, *Fertil. Steril.,* 57, 626, 1992.
38. **Testart, J.,** Cleavage stage of human embryos two days after fertilization in vitro and their developmental ability after transfer into the uterus, *Hum. Reprod.,* 1, 29, 1986.
39. **Puissant, F., Rysselberge, M.V., Barlow, P., Deweze, J., and Leroy, F.,** Embryo scoring as a prognostic tool in IVF treatment, *Hum. Reprod.,* 2, 705, 1987.
40. **Grillo, J. M., Gamerre, M., Lacroix, O., Noizet, A., and Vitry, G.,** Influence of the morphological aspect of embryos obtained by in vitro fertilization on their implantation rate, *J. In Vitro Fertil. Embryo Transfer,* 8, 317, 1991.
41. **Scott, R. T., Hofmann, G. E., Veek, L. L., Jones, H. W., and Muasher, S. J.,** Embryo quality and pregnancy rates in patients attempting pregnancy through in vitro fertilization, *Fertil. Steril.,* 55, 426, 1991.
42. **Erenus, M., Zouves, C., Rajamahendran, P., Leung, S., Fluker, M., and Gomel, V.,** The effect of embryo quality on subsequent pregnancy rates after in vitro fertilization, *Fertil. Steril.,* 56, 707, 1991.
43. **Bolton, V.N., Hawes, S.M., Taylor, C.T., and Parsons, J.H.,** Development of spare human preimplantation embryos in vitro: an analysis of the correlations among gross morphology, cleavage rates, and development to the blastocyst, *J. In Vitro Fertil. Embryo Transfer,* 6, 30, 1989.
44. **Winston, N.J., Braude, P.R., Pickering, S.J., George, M.A., Cant, A., Currie, J., and Johnson, M.H.,** The incidence of abnormal morphology and nucleocytoplasmic rations in 2-, 3- and 5-day human pre-embryos, *Hum. Reprod.,* 6, 17, 1991.
45. **Trounson, A. O. and Sathananthan, A. H.,** The application of electron microscopy in the evaluation of 2-4 cell human embryos cultured in vitro for embryo transfer, *J. In Vitro Fertil. Embryo Transfer,* 3, 153, 1984.
46. **Tesarik, J., Kopecny, V., Plachot, M., and Mandelbaum, J.,** Ultrastructural and autoradiographic observations on multinucleated blastomeres of human cleaving embryos obtained by in vitro fertilization, *Hum. Reprod.,* 2, 127, 1987.
47. **Sathananthan, A. H. and Trounson, A. O.,** The human pronuclear ovum: fine structure of monospermic and polyspermic fertilization in vitro, *Gamete Res.,* 12, 385, 1985.
48. **Balakier, H. and Casper, R.F.,** A morphologic study of unfertilized oocytes and abnormal embryos in human in vitro fertilization, *J. In Vitro Fertil. Embryo Transfer,* 8, 73, 1991.
49. **Hartshorne, G. M., Elder, K., Crow, J., Dyson, H., and Edwards, R. G.,** The influence of in vitro development upon post-thaw survival and implantation of cryopreserved human blastocysts, *Hum. Reprod.,* 6, 136, 1991.
50. **Hardy, K., Handyside, A. H., and Winston, R. M. L.,** The human blastocyst: cell number, death and allocation during late preimplantation development in vitro, *Development,* 107, 597, 1989.
51. **Bolton, V. N., Wren, M. E., and Parsons, J. H.,** Pregnancies following in vitro fertilization and transfer of human blastocysts, *Fertil. Steril.,* 55, 830, 1991.
52. **Sjögren, A., Sjöblom, P., and Hamberger, L.,** Culture of human spare embryos: association between blastocyst formation and pregnancy, *J. Assisted Reprod. Genet.,* 9, 41, 1992.

53. **Dorkras, A., Sargent, I. L., Ross, C., Gardner, R. L., and Barlow, D. H.,** The human blastocyst: morphology and human chorionic gonadotrophin secretion in vitro, *Hum. Reprod.,* 6, 143, 1991.
54. **Bongso, A., Ng, S.-C, Fong, C.-Y, and Ratnam, S.,** Cocultures: a new lead in embryo quality improvement for assisted reproduction, *Fertil. Steril.,* 56, 179, 1991.
55. **Fitzgerald, L. and DiMattina, M.,** An improved medium for long-term culture of human embryo overcomes the in vitro developmental block and increases blastocyst formation, *Fertil. Steril.,* 57, 641, 1992.
56. **Menezo, Y. J. R., Guerin, J. F., and Czyba, J. C.,** Improvement of human early embryo development in vitro by co-culture on monolayers of Vero cells, *Biol. Reprod.,* 42, 301, 1990.
57. **Zolti, M., Ben-Rafael, Z., Meirom, R., Shemesh, M., Bider, D., Mashiach, S., and Apte, R.N.,** Cytokine involvement in oocytes and early embryos, *Fertil. Steril.,* 56, 265, 1991.
58. **Svalander, P.C., Holmes, P.V., Olovsson, M., Wikland, M., Gemzell-Danielsson, K., and Bygdeman, M.,** Platelet-derived growth factor is detected in human blastocyst culture medium but not in human follicular fluid— a preliminary report, *Fertil. Steril.,* 56, 367, 1991.
59. **Cohen, J., Elsner, C., Kort, H., Malter, H., Massey, J., Mayer, M.P., and Wimer, K.,** Impairment of the hatching process following IVF in the human and improvement of implantation by assisting hatching using micromanipulation, *Hum. Reprod.,* 5, 7, 1990.
60. **Cohen, J., Alikani, M., Trowbridge, J., and Rosenwaks, Z.,** Implantation enhancement by selective assisted hatching using zona drilling of human embryos with poor prognosis, *Hum. Reprod.,* 7, 685, 1992.
61. **Bustillo, M. and Schulman, J.D.,** Transcervical ultrasound guided intrafallopian replacement of gametes, zygotes and embryos, *J. In Vitro Fertil. Embryo Transfer,* 6, 321, 1989.
62. **Yovich, J. L., Draper, R. R., Turner, S. R., and Cummins, J. M.,** Transcervical tubal embryo-stage transfer (TC-TEST), *J. In Vitro Fertil. Embryo Transfer,* 7, 137, 1990.
63. **Patton, P. E., Hickok, L. R., and Wolf, D. P.,** Successful hysteroscopic cannulation and tubal transfer of cryopreserved embryos, *Fertil. Steril.,* 55, 640, 1991.
64. **Kerin, J. F.,** Nonhysteroscopic falloposcopy: a proposed method for visual guidance and verification of tubal cannula placement for endotuboplasty, gamete and embryo transfer procedures, *Fertil. Steril.,* 57, 1133, 1992.
65. **Balmaceda, J. P., Alam, V., Roszjtein, D., Ord, T., Snell, K., and Asch, R. H.,** Embryo implantation rates in oocyte donation: a prospective comparison of tubal versus uterine transfers, *Fertil. Steril.,* 57, 362, 1992.
66. **Hurley, V.A., Osborn, J.C., Leoni, M.A., and Leeton, J.,** Ultrasound-guided embryo transfer: a controlled trial, *Fertil. Steril.,* 55, 559, 1991.
67. **Knutzen, V., Stratton, C.J., Sher, G., McNamee, P.I., Huang, T.T., and Soto-Albors, C.,** Mock embryo transfer in early luteal phase, the cycle before in vitro fertilization and embryo transfer; a descriptive study, *Fertil. Steril.,* 57, 156, 1992.
68. **Gonen, Y., Dirnfeld, M., Goldman, S., Koifman, M., and Abramovici, H.,** Does the choice of catheter for embryo transfer influence the success rate of in-vitro fertilization? *Hum. Reprod.,* 6, 1092, 1991.
69. **Danasouri, I.E. and Milki, A.,** A new cervical introducer for embryo transfer with soft open-ended catheters, *Fertil. Steril.,* 57, 939, 1992.
70. **Vaught, L.K., Stratton, C.J., Julian, P., Vaught, W.G., Sher, G., Knutzen, V., and Marriage, V.,** An improved system for catheter loading during embryo transfer, *J. In Vitro Fertil. Embryo Transfer,* 4, 346, 1987.
71. **Feichtinger, W., Kemeter, P., and Menezo, Y.,** The use of synthetic culture medium and patients' serum for human in vitro fertilization and embryo replacement, *J. In Vitro Fertil. Embryo Transfer,* 3, 87, 1986.

72. **Khan, I., Staessen, C., Devroey, P., and Van Steirteghem, A.C.,** Human serum albumin verses serum: a comparative study on embryo transfer medium, *Fertil. Steril.,* 56, 98, 1991.
73. **Bollen, N., Camus, M., Staessen, C., Tournaye, H., Devroey, P., and Van Steirteghem, A.C.,** The incidence of multiple pregnancy after in vitro fertilization and embryo transfer, gamete, or zygote intrafallopian transfer, *Fertil. Steril.,* 55, 314, 1991.

Chapter 5

EMBRYO CULTURE SYSTEMS

David K. Gardner and Michelle Lane

TABLE OF CONTENTS

I. Introduction 86
  A. Problems Associated with Embryo Culture 87
  B. Development of Embryo Culture Systems 87
    1. Simple Salt Solutions with Added Energy Substrates 87
    2. Complex Tissue Culture Media 89

II. Composition of Embryo Culture Media 89
  A. Water 90
  B. Ions 92
  C. Energy Substrates 92
  D. Amino Acids 93
  E. Vitamins 94
  F. Nucleic Acid Precursors 94
  G. Protein 95
  H. Hormones and Growth Factors 96
  I. Buffer System 96
  J. Gas Phase 97
  K. Summary 97

III. Preparation of Culture Media 98
  A. Water Source 98
  B. Glassware 98
  C. Media Preparation 99
    1. "Simple" Type Culture Medium: Human Tubal Fluid 99
    2. "Complex" Type Culture Medium: Ham's F-10 100
    3. Flushing and Collecting Medium 100
    4. pH Standards 101
    5. Protein Supplementation 101

IV. Screening of Media: Mouse Embryo Bioassay 102
  A. Suitability of the Mouse Bioassay 102
  B. Performing the Mouse Bioassay 104
    1. The Zygote Test 104
    2. The Two-Cell Test 104

V. Culture Systems 105

VI. Co-Culture 105
    A. Fetal Bovine Fibroblasts 106
    B. Fallopian Tube Epithelial Cells 106
    C. Vero Cells 106

VII. Future Directions 107

References 107

I. INTRODUCTION

The success of clinical IVF is compromised by sub-optimal culture conditions, resulting in impaired embryo development[1-3] and a subsequent loss of viability.[4] Relatively few human embryos conceived through IVF develop to term after transfer to the mother or develop to the blastocyst stage if left in culture.[5] Improvements in culture conditions would elevate the viability of embryos, resulting in an increase in pregnancy rates. Furthermore, improvements in culture conditions would also increase the number of embryos reaching the blastocyst stage, which has several advantages. First, it would permit the transfer of later stage embryos to the uterus of the mother, where they normally reside *in vivo*; second, there would be more time to assess the viability of the embryo before transfer (see Chapter 10); and third the generation of blastocysts would facilitate the introduction of trophectoderm biopsy for the screening of genetic diseases (see Chapter 6).

The culture media employed for clinical IVF vary greatly in their composition, yet there is little difference between media in their ability to support development *in vitro* or in subsequent pregnancy rates after transfer. This has led to a great deal of confusion concerning the formulation of embryo culture media and the role of their components in embryo development.

Optimization of embryo development *in vitro* is not only dependent upon the composition of the culture medium but is also affected by physical parameters, such as the incubation environment or the presence of somatic cells. Therefore, it is more appropriate to consider improving "embryo culture systems", than culture media alone. The primary aim of this chapter is to detail the known effects of media components and incubation systems on embryo development in culture and on subsequent viability after transfer. This is followed by a detailed description of media preparation, using two different types of culture media as examples, and sections on culture conditions and co-culture with somatic cells.

A. PROBLEMS ASSOCIATED WITH EMBRYO CULTURE

Development of the mammalian preimplantation embryo *in vitro* is fraught with problems. Present culture systems do not mimic either the physical or environmental conditions of the female reproductive tract. An apparent disregard of maternal physiology has contributed to the slow improvement of culture conditions. Within the lumen of the female reproductive tract, the developing embryo is exposed to microliter volumes of fluid.[6] In contrast, the embryo grown *in vitro* is subject to relatively large volumes of medium, up to 1 ml. Consequently, any autocrine factor(s) produced by the developing embryo will be diluted and may therefore become ineffectual. It has been demonstrated in the mouse that cleavage rate and blastocyst formation increase when embryos are grown in groups or reduced volumes,[7,8] and that decreasing the incubation volume can significantly increase embryo viability.[8] Similar results have been obtained with sheep embryos (Gardner and Lane, unpublished observations). Furthermore, any paracrine factor(s) produced by the female reproductive tract will also be absent from the system.

In contrast to the female reproductive tract, most conventional embryo culture systems are static, employing a single medium for the entire preimplantation period. *In vivo*, the embryo is exposed to a dynamic environment, constantly changing as the embryo passes along the oviduct to the uterus. Concomitantly, the embryo itself exhibits a changing nutrient preference,[9,10] reflecting the changes in energy metabolism which occur between fertilization and the blastocyst.[11,12]

Mammalian embryos exhibit a species specific arrest in development if the zygote is grown in sub-optimal culture conditions. Such cleavage arrest usually occurs during the cell cycle of embryonic genome activation. In the human this occurs at the late 4- to early 8-cell stage[13] and in the mouse it occurs at the 2-cell stage.[14] These developmental blocks in culture can best be regarded as *in vitro* artifacts, induced by the inadequacies of the culture conditions. Many such culture-induced blocks have recently been overcome by the development of more suitable conditions.[15-18]

B. DEVELOPMENT OF EMBRYO CULTURE SYSTEMS

Media used to culture the mammalian preimplantation embryo, are of two types.

1. Simple Salt Solutions with Added Energy Substrates

These media were originally formulated to support the development of zygotes from certain inbred strains of mice and their F1 hybrids.[19] Examples of this type of medium used in clinical IVF are M16,[20] T6,[20] Earle's,[21] HTF,[22] and CZB.[15] As shown in Table 1, there has been little change in the formulation of such media over the past 30 years. Such "simple" media are usually supplemented with either serum or serum albumin.

TABLE 1
Composition (mM) of "Simple" Embryo Culture Media

Component	Whitten (1957)[23]	Brinster (1965)[24]	Whitten & Biggers (1968)[19]	BWW (1971)[25]	M16[a] (1971)[20]	T6[a] (1971)[20]	Earle's[a] (1981)[21]	HTF[a] (1985)[22]	CZB[a] (1989)[15]	MTF (1990)[26]
NaCl	118.46	119.23	68.49	94.59	94.66	99.23	116.30	101.60	81.62	114.19
KCl	4.74	4.78	4.78	4.78	4.78	2.68	5.36	4.69	4.83	4.78
KH_2PO_4	1.18	1.19	1.19	1.19	1.19	0.00	0.00	0.37	1.18	1.19
$NaH_2PO_4 \cdot 2H_2O$	0.00	0.00	0.00	0.00	0.00	0.36	1.02	0.00	0.00	0.00
$CaCl_2 \cdot 2H_2O$	0.00	1.71	0.00	0.00	1.71	1.80	1.80	2.02	1.70	1.71
$MgCl_2 \cdot 6H_2O$	0.00	0.00	0.00	0.00	0.00	0.47	0.00	0.00	0.00	0.00
$MgSO_4 \cdot 7H_2O$	1.18	1.19	1.19	1.19	1.19	0.00	0.00	0.20	1.18	1.19
$NaHCO_3$	24.88	25.00	25.07	25.07	25.00	25.00	26.18	25.00	25.12	25.00
Ca Lactate	2.54	0.00	1.71	1.71	0.00	0.00	0.00	0.00	0.00	0.00
Na Lactate	0.00	25.00	21.58	21.58	23.28	25.00	0.00	21.40	31.30	4.79
Na Pyruvate	0.00	0.25	0.33	0.25	0.33	0.25	0.10	0.33	0.27	0.37
Glucose	5.55	0.00	5.56	5.56	5.56	5.56	5.55	2.78	0.00	3.40
BSA (mg/ml)	1.00	1.00	4.00	1.00	4.00	3.00	[b]	5.00	5.00	4.00
Ratios										
Na/K	30.24	35.46	19.34	23.70	24.05	55.91	26.79	27.52	23.01	24.18
Ca/Mg	2.15	1.44	1.44	1.44	1.44	2.25	2.22	10.0	1.44	1.44
L/P	—	100.00	70.58	93.16	70.55	100.00	—	64.85	115.93	12.95

Notes: Penicillin present in all media at 100 U/ml. Streptomycin present in all media at 50 μg/ml. CZB contains 110 μM EDTA and 1.0 mM Glutamine.

[a] Used in clinical IVF.
[b] Medium supplemented with serum.

TABLE 2
Composition of Ham's F-10 Medium

Component	Concentration (mM)	Component	Concentration (mM)
NaCl	126.60	Leucine	0.10
KCl	3.82	Lysine	0.20
MgSO$_4$·7H$_2$O	0.62	Methionine	0.03
Na$_2$HPO$_4$	1.31	Phenylalanine	0.03
KH$_2$PO$_4$	0.61	Proline	0.10
NaHCO$_3$	14.28	Serine	0.10
CaCl$_2$·2H$_2$O	0.30	Threonine	0.03
CuSO$_4$·5H$_2$O	0.00001	Tryptophan	0.003
FeSO$_4$·7H$_2$O	0.0030	Tyrosine	0.12
ZnSO$_4$·7H$_2$O	0.0001	Valine	0.03
Phenol Red	0.034		
		Biotin	0.0001
Sodium pyruvate	1.00	Ca pantothenate	0.0015
Calcium lactate	2.23	Choline chloride	0.005
Glucose	6.11	Cyanocobalamine	0.001
		Folic acid	0.003
Alanine	0.10	Inositol	0.003
Arginine	1.21	Nicotinamide	0.005
Asparagine	0.11	Pyridoxine	0.001
Aspartic acid	0.10	Riboflavin	0.001
Cysteine	0.26	Thiamine	0.003
Glutamate	0.1		
Glutamine	1.0	Hypoxanthine	0.03
Glycine	0.1	Lipoic acid	0.001
Histidine	0.14	Thymidine	3.00
Isoleucine	0.02		

Note: Penicillin present at 100 U/ml. Streptomycin present at 50 µg/nl.

2. Complex Tissue Culture Media

These media are commercially available, designed to support the growth of somatic cells in culture, e.g., Hams' F-10[27] (Table 2). Such media are far more complex, containing amino acids, vitamins, and nucleic acid precursors and are usually supplemented with 5 to 10% serum. There have been limited attempts to formulate complex media specifically for embryo culture[28] (Table 3). However, such media bear little homology to the levels of ions and metabolites within the female tract (Table 4).

II. COMPOSITION OF EMBRYO CULTURE MEDIA

The composition of embryo culture systems can be broken down into the following components:

1. Water
2. Ions

TABLE 3
Composition of Menezo's B3 Medium

Component	Concentration (mM)	Component	Concentration (mM)
NaCl	104.36	Serine	0.14
KCl	9.39	Taurine	0.10
MgSO$_4$.7H$_2$O	0.81	Threonine	0.21
Na$_2$HPO$_4$	0.46	Tryptophan	0.12
KH$_2$PO$_4$	0.44	Tyrosine	0.14
NaHCO3	21.42	Valine	0.64
Phenol Red	0.042		
		Biotin	0.0041
Sodium pyruvate	2.27	Ca pantothenate	0.0021
Calcium lactate	0.56	Cyanocobalamine	0.00074
Glucose	6.67	Folic acid	0.0068
		Nicotinic acid	0.0081
Alanine	0.76	Pyridoxine	0.0049
Aspartic acid	0.19	Riboflavin	0.0027
Arginine	0.29	Thiamine	0.0030
Cysteine	0.083		
Cysteine S	0.073	Adenine	0.037
Glutamate	1.0	Cytosine	0.045
Glutamine	0.17	Guanine	0.033
Glycine	5.33	Thymine	0.040
Histidine	0.16	Uracil	0.045
Isoleucine	0.19		
Leucine	0.23	Cholesterol	0.065
Lysine	0.24	Sodium acetate	0.036
Methionine	0.084	Citrulline	0.20
Phenylalanine	0.15	Ornithine	0.113
Proline	0.17		

Note: Penicillin present at 100 U/ml. Streptomycin present at 50 µ/nl.

3. Energy substrates
4. Amino acids
5. Vitamins
6. Nucleic acid precursors
7. Protein
8. Growth factors/hormones
9. Buffer system
10. Gas phase

The effects of each component on embryo development in culture will be discussed in turn.

A. WATER

Water is the major component of any medium, making up about 99% of the contents. The source and purity of water used for media preparation is therefore a major factor in assuring the quality of the medium. The ability of embryos to develop in culture is positively correlated to water quality. Whittingham[20] demonstrated that the development of 2-cell mouse embryos to the blastocyst

TABLE 4
Composition (mM) of Mammalian Fluids and Embryo Culture Media

Component	Human oviduct fluid[29,30]	Human uterine fluid[31]	Human serum[29]	Mouse oviduct fluid[26,32]	HTF medium[22]	Ham's F-10[27]	Menezo's B3 medium[28]
Na	130	nd	145	139	148	143	129
Cl	132	nd	nd	165	110	131	114
K	21.2	nd	5.0	23.4	5.1	4.4	9.8
Ca	1.13	nd	1.13	1.71	2.02	0.30	0.56
Mg	1.42	nd	2.00	1.04	0.20	0.62	0.81
S	12.3	nd	nd	8.45	0.20	0.62	0.17
P	8.69	nd	nd	8.93	0.37	1.92	0.90
Pyruvate	0.24	0.10	0.10	0.37	0.33	1.00	2.27
Lactate	1.98	5.87	0.60	4.79	21.4	2.23	0.56
Glucose	1.11	3.15	5.00	3.40	2.78	6.11	6.67
Glutamine	0.30	nd	nd	0.20	0.00	0.30	0.17
Ratios								
Na/K	6.1	—	29.0	5.9	29.0	32.3	13.1
Ca/Mg	0.80	—	0.57	1.64	10.10	0.48	0.69
L/P	8.25	25.22	6.00	12.95	64.85	0.30	0.25

in culture was enhanced when the medium was prepared using triple distilled water as opposed to double or single distilled water. However, the process of distillation has inherent problems, due to the possible leaching of ions and pyrogens from the glassware. A more reliable water purification system is Millipore-Q, which produces pyrogen-free water, with a resistance greater than 18 megΩ. Depending upon the local water source, however, it may be necessary to distill the original supply.

B. IONS

The ionic basis of culture media used for clinical IVF vary markedly (Tables 1, 2, and 3). Surprisingly little is known about the role of ions during pre-implantation embryo development. The ionic composition of oviduct fluid from the human and mouse have been sampled by micropuncture and analyzed using an electron probe[29,32] (Table 4). Mammalian oviduct fluid is characterized by high potassium and chloride concentrations.

High potassium levels in culture media have been reported to have a beneficial effect on sperm capacitation[33] and embryo development.[34] However, there is conflicting data on the positive effects of potassium on embryo cleavage.[35-37] It is difficult to interpret the effects of single ions in culture medium, when there appear to be many subtle interactions between embryo function, ions, and metabolites.

Optimization of the ionic component of media is compounded by the ability of embryos in culture to develop apparently normally in a wide range of ion concentrations. Wales[38] used the development of 2-cell mouse embryos to the blastocyst in order to determine the range of ion concentrations capable of supporting development *in vitro*. Embryos formed blastocysts in medium with a potassium concentration ranging between 0.4 to 48 mM, a magnesium concentration between 0 to 9.6 mM, a calcium concentration between 0.1 to 10.2 mM, and a phosphate concentration between 0 to 7.2 mM, with a narrower range of optima for all ions. Studies on the hamster have shown that the first cleavage and development of 2-cell embryos to the blastocyst occur in a wide range of sodium, magnesium, calcium, and potassium concentrations.[39,40]

Further to their specific functions, the ions in any medium make the largest single contribution to osmotic pressure. The optimal osmolarity for the development of human embryos in culture has not been determined. However, mouse[41] and hamster[39] embryos will develop in a wide range of osmolarities (200 to 350 mOsmols). Although conventional embryo culture media have an osmolarity of between 275 to 295 mOsmols, enhanced development of mouse embryos appears to occur at reduced osmolarities.[19,42]

C. ENERGY SUBSTRATES

The energy requirements of the preimplantation human embryo have yet to be fully determined. However, analyses of nutrient uptakes *in vitro* (see Chapter 10) have revealed that the human embryo has an initial preference for pyruvate, with increasing glucose uptake as development proceeds.[43-45]

Such data suggests that glycolysis is a pathway not used preferentially by the early human embryo prior to the blastocyst.

The pattern of nutrient utilization by human embryos is very similar to that reported for the mouse. The mouse oocyte and zygote take up little glucose compared to pyruvate. Around the time of compaction, there is a decline in pyruvate utilization, with glucose becoming the preferred nutrient at the blastocyst.[9,10] These studies on nutrient uptakes reflect the findings of earlier culture experiments, which found that the mouse oocyte and zygote exhibit an absolute requirement for pyruvate as an energy source.[46] Lactate can be utilized as an energy source from the 2-cell stage and acts synergistically with pyruvate.[47] Surprisingly, glucose as the sole substrate cannot support mouse embryo development prior to the late 4-/early 8-cell stage.[24,48] This inability to utilize glucose as an energy source during the first three cell cycles was subsequently attributed to a blockade in glycolysis.[49,50] Recent studies on the mouse,[15] hamster,[51-53] and sheep[54] embryos have demonstrated that glucose is involved in cleavage arrest *in vitro*. This has been attributed to the premature stimulation of glycolysis,[55] a pathway not preferentially used by the embryo prior to blastocoel formation.[12] This inhibition of embryo development by glucose should be considered an *in vitro*-induced artifact, as glucose is present at relatively high levels (around 3 mM) in the oviduct lumen (Table 4).[26,30]

Most embryo culture media contain the nutrients pyruvate, lactate, and glucose. If one or more of these nutrients are absent from the medium formulation, then they are added as a component of serum. The levels of energy substrates in most culture media (Table 4), are present at the concentrations found to be optimal for the development of 2-cell mouse embryos to blastocysts *in vitro*.[24] Analysis of the composition of luminal fluid from the mammalian oviduct reveals two striking points: (1) the levels of nutrients are similar in the species studied;[26,30,56,57] (2) the levels are markedly different from those present in embryo culture media (Table 4). The concentration of metabolites in culture media have a direct effect on the embryo and the activity of its metabolic pathways.[26,37,58]

D. AMINO ACIDS

Mouse oocytes and embryos maintain an endogenous pool of amino acids[59] and possess specific transport systems for amino acids during development.[60,61] Furthermore, oviduct and uterine fluids contain significant levels of free amino acids.[26,62] Therefore it would appear that amino acids have a physiological role in the pre-/peri-implantation period of mammalian development. Although it is possible to get complete development of the human and mouse zygote to the blastocyst in culture in the absence of amino acids,[44] it has been shown that mouse and hamster embryo development *in vitro* is improved when amino acids are included in the culture medium. Oviduct fluid, obtained from the rabbit, is characterized by relatively high levels of glycine, alanine, threonine, taurine, glutamate, and serine. Analysis of human and mouse oviduct fluids has shown that there are also significant levels of glutamine present (Table 4).[26,30]

Gardner and Lane[63] have examined the effects of amino acids on the development of mouse zygotes in culture. It was found that cleavage rate, blastocyst formation, and hatching were all significantly increased by the inclusion of those amino acids present at high levels in the oviduct. In contrast, the inclusion of amino acids which are present at low levels in oviduct fluid, Eagle's essential amino acids, caused a significant reduction in cleavage and hatching rates.

The effects of single amino acids on hamster embryos in culture have been reported by Bavister and co-workers.[17,64] Asparagine, aspartate, glycine, histidine, serine, and taurine were all found to be stimulatory, while cysteine, isoleucine, leucine, phenylalanine, threonine, and valine were inhibitory.

As well as enhancing development in culture, amino acids have been implicated in elevating the viability of embryos in culture.[37,65,66]

The mechanism by which amino acids confer their benefit to embryos in culture has yet to be resolved.

Although there is an enhancement of embryo development *in vitro* when certain amino acids are included in the media formulation, there are problems associated with prolonged culture. Embryos metabolize amino acids with the release of ammonia. Furthermore, amino acids in solution at 37°C, particularly glutamine, spontaneously break down and release ammonia, with the resultant build up of ammonium ions in the medium. Ammonium ions are highly detrimental to embryo development in culture. Therefore, if amino acids are included in the medium formulation, then it is important not to store media at 37°C and to ensure that embryos are transferred to fresh media after around 48 h of culture.[63]

E. VITAMINS

Although vitamins are present in complex media formulations, their effects on embryo development are unknown. Human[44] and mouse[19] zygotes will form blastocysts in culture in the absence of vitamins. In contrast, the rabbit blastocyst requires vitamins for expansion.[67] However, Kane[67] found that one of the vitamins present in Ham's F-10, B12, caused a decrease in blastocyst expansion. B-group vitamins are an integral part of carbohydrate and amino acid metabolism, and may therefore have an important role to play in embryo development, but at present their function is unclear.

F. NUCLEIC ACID PRECURSORS

The development of human[44] and mouse[19] zygotes to blastocysts in culture does not require the presence of nucleic acid precursors in the medium. Mouse embryos can incorporate exogenous radiolabelled nucleosides into their RNA and DNA.[2] The ability of embryos to grow in the absence of nucleosides indicates that *de novo* pathways of nucleic acid synthesis are active at this stage.

Loutradis et al.[68] observed that hypoxanthine, present in Ham's F-10, induced a block in mouse embryo development at the 2-cell stage *in vitro*.

Hypoxanthine is thought to inhibit the purine salvage pathway.[69] It is now possible to purchase Ham's F-10 without hypoxanthine. Subsequent studies have revealed that both adenosine and inosine are detrimental to the development of mouse embryos after the first cleavage division.[70] Without further research into the role of nucleotides in embryo development, their omission from media formulations would seem advisable.

G. PROTEIN

The most commonly used protein source in human IVF and embryo culture is patient's serum, added to the medium at a concentration of 5 to 10%. The use of serum in embryo culture medium has several inherent drawbacks apart from the considerable expense and time required for its collection. Serum contains many components which are poorly characterized. Proteins in serum have macromolecules attached, such as hormones, vitamins, and fatty acids, as well as chelated metal ions and pyrogens.[71,72] The concentration of such macromolecules may vary between patients and within the menstrual cycle. This makes any comparison between batches of medium which contain serum almost impossible. Furthermore, there is evidence that serum itself contains properties that are toxic to embryos *in vitro*.[73]

If serum is not included in culture medium, protein can be added in the form of serum albumin. Both Human Serum Albumin (HSA)[74-76] and Bovine Serum Albumin (BSA)[77] have been used successfully in the culture of human embryos. The use of HSA requires adequate screening for HIV, hepatitis, etc. Although serum albumin is a relatively pure fraction, it is still contaminated with fatty acids and other small molecules. The latter includes an embryotrophic factor, which stimulates cleavage and growth in rabbit morulae and blastocysts. This has recently been determined to be citrate.[78] Not only are there significant differences between sources of serum albumin,[79] but also between batches from the same source.[80,81] Therefore, when using serum albumin, it is essential that each batch is screened for its ability to adequately support embryo development in the mouse prior to clinical use (see Section IV).

The role of protein in embryo culture medium may not only be as a fixed nitrogen source, but also as a chelator of toxic metal ions. Fissore et al.[82] demonstrated that, in the absence of protein, the chelating agent ethylenediaminetetraacetic acid (EDTA) at a concentration of 10 μM, enabled the development of mouse zygotes to the blastocyst. In the absence of EDTA, embryo development was significantly reduced. Caro and Trounson[83] found no difference in fertilization rates, embryo cleavage, or pregnancy rates when human embryos were cultured in medium T6 with or without 10% maternal serum. This study questions the role of serum in embryo culture medium. It is probable that serum and serum albumin exert a beneficial effect when culture conditions are sub-optimal, e.g., when toxic metal ions are present either in the water or leached from a glass or plastic container.

A practical benefit of having a protein source or other macromolecule, such as PolyVinyl Alcohol (PVA),[84] present in the medium is for ease of embryo manipulation. In the absence of protein, PVA, or other surfactants, embryos are difficult to handle and tend to stick to both plastic culture dishes and glass pipettes.

The drawbacks of using serum in media have led to the development of synthetic serum substitutes. Unfortunately, these serum replacements have been developed for tissue culture and not specifically for embryo culture. Holst et al.[85] used MediCult synthetic serum replacement, supplemented with HSA, in a clinical trial. Using this system, they obtained equivalent rates of fertilization, cleavage, and implantation compared to serum supplementation. In a separate trial, Psalti et al.[86] found that using UltroSer G as the serum replacement resulted in a decrease in sperm survival, fertilization, and embryo viability. Disadvantages of these commercially available serum supplements are their cost and undisclosed composition.

H. HORMONES AND GROWTH FACTORS

Although the mouse blastocyst is capable of metabolizing exogenous steroid hormones,[87] there is little evidence in the literature of the direct action of hormones on the early embryo.[88-91] However, prolactin at a concentration of 300 ng/ml, has been shown to improve the rate of blastocyst formation from cultured 2-cell mouse embryos.[92] Available evidence indicates that the effects of maternal hormones on the developing embryo are mediated by the cells of the reproductive tract.[93]

The role of growth factors in the development of the preimplantation mammalian embryo is the subject of extensive research. Studies on the mouse embryo have revealed receptors for insulin-like growth factor-II (IGF-II)[94] and insulin[95] from the 2-cell and morula stages respectively. Insulin has been shown to have mitogenic effects on the blastocyst,[96] and to stimulate RNA,[97] and protein[98] synthesis in compacted embryos and blastocysts. Epidermal growth factor (EGF) has also been shown to increase protein synthesis in the mouse blastocyst; its effects however are limited to the trophectoderm.[99] Paria and Dey[7] found that both EGF and transforming growth factor-α (TGF-α) have mitogenic effects on mouse embryos cultured from the 2-cell stage. In the mouse, receptors for EGF appear at the blastocyst stage. It is therefore plausible that the preimplantation human embryo possesses specific receptors for growth factors. As most human embryos are transferred around the 2- to 8-cell stage, it is likely that expression of growth factor receptors occurs after the embryo is transferred to the female tract. Due to the high costs of growth factors for media supplementation and the lack of data on their role in human embryo development, it is considered prudent that they are not included in current media formulations for clinical IVF.

I. BUFFER SYSTEM

Most embryo media utilize a bicarbonate/CO_2 buffer system to maintain a physiological pH of around 7.2 to 7.4 in the medium. The inclusion of sodium bicarbonate in the medium requires the use of a gassing incubator to maintain a 5% CO_2 atmosphere. An advantage of the bicarbonate/CO_2 system is that it is the physiological buffer in the fluid surrounding mammalian cells. A major drawback, however, is the rapid pH increase that occurs when the medium is exposed to air, resulting in embryo damage or necrosis if prolonged. One solution to this problem is the use of an oil overlay to slow gas exchange when culture dishes are taken out of the incubator, e.g., for embryo scoring. This approach is not feasible, however, for oocyte collection or prolonged embryo manipulation. A possible alternative is the use of phosphate-buffered medium, which does not require a CO_2 environment to maintain its pH in air. Unfortunately, phosphate-buffered media appear to be detrimental to embryo development *in vitro*.[100-102] A suitable alternative to phosphate is N-2-hydroxyethylpiperazine-N'-2-ethanesulphonic acid (HEPES),[103] with a pKa of 7.55 at 20°C. HEPES has been used successfully as a buffer in media for human oocyte collection and embryo handling. In such media, it is usual to replace 20 m*M* bicarbonate with HEPES, leaving 5 m*M* bicarbonate.[104] The rationale for this is that embryos require bicarbonate for development.[46,102] At low concentrations of HEPES (< 20 m*M*), the bicarbonate competes with the HEPES, which subsequently loses its buffering capacity as the bicarbonate dissociates, and consequently increases the pH.[105] Although there have been some concerns about the toxicity of HEPES, it is possible to get complete mouse embryo development *in vitro* in the presence of this buffer in the medium.[102]

J. GAS PHASE

The two active gases employed in embryo culture systems are oxygen and carbon dioxide. Most IVF clinics use a gas phase of 5% CO_2 in air. Studies on the mouse,[106,107] sheep,[108] cattle,[108], and goat,[81] have all demonstrated that a reduced oxygen level, between 5 to 7%, is far superior in supporting embryo development than the 20% present in air. The benefit conferred by a reduced oxygen concentration may be attributed to a decrease in the formation of superoxide radicals, which have been associated with developmental arrest in the mouse.[109,110] Even a transient exposure to high oxygen levels, i.e., 20% for 1 h, can significantly reduce subsequent development in lower oxygen tensions.[107,111] Although there is little data on the effects of oxygen on the human embryo, it would seem advisable to use a reduced oxygen tension (around 5%).

Carbon dioxide is not only required to maintain the pH of bicarbonate buffered media, but is readily incorporated into protein and nucleic acids by the mouse embryo at all stages prior to implantation.[112] The optimum concentration of CO_2 for human embryo development is yet to be determined.

K. SUMMARY

It is evident from the above review that the effects and roles of media components on embryo development *in vitro* are far from understood. Complex interactions between media components and the embryo make determination of the optimal component concentrations a difficult task. This is reflected by the markedly different composition of culture media used in clinical IVF, although their apparent ability to support embryo development is similar. Certain components of culture systems appear to be detrimental to embryo development, such as nucleotides in the medium and high oxygen in the atmosphere. It is, therefore, important to be aware of the precise composition of the embryo culture system employed and the effect that the individual components have on embryo development.

It is not surprising that there is a lack of consensus as to which culture system or medium is the most suitable for clinical IVF. Consequently, in the following section, the preparation of two types of culture media (simple and complex) are described in detail. The role of the physical environment is also considered.

III. PREPARATION OF CULTURE MEDIA

Sterile technique should be observed during media preparation, and apart from the weighing of components, should be performed in a Laminar flow. All components of the medium must be of the highest grade, e.g., Analar (BDH), Tissue Culture tested (Sigma).

A. WATER SOURCE

In our IVF program at the Monash IVF Clinic, Melbourne, a Millipore-Q system is used to produce high quality pyrogen-free water (Milli-Q) for media preparation and for washing of all glassware and equipment. Weekly maintenance of the water system is essential and has been well described by May and Hanshew.[113] Water for media preparation and glassware washing should have a resistance of >18 megΩ.

B. GLASSWARE

Glassware for media preparation should be designated solely for this purpose. Cleanliness of glassware is of the utmost importance. No detergents are used in the treatment of glassware at Monash IVF. After use, the glassware is cleaned of any marks with acetone, and the glassware is subsequently washed several times in water purified by Reverse Osmosis (RO); the glassware is then left to soak overnight in an RO water bath. The following morning, the glassware is rinsed at least six times with Milli-Q water, filled and submerged in a sonicator. Cleaning by sonication takes around 3 h in hot water. After sonication, glassware is rinsed at least six times with fresh Milli-Q water and subsequently dried inverted, by heating at 120°C for 12 h. Glassware is then packaged separately and sterilized by heating overnight at 120°C.

Heavily soiled glassware is soaked overnight in a 5% solution of 7X detergent, and subsequently rinsed in hot tap water, followed by washing in RO water and an overnight soak in RO bath for normal washing the next day.

TABLE 5
Composition of Medium HTF

Component	mM	g/liter
NaCl	101.60	5.938
KCl	4.69	0.350
KH_2PO_4	0.37	0.050
$CaCl_2.2H_2O$	2.02	0.300
$MgSO_4.7H_2O$	0.20	0.049
$NaHCO_3$	25.00	2.101
NaPyruvate	0.33	0.036
NaLactate	21.40	4.000
Glucose	2.78	0.501

Note: Penicillin present at 100 U/ml. Streptomycin present at 50 μ/nl. Phenol red present at 0.01 g/l.

All new glassware is pre-washed in 3% HCl for 24 h. Glassware is then rinsed in RO water and placed in the RO soak overnight.

All metal items are treated separately from the glassware.

C. MEDIA PREPARATION

Numerous media have been used in clinical IVF, including T6,[20] Earle's,[21] HTF,[22] CZB,[15] Ham's F-10,[27] and Menezo's B3 medium.[28] At Monash IVF, HTF supplemented with patient's serum is used routinely. Although it is possible to purchase ready-made media, at Monash IVF the media is prepared in the laboratory. This has the advantage that a stringent quality control can be supervised and changes in medium formulations can be implemented easily. A drawback of this approach is the time of preparation.

1. "Simple" Type Culture Medium: Human Tubal Fluid

The components of medium HTF are shown in Table 5. The following describes the preparation of one liter of medium.

1. Weigh out the salts and metabolites, except lactate, and calcium chloride individually into a one liter volumetric flask;
2. Weigh out lactate, calcium chloride and the antibiotics, individually into separate beakers;
3. Add 500 ml of water to the volumetric flask to dissolve the salts and metabolites;
4. Dissolve the antibiotics with water, and pour into the flask; rinse the beaker several times with water and add contents to the flask; the same procedure is followed for lactate and calcium chloride; care must be taken to ensure that all the components are dissolved and transferred to the volumetric flask;
5. Once everything in the volumetric flask has dissolved, make up to a volume of one liter with water; filter the medium using a vacuum pump,

through a 0.2 μm disposable filter, into sterile tubes; the first 10 ml filtered should not be used for embryo culture but can be used to determine osmolarity before being discarded;
6. If the osmolarity of the medium is not between 285 and 295, it should be discarded and prepared again; if the osmolarity is too high do not add water to bring the osmotic pressure down, as it will also dilute the medium components; the measured osmolarity of a medium is less than the calculated value; this can be attributed to the incomplete dissociation of ions once they reach mM concentrations.

2. "Complex" Type Culture Medium: Ham's F-10

The components of medium Ham's F-10 are shown in Table 2. The following describes the preparation of one liter of medium. This medium is purchased as a powder where one sachet makes one liter of medium. It is necessary to add extra components to this medium which are required for embryo culture.

1. Weigh out antibiotics, lactate, calcium chloride, and sodium bicarbonate into separate beakers;
2. Add 500 ml of water to the volumetric flask;
3. Pour the contents of the sachet of Ham's F-10 medium into the volumetric flask; rinse the sachet several times with water to ensure that all the contents are transferred to the volumetric flask;
4. Dissolve the antibiotics with water and pour into the volumetric flask; rinse the beaker several times with water and empty into the volumetric flask; use the same procedure for dissolving the lactate, calcium chloride, and sodium bicarbonate; addition of bicarbonate to the medium will change the color from yellow to pink;
5. Add water to a volume of about 950 ml;
6. Determine the pH of the medium, which should be in the range of 7.4; if the pH is less than this, it should be adjusted using a 0.2 M solution of sodium hydroxide, added using a finely pulled Pasteur pipette;
7. Once the pH of the medium is 7.4, make up to one liter with water;
8. Filter the medium using a vacuum pump, through a 0.2 μm disposable filter, into sterile flasks. The first 10 ml of medium filtered should not be used for embryo culture but can be used to determine osmolarity before being discarded.

The osmolarity of the medium should be in the range of 280 to 290 mOsmol. If the medium is not within this range, it should be discarded and the process repeated. If the osmolarity is too high, do not add water to bring the osmotic pressure down, as this will also dilute the medium components.

3. Flushing and Collecting Medium

Embryo culture media are buffered by bicarbonate and therefore require a 5% CO_2 atmosphere to maintain a physiological pH (7.3 to 7.4). Outside an enriched CO_2 environment, embryo culture media becomes alkaline rapidly and turns bright pink. Therefore, for oocyte collection and manipulation, an alternative buffering system is required. Dulbecco's Phosphate-Buffered Saline can be used for this purpose. However, in light of the known adverse effects of phosphate on the mammalian embryo, HEPES has become the preferred buffer in medium. Monash IVF routinely use a HEPES-buffered modification of HTF as the flushing medium, in which 20 mM bicarbonate is replaced with 20 mM HEPES, adjusted to pH 7.4. Ideally, the collection medium and the culture medium should have the same composition (with the exception of the buffer) to minimize the stress placed on the oocyte.

It is advisable to prepare an excess of this medium, as it should be used to flush-out all equipment/catheters before use. The following describes preparation of this medium.

1. Weigh the salts and metabolites except the antibiotics, lactate, calcium chloride, and HEPES into a one liter volumetric flask; weigh the antibiotics, lactate, calcium chloride and HEPES into separate beakers;
2. Add 500 ml of water to the volumetric flask to dissolve the salts and metabolites;
3. Dissolve the antibiotics with water and pour into the volumetric flask; rinse the beaker several times with water and add the contents to the flask; the same procedure is followed for lactate, calcium chloride, and HEPES;
4. Add water to a volume of around 850 ml;
5. Determine the pH of the medium; this can be done with color standards (see below). Adjust the pH to 7.4 with a 0.2 M solution of sodium hydroxide, added dropwise; make up to volume of 1 liter with water;
6. Filter the medium using a vacuum pump, through a 0.2 µm disposable filter, into sterile flasks; the first 10 ml of the medium should not be used for embryo handling but can be used to determine osmolarity before being discarded; the osmolarity of the handling medium should be within the same range as the basal bicarbonate medium.

4. pH Standards

A simple and reliable method of checking the pH of a medium is to use color standards. The color standards use 0.067 M solutions of potassium phosphate and sodium phosphate. These solutions are then added together in varying quantities to produce solutions of the required pH. The preparation of such standards is shown in Table 6.

5. Protein Supplementation

The following describes preparation of serum.

1. Once the patient's blood has been collected, it should not be allowed to clot, but rather centrifuged immediately (around 10 min at about 1000 g) in sterile plastic tubes;

TABLE 6
Color Standards for pH of Media

Stock A: 9.08 g KH_2PO_4 (0.067 M), 10 mg phenol red in 1 liter of water.
Stock B: 9.46 g Na_2HPO_4 (0.067 M), 10 mg phenol red in 1 liter of water.

pH at 18°C	Solution A (ml)	Solution B (ml)
6.6	62.7	37.3
6.8	50.8	49.2
7.0	39.2	60.8
7.2	28.5	71.5
7.4	19.6	80.4
7.6	13.2	86.8

Notes: Measure the pH with meter, and adjust pH as required; i.e., add solution A to lower the pH (make more acidic), add solution B to increase the pH (make more alkaline). The pH standards should be filter-sterilized and can then be kept for up to six months.

2. After centrifugation, pipette the plasma into a second sterile tube;
3. Leave the plasma to clot;
4. Remove the coagulate and heat-inactivate the remaining serum by incubating at 56°C for 30 min;
5. Serum can then be sterilized by filtration (0.2 μm) and frozen.

Serum albumin requires very little preparation. Albumin can be used from the bottle, as it is filter-sterilized in the medium. All batches of albumin should be screened by the mouse bioassay prior to use. For a medium supplemented with serum albumin, the media is poured into a beaker, and the serum albumin is weighed and placed on top and allowed to dissolve. This usually takes around 5 min and can be facilitated by gentle stirring. The medium should be filtered immediately.

IV. SCREENING OF MEDIA: MOUSE EMBRYO BIOASSAY

A. SUITABILITY OF THE MOUSE BIOASSAY

The preimplantation mouse embryo is the most widely used bioassay for culture media and equipment used in clinical IVF. Using mice for testing media for human embryos has been the focus of much discussion[114,115] due to conflicting reports in the literature of its suitability as a bioassay.[116,117] Fukuda et al.[116] reported that, for the mouse, *in vitro* fertilization and the development of zygotes and 2-cell embryos in culture were positively correlated with the purity of the water source used in the preparation of media. In contrast, Silverman et al.[117] found that media prepared with tap water could support adequate development of 2-cell mouse embryos to one blastocyst stage, compared to media prepared with ultrapure water. The apparent contradiction of these studies can possibly be resolved by taking into account the different types of media used. Fukuda et al.[116] used BWW, a "simple-type" medium, whereas Silverman et al.[117] used Ham's F-10. The latter medium contains amino acids, which may chelate any possible toxins present in the tap water, e.g., heavy metals.

The sensitivity of mouse embryos to their environment is inversely proportional to the age of the embryo at recovery, i.e., 1-cell embryos are more susceptible to toxins in the medium than embryos collected at the 2-cell stage.[118] Removal of the zona pellucida from the zygote further increases the sensitivity of the embryo to the culture conditions.[119]

A common mouse embryo bioassay is to culture the zygote for 24 h in medium with BSA (4 mg/ml) followed by 72 h in protein-free medium. The rationale for using protein-free medium is that serum or serum albumin can chelate toxins, such as heavy metal ions, present in the medium. The presence of proteins would therefore hide any potential detrimental effects of the medium. The percentage of zygotes forming blastocysts at 96 h of culture is used as the end point of the bioassay, media supporting greater than 85% development being considered acceptable for clinical use. However, such an end-point is very subjective. A more objective approach would be to determine cell numbers. Unfortunately, this is very time consuming and probably beyond the capacity of most IVF centers. Furthermore, weekly screening of media by mouse bioassay is not without expense, both in terms of technical time and animals. There are no conclusive studies on the usefulness of the mouse bioassay in screening each batch of media. However, the bioassay has proved most useful in screening several potential embryo toxins present in the equipment used in clinical work, e.g., catheters.[120]

In our IVF unit, we routinely use the 1-cell mouse embryo test to screen new batches of oil, new batches of consumables, and each component of the medium. However, we no longer advocate the screening of each batch of medium prepared, since we ensure a high degree of care is taken when medium is prepared.

With regards to alternative assays, such as hybridoma cell lines, although such cells in culture can be particularly sensitive to toxins in the medium, they are not embryonic cells and therefore may not detect potential embryo toxins. Rinehart et al.[121] used a hamster sperm motility assay to quantitate differences in water supply. Although potentially very sensitive, there is little clinical data on the applicability of this test. Unfortunately, in Australia it is not possible to use this bioassay, and we therefore have to rely on the mouse. Although the mouse embryo bioassay does have a role in clinical IVF, at best it is only a test of the ability of the mouse embryo to develop. There is no guarantee that factors that do not affect the mouse will not be detrimental to the human. The ultimate quality control on all media for IVF is their ability to support human embryo growth. It is obviously unethical to use human embryos for this purpose. A possible solution would be to use triploid embryos as an assay of medium quality, as these cannot be replaced in the prospective mother.

B. PERFORMING THE MOUSE BIOASSAY

The type of mouse bioassay performed to screen components for human IVF depends upon the strain of mouse used. Inbred strains and their F1 hybrids are less sensitive to their environment, and therefore the embryos are collected at the zygote. Embryos from outbred strains of mouse are more sensitive to environmental factors. These embryos exhibit the 2-cell block in culture and therefore are collected at the 2-cell stage. Multiple ovulations are induced by injecting 4 to 6 week old virgin females with 5 IU pregnant mares serum (PMS), followed 48 h with 5 IU human chorionic gonadotrophin (hCG). Females are placed with males immediately following the second injection, and mating is assessed the following morning by the presence of a vaginal plug. Embryos are cultured in groups of ten in 20 µl drops of medium under an oil overlay at 37°C.[8] Culture dishes should be set up and allowed to equilibrate overnight in a 5% CO_2 atmosphere. To overcome any donor variation, embryos from each female should be allocated equally to each treatment group.

1. The Zygote Test

On the day of plug, females are sacrificed and the oviducts excised and placed into warm collecting medium in a petri dish. The swollen ampullary region of the oviduct is torn open close to the cumulus mass, which is then expelled under positive pressure into the medium. The cumulus is disaggregated by the addition of hyaluronidase (1 mg/ml) to the collecting medium. After around one minute the cumulus disperses, leaving denuded zygotes. The embryos are then washed twice in collecting medium and once in the culture medium and placed into culture.

Zygotes are initially cultured in a medium containing BSA. After 24 h, the embryos are transferred to a fresh drop of equilibrated protein-free medium and cultured for a further 72 h. Embryo morphology is assessed and blastocyst formation determined. If more than 85% of the zygotes have reached the blastocyst stage, the medium or equipment tested are considered suitable for clinical use.

2. The Two-Cell Test

Forty-eight hours after the hCG injection, females are sacrificed and the oviducts placed into warm handling medium. Two-cell embryos are flushed from the oviduct using a blunt 32-gauge hypodermic needle attached to a 1 ml syringe filled with collecting medium. The 2-cells are collected, washed twice in collecting medium and once in culture medium, and placed into culture. Two-cell embryos are cultured for 72 h in a protein-free medium, and morphology is assessed for blastocyst stage, formation. If more than 85% of the 2-cells have reached the blastocyst stage, the medium or equipment tested are considered suitable for clinical use.

V. CULTURE SYSTEMS

Human embryos are routinely cultured in either microliter volumes of medium under a layer of oil, usually paraffin or silicone, or in relatively large volumes of medium (up to 1 ml) without an oil overlay.

The benefits of a reduced incubation volume and increased embryo density on the development and viability of mouse embryos in culture has been discussed.[8] However, the effect of incubation volume and embryo density on human embryo development has yet to be determined.

Although the use of an oil overlay is time-consuming and can be messy, it prevents the evaporation of media, thereby reducing the harmful effects of increases in osmolarity. Furthermore, the use of an oil overlay reduces changes in pH caused by a loss of CO_2 from the medium when culture dishes are taken out of the incubator for embryo examination.

If oil is to be used, then paraffin or silicone is recommended. Embryo development has been obtained using both types of oil; unfortunately paraffin has the disadvantage of being highly labile. As a result of this, paraffin oil has a shorter shelf life than silicone oil. However, in a busy laboratory, the oil is used before it has a chance to become toxic. It is advisable to purchase paraffin oil in small bottles (500 ml) to ensure rapid use once they are opened. If a bottle of oil is unused after 4 weeks, it should be retested using the mouse bioassay. Whichever oil is chosen, it should first be washed with medium prior to use. This is accomplished by adding oil to protein-free culture medium (2:1) in a sterile tissue culture flask and shaking vigorously. The mixture is left to separate, and the oil is removed and aliquoted ready for use. It is essential that each bottle of oil purchased is tested using the mouse bioassay prior to clinical use. In our experience, bottle to bottle variation is as great as batch to batch.

If it is decided to avoid the use of oil, then 4-well plates or organ dishes can be used. One well in a 4-well plate can hold 0.8 ml of medium. If 4-well plates are used, care must be taken to reduce the changes in pH caused by loss of CO_2 from the medium. One way of achieving this is to "work" in a 5% CO_2 environment, made possible by the use of humidicribs, which can maintain the desired atmosphere. An alternative to using dishes for embryo culture is the use of tubes. Using tubes it is possible to minimize pH changes due to the loss of CO_2 by gassing tubes immediately after oocyte/embryo manipulation. However, both 4-well plates and tubes necessitate the use of large incubation volumes.

VI. CO-CULTURE

Prior to the development of more suitable culture conditions, mouse zygotes in culture exhibited a block at the 2-cell stage. However, this culture-induced block could be overcome if embryos were transferred into the ampulla region of explanted oviducts.[122] Such experiments have highlighted the special environment created by the oviduct, which provides a factor(s) otherwise absent from the culture system. The explanted oviduct has subsequently facilitated the development of embryos from several other mammals which exhibit embryonic arrest in culture.[123,124] More recently, however, the inadequacies of media formulations have been alleviated by co-culturing embryos with somatic cells, either in suspension or as a monolayer.[125,126]

It is not in the scope of this section to review all aspects of co-culture, as this has been dealt with in several articles and reviews.[127,128] Rather, it is the aim of this section to discuss the relevance of specific co-culture systems for clinical IVF.

Of the cell types that have been employed in clinical work, three will be discussed here: fetal bovine fibroblasts, fallopian tube epithelial cells, and Vero cells.

A. FETAL BOVINE FIBROBLASTS

The use of fetal uterine fibroblasts for clinical application was pioneered by Wiemer and coworkers. Using a monolayer of fibroblasts, Wiemer et al.[129,130] obtained significantly better embryo development *in vitro* and a doubling of pregnancy rates after transfer. Although there appear to be major advantages in using this co-culture system, rigorous screening of the bovine uterine cells must be performed for many potentially infectious viruses, including bovine rhinotracheitis virus, bovine parainfluenza virus, bovine diarrhea virus, bovine leukemia virus, and bovine syncytial virus. This may not be a feasible procedure for most clinical IVF programs.

B. FALLOPIAN TUBE EPITHELIAL CELLS

Of the cell types used, fallopian tube epithelial cells are the ones most expected to have a stimulatory effect on embryo development in culture. The use of fallopian tube epithelial cells in clinical IVF has been pioneered by Bongso et al.,[131-133] who showed that development of human embryos *in vitro* was significantly improved by co-culture on a monolayer of cells obtained from the ampullary region of the fallopian tube, 69% of embryos forming a blastocele compared to only 33% in the control group. Subsequently, it was found that fertilization rates were increased in the presence of ampullary epithelial cells.[134]

Unfortunately, the use of human fallopian tube epithelial cells has two practical limitations. First, it is essential to screen each fallopian tube donor for viruses, hepatitis B, etc. Second, human ampullary cell lines differentiate after around four to five passages, becoming fibroblast-like. A continual source of fallopian tubes may therefore be required to produce new cell lines. In a routine clinical IVF program, this becomes impractical.

C. VERO CELLS

Vero cells are derived from the green monkey kidney and they have been used in embryo co-culture systems because they share a common embryonic origin with cells of the genital tract. Although human embryo development *in vitro* is enhanced in the presence of Vero cells,[135] there is little data on the viability of such embryos. From initial studies, it appears that Vero cells could "rescue" embryos from degenerating in culture.

A practical benefit of using Vero cells is that they are readily available and relatively easy to culture, passage, and cryopreserve. Furthermore, they are readily screened for viral contamination. The use of Vero cells is therefore not beyond the limits of most IVF clinics.

How the beneficial effects of somatic cells are conferred on the developing embryo has yet to be resolved. Whatever the mechanism, it is apparent that it is not tissue or species specific. The benefits conferred on embryos of other mammals, such as the cow, by conditioned medium (medium in which oviductal cells had grown) would indicate that somatic cells act via a secreted product, possibly a protein capable of chelating toxins (such as heavy metals) in the medium. Alternatively, the oviduct cells could produce specific growth factors which stimulate embryo development. However, conditioned medium cannot substitute for cell co-culture in all species.[131] It has recently been proposed that the benefit of the somatic cell monolayer can be attributed to its ability to reduce the oxygen tension in the vicinity of the embryo, thereby reducing the production of superoxide radicals.[136]

A problem with co-culture that has received little attention is the choice of which medium to use. In a co-culture system, one is faced with the dilemma of having to satisfy the requirements of two very different cell types in culture. If the medium is chosen to fulfill the requirements of the somatic cells, then the embryo may be compromised by the inclusion of such components as nucleotides, essential amino acids, etc. In contrast, if the medium is chosen to fulfill the requirements of the embryo, it may be too simple in composition to maintain the viability of the somatic cells, resulting in cellular necrosis after a short period of time, which may in turn adversely affect embryo development.

To resolve the apparent paradox, somatic cells can be cultured in a complete medium with serum until confluent, after which they can be "weaned" onto a simpler medium which has been shown not to compromise embryo development but which can support somatic cell development for several days.[36]

VII. FUTURE DIRECTIONS

It is clear from this chapter that the only consensus regarding embryo culture systems is that there is no consensus. It is fortuitous that the human embryo, more so than those of other mammals, can tolerate such a wide range of media (Tables 1 through 3). The composition of most media currently used in clinical IVF appear, in theory at least, to be potentially detrimental to embryo development.

Presently, there is a much needed resurgence in research on the mammalian preimplantation embryo, which will help clarify the current confusion regarding culture systems. Improvements in embryo culture systems probably will be made in two distinct ways:

1. As our understanding of embryo and maternal physiology increases, we will be able to formulate media to cater to the changing requirements of the oocyte and resultant embryo; this will almost certainly require the formulation of several media, each designed to cater to a specific time/stage of development, in order to maintain embryo viability;
2. Not only is it important to fulfill the embryo's requirements during the preimplantation period, but it is also important to protect the embryo from the stress induced by removing it from the female tract; embryo "protectants" will therefore be included in media formulations to minimize embryo trauma; such protectants may include chelators, such as EDTA and Transferrin;[137] antioxidants, such as glutathione; ascorbic acid; dissipaters of superoxide radicals, such as superoxide dismutase; and osmolytes, such as glycine.[138]

REFERENCES

1. **Bowman, P. and McLaren, A.,** Cleavage rate of mouse embryos *in vivo* and *in vitro*, *J. Embryol. Exp. Morphol.*, 24, 203, 1970.
2. **Streffer, C., van Beuningen, D., Molls, M., Zamboglou, N., and Schulz, J.,** Kinetics of cell proliferation in the preimplantation mouse embryo *in vivo* and *in vitro*, *Cell Tissue Kinet.*, 13, 135, 1980.
3. **Harlow, G. M. and Quinn, P.,** Development of preimplantation mouse embryos *in vivo* and *in vitro*, *Aust. J. Biol. Sci.*, 35, 187, 1982.
4. **Biggers, J. D.,** *In vitro* fertilization and embryo transfer in human beings, *New Engl. J. Med.*, 304, 336, 1981.
5. **Steptoe, P. C., Edwards, R. G., and Walters, D. E.,** Observations on 767 clinical pregnancies and 500 births after human *in vitro* fertilization, *Hum. Reprod.*, 1, 89, 1986.
6. **Leese, H. J.,** The formation and function of oviduct fluid, *J.Reprod. Fertil.*, 82, 843, 1988.
7. **Paria, B. C. and Dey, S. K.,** Preimplantation embryo development *in vitro*: cooperative interactions among embryos and role of growth factors, *Proc. Natl. Acad. Sci. U.S.A.*, 87, 4756, 1990.
8. **Lane, M. and Gardner, D. K.,** Effect of incubation volume and embryo density on the development and viability of mouse embryos *in vitro*, *Hum. Reprod.*, 7, 558, 1992.
9. **Leese, H. J. and Barton, A. M.,** Pyruvate and glucose uptake by mouse ova and preimplantation embryo, *J. Reprod. Fertil.* 71, 9, 1984.
10. **Gardner, D. K. and Leese, H. J.,** Non-invasive measurement of nutrient uptake by single cultured pre-implantation mouse embryos, *Hum. Reprod.*, 1, 25, 1986.
11. **Biggers, J. D., Gardner, D. K., and Leese, H. J.,** Control of carbohydrate metabolism on preimplantation embryos, in *Growth Factors in Mammalian Development*, Rosenblum, I.Y. and Heyner, S., Eds., CRC Press, Boca Raton, FL, 1989, 19.
12. **Leese, H. J.,** Metabolism of the preimplantation mammalian embryo, in *Oxford Reviews of Reproductive Biology*, Milligan, S. R., Ed., Oxford University Press, Oxford, 1992, 35.

13. **Braude, P. R., Bolton, V. N., and Moore, S.,** Human gene expression first occurs between the four- and eighth-cell stages of preimplantation development, *Nature,* 332, 459, 1988.
14. **Flach, G., Johnson, M. H., Braude, P. R., Taylor, R. A. S., and Bolton, V. N.,** The transition from maternal to embryonic control in the 2-cell mouse embryo, *EMBO J.,* 1, 681, 1982.
15. **Chatot, C. L., Ziomek, C. A., Bavister, B. D., Lewis, J. L., and Torres, I.,** An improved culture medium supports development of random-bred 1-cell mouse embryos *in vitro, J. Reprod. Fertil.,* 86, 679, 1989.
16. **Kishi, J., Noda, Y., Narimoto, K., Umaoka, Y., and Mori, T.,** Block to development in cultured rat 1-cell embryos is overcome using medium HECM-1, *Hum. Reprod.,* 6, 1445, 1991.
17. **Bavister, B. D. and McKiernan, S. H.,** Regulation of hamster embryo development *in vitro* by amino acids, in *Preimplantation Embryo Development,* Bavister, B. D., Ed., Plenum Press, New York, 1992, in press.
18. **Petters, R. M., Johnson, B. H., Reed, M. L., and Archibong, A. E.,** Glucose, glutamine and inorganic phosphate in early development of the pig embryo in vitro, *J. Reprod. Fertil.,* 89, 269, 1990.
19. **Whitten, W. K. and Biggers, J. D.,** Complete development *in vitro* of the preimplantation stages of the mouse in a simple chemically defined medium, *J. Reprod. Fertil.,* 17, 399, 1968.
20. **Whittingham, D. G.,** Culture of mouse ova, *J. Reprod. Fertil. Suppl.,* 14, 7, 1971.
21. **Edwards, R. G.,** Test-tube babies, *Nature,* 293, 253, 1981.
22. **Quinn, P., Kerin, J. F., and Warnes, G. M.,** Improved pregnancy rate in human *in vitro* fertilization with the use of a medium based on the composition of human tubal fluid, *Fertil. Steril.,* 44, 493, 1985.
23. **Whitten, W. K.,** The effect of progesterone on the development of mouse eggs *in vitro, J. Endocrinol.,* 16, 80, 1957.
24. **Brinster, R. L.,** Studies on the development of mouse embryos *in vitro.* IV. Interaction of energy sources, *J. Reprod. Fertil.,* 10, 227, 1965.
25. **Biggers, J. D., Whitten, W. K., and Whittingham, D. G.,** The culture of mouse embryos *in vitro,* in *Methods of Mammalian Embryology,* Daniel, J. C., Jr., Ed., W. H. Freeman, San Francisco, 1971, 86.
26. **Gardner, D. K. and Leese, H. J.,** Concentrations of nutrients in mouse oviduct fluid and their effects on embryo development and metabolism *in vitro, J. Reprod. Fertil.,* 88, 361, 1990.
27. **Ham, R. G.,** An improved nutrient solution for diploid chinese hamster and human cell lines, *Exp. Cell Res.,* 29, 515, 1963.
28. **Menezo, Y. J. R., Testart, J., and Perrone, D.,** Serum is not necessary in human *in vitro* fertilization, early embryo culture, and transfer, *Fertil. Steril.,* 42, 750, 1984.
29. **Borland, R. M., Biggers, J. D., Lechene, C. P., and Taymour, M. L.,** Elemental composition of fluid in the human fallopian tube, *J. Reprod. Fertil.,* 58, 479, 1980.
30. **Gott, A. L., Hardy, K., Winston, R. M. L., and Leese, H. J.,** The nutrition and environment of the early human embryo, in *Proceedings of the Nutritional Society,* London, 2A(Abstr.), 1990.
31. **Gardner, D. K., Lane, M., Leeton, J., and Calderon, I.,** unpublished data, 1993.
32. **Borland, R. M., Hazra, S., Biggers, J. D., and Lechene, C. P.,** The elemental composition of the environment of the gametes and preimplantation embryo during the initiation of pregnancy, *Biol. Reprod.,* 16, 147, 1977.
33. **Roblero, L. S., Guadarrama, A., Ortiz, M. E., Fernandez, E., and Zegers-Hochschild, F.,** High potassium concentration and the cumulus corona oocyte complex stimulate the fertilizing capacity of human spermatozoa, *Fertil. Steril.,* 54, 328, 1990.
34. **Roblero, L. S. and Riffo, M. D.,** High potassium concentration improves preimplantation development of mouse embryo *in vitro, Fertil. Steril.,* 45, 412, 1986.

35. **Wiley, L. M., Yamami, S., and Van Muyden, D.**, Effect of potassium concentration, type of protein supplement, and embryo density on mouse preimplantation development *in vitro*, *Fertil. Steril.*, 45, 111, 1986.
36. **Sakkas, D. and Trounson, A. O.**, Formulation of a complex serum-free medium (CSM) for use in the co-culture of mouse embryos with cells of the female reproductive tract, *Reprod. Fertil. Dev.*, 3, 99, 1991.
37. **Gardner, D. K. and Sakkas, D.**, Mouse embryo cleavage, metabolism and viability: role of medium composition, *Hum. Reprod.*, in press.
38. **Wales, R. G.**, Effects of ions on the development of the pre-implantation mouse embryo *in vitro*, *Aust. J. Biol. Sci.*, 23, 421, 1970.
39. **Bavister, B. D. and Golden, M.**, Alteration of extracellular cation concentrations and ratios in culture medium does not affect first cleavage division of hamster zygotes *in vitro* nor overcome the "two-cell block", *Reprod. Fertil. Dev.*, 1, 231, 1989.
40. **McKiernan, S. H. and Bavister, B. D.**, Environmental variables influencing *in vitro* development of hamster 2-cell embryos to the blastocyst stage, *Biol. Reprod.*, 43, 404, 1990.
41. **Brinster, R. L.**, Studies on the development of mouse embryos *in vitro*. I. The effect of osmolarity and hydrogen ion concentration, *J. Exp. Zool.*, 158, 49, 1965.
42. **Lawitts, J. A. and Biggers, J. D.**, Overcoming the 2-cell block by modifying standard components in a mouse embryo culture medium, *Biol. Reprod.*, 45, 245, 1991.
43. **Leese, H. J., Hooper, M. A. K., Edwards, R. G., and Ashwood-Smith, M. J.**, Uptake of pyruvate by early human embryos determined by a non-invasive technique, *Hum. Reprod.*, 1, 181, 1986.
44. **Hardy, K., Hooper, M. A. K., Handyside, A. H., Rutherford, A. J., Winston, R. M. L., and Leese, H. J.**, Non-invasive measurement of glucose and pyruvate uptake by individual human oocytes and preimplantation embryos, *Hum. Reprod.*, 4, 188, 1989.
45. **Gott, A. L., Hardy, K., Winston, R. M. L., and Leese, H. J.**, Non-invasive measurement of glucose and pyruvate uptake by individual human oocytes and preimplantation embryos, *Hum. Reprod.*, 5, 104, 1990.
46. **Biggers, J. D., Whittingham, D. G., and Donahue, R. P.**, The pattern of energy metabolism in the mouse oocyte and zygote, *Proc. Natl. Acad. Sci. U.S.A*, 58, 560, 1967.
47. **Cross, P. C. and Brinster, R. L.**, The sensitivity of one-cell mouse embryos to pyruvate and lactate, *Exp. Cell Res.*, 77, 57, 1973.
48. **Brinster, R. L. and Thomson, J. L.**, Development of eight-cell mouse embryos *in vitro*, *Exp. Cell Res.*, 42, 308, 1966.
49. **Barbehenn, E. K., Wales, R. G., and Lowry, O. H.**, The explanation for the blockade in glycolysis in early mouse embryos, *Proc. Natl. Acad. Sci. U.S.A.*, 71, 1056, 1974.
50. **Barbehenn, E. K., Wales, R. G., and Lowry, O. H.**, Measurement of metabolites in single preimplantation embryos; a new means to study metabolic control in early embryos, *J. Embryol. Exp. Morphol.*, 43, 29, 1978.
51. **Schini, S. A. and Bavister, B. D.**, Two-cell block to development of cultured hamster embryos is caused by phosphate and glucose, *Biol. Reprod.*, 39, 1183, 1988.
52. **Seshagiri, P. B. and Bavister, B. D.**, Glucose inhibits development of hamster 8-cell embryos *in vitro*, *Biol. Reprod.*, 40, 599, 1989.
53. **Seshagiri, P. B. and Bavister, B. D.**, Phosphate is required for inhibition by glucose of hamster 8-cell embryos *in vitro*, *Biol. Reprod.*, 40, 607, 1989.
54. **Thompson, J. G. E., Simpson, A. C., Pugh, P. A., and Tervit, H. R.**, An examination of the requirement for glucose in preimplantation sheep embryos during *in vitro* culture, in *Preimplantation Embryo Development*, Bavister, B. D., Ed., Plenum Press, New York, 1992, in press.
55. **Seshagiri, P. B. and Bavister, B. D.**, Glucose and phosphate inhibit respiration and oxidative metabolism in cultured hamster eight-cell embryos: evidence for the "Crabtree effect," *Molec. Reprod. Devel.*, 30, 105, 1991.

56. **Leese, H. J. and Barton, A. M.,** Production of pyruvate by isolated mouse cumulus cells, *J. Exp. Zool.*, 234, 231, 1985.
57. **Nichol, R., Hunter, R. H. F., Gardner, D. K., Leese, H. J., and Cooke, G. M.,** Concentrations of energy substrates in oviductal fluid and blood plasma of pigs during the peri-ovulatory period, *J. Reprod. Fertil.*, 96, 699, 1992.
58. **Menke, T. M. and McLaren, A.,** Mouse blastocysts grown *in vivo* and *in vitro*: carbon dioxide production and trophoblast outgrowth, *J. Reprod. Fertil.*, 23, 117, 1970.
59. **Schultz, G. A., Kaye, P. L., McKay, D. J., and Johnson, M. H.,** Endogenous amino acids pool sizes in mouse eggs and preimplantation embryos, *J. Reprod. Fertil.*, 61, 387, 1981.
60. **Van Winkle, L. J.,** Amino acid transport in developing animal oocytes and early conceptuses, *Biochim. Biophys. Acta*, 947, 173, 1988.
61. **Kaye, P. L.,** Metabolic aspects of the physiology of the preimplantation embryo, in *Experimental Approaches to Mammalian Embryonic Development*, Rossant, J. and Pedersen, R. A., Eds., Cambridge University Press, New York., 1986, 267.
62. **Miller, J. G. O. and Schultz, G. A.,** Amino acid content of preimplantation rabbit embryos and fluids of the reproductive tract, *Biol. Reprod.*, 36, 125, 1987.
63. **Gardner, D. K. and Lane, M.,** Amino acids and ammonium regulate the development of preimplantation mouse embryos in culture, *Biol Reprod.*, 48, 377, 1993.
64. **Bavister, B. D. and Arlotto, T.,** Influence of single amino acids on the development of hamster one-cell embryos *in vitro*, *Mol. Reprod. Devel.*, 25, 45, 1990.
65. **Mehta, T. S. and Kiessling, A. A.,** Development potential of mouse embryos conceived *in vitro* and cultured in ethylenediamineetraacetic acid or without amino acids or serum, *Biol. Reprod.*, 43, 600, 1990.
66. **Zhang, X. and Armstrong, D. T.,** Presence of amino acids and insulin in a chemically defined medium improves development of 8-cell rat embryos *in vitro* and subsequent implantation *in vivo*, *Biol. Reprod.*, 42, 662, 1990.
67. **Kane, M. T.,** The effects of water-soluble vitamins on the expansion of rabbit blastocysts *in vitro*, *J. Exp. Zool.*, 245, 220, 1988.
68. **Loutradis, D., John, D., and Kiessling, A. A.,** Hypoxanthine causes a 2-cell block in random-bred mouse embryos, *Biol. Reprod.*, 37, 311, 1987.
69. **Downs, S. M. and Dow, M. P.,** Hypoxanthine-maintained two-cell block in mouse embryos: dependence on glucose and effect of hypoxanthine phosphoribosyltransferase inhibitors, *Biol. Reprod.*, 44, 1025, 1991.
70. **Nureddin, A., Epsaro, E., and Kiessling, A. A.,** Purines inhibit the development of mouse embryos *in vitro*, *J. Reprod. Fertil.*, 90, 455, 1990.
71. **Barnes, D. and Sato, G.,** Methods for growth of cultured cells in serum-free medium, *Anal. Biochem.*, 102, 255, 1980.
72. **Barnes, D. and Sato, G.,** Serum-free cell culture: a unifying approach, *Cell*, 22, 649, 1980.
73. **Ogawa, T. and Marrs, R. P.,** The effect of protein supplementation on single-cell mouse embryos *in vitro*, *Fertil. Steril.*, 47, 156, 1987.
74. **Ashwood-Smith, M. J., Hollands, P., and Edwards, R. G.,** The use of albuminar 5 (TM) as a medium supplement in clinical IVF, *Hum. Reprod.*, 4, 702, 1989.
75. **Khan, I., Staessen, C., Devroey, P., and Van Steirteghem, A. C.,** Human serum albumin versus serum: a comparative study on embryo transfer medium, *Fertil. Steril.*, 56, 98, 1991.
76. **Staessen, C., Van den Abbeel, E., Carle, M., Khan, I., Devroey, P., and Van Steirteghem, A. C.,** Comparison between human serum and albuminar-20 (TM) supplement for *in vitro* fertilization, *Hum. Reprod.*, 5, 336, 1990.
77. **Benadiva, C. A., Kuczynski-Brown, B., Maguire, T. G., Mastroianni, L., Jr., and Flickinger, G. L.,** Bovine serum albumin (BSA) can replace patient serum as a protein source in an *in vitro* fertilization (IVF) program, *JIVET*, 6, 164, 1989.
78. **Kane, M. T. and Fahy, M. M.,** Blastocyst growth and development, in *Preimplantation Embryo Development*, Bavister, B.D., Ed., Plenum Press, New York, 1992, in press.

79. **Caro, C. M. and Trounson, A. O.**, The effect of protein on preimplantation mouse embryo development *in vitro*, *JIVET*, 1, 183, 1984.
80. **Kane, M. T.**, Variability in different lots of commercial bovine serum albumin affects cell multiplication and hatching of rabbit blastocysts in culture, *J. Reprod. Fertil.*, 69, 555, 1983.
81. **Batt, P. A., Gardner, D. K., and Cameron, A. W. N.**, Oxygen concentration and protein source affect the development of preimplantation goat embryos *in vitro*, *Reprod. Fertil. Dev.*, 3, 601, 1991.
82. **Fissore, R. A., Jackson, K. V., and Kiessling, A. A.**, Mouse zygote development in culture medium without protein in the presence of ethylenediaminetetraacetic acid, *Biol. Reprod.*, 41, 835, 1989.
83. **Caro, C. M. and Trounson, A. O.**, Successful fertilization, embryo development, and pregnancy in human *in vitro* fertilization (IVF) using a chemically defined culture medium containing no protein, *JIVET*, 3, 215, 1986.
84. **Bavister, B. D.**, Substitution of a synthetic polymer for protein in a mammalian gamete culture system, *J. Exp. Zool.*, 217, 45, 1981.
85. **Holst, N., Bertheussen, K., Forsdahl, F., Hakonsen, M. B., Hansen, L. J., and Nielsen, H. I.**, Optimization and simplification of culture conditions in human *in vitro* fertilization (IVF) and preembryo replacement by serum-free media, *JIVET*, 7, 47, 1990.
86. **Psalti, I., Loumaye, E., Pensis, M., Depreester, S., and Thomas, K.**, Evaluation of a synthetic serum substitute to replace fetal cord serum for human oocyte fertilization and embryo growth *in vitro*, *Fertil. Steril.*, 52, 807, 1989.
87. **Wu, J.-T.**, Metabolism of progesterone by preimplantation mouse blastocysts in culture, *Biol. Reprod.*, 36, 549, 1987.
88. **Edirisinghe, W. R. and Wales, R. G.**, Effect of parental administration of oestrogen and progesterone on the glycogen metabolism of mouse morulae-early blastocysts *in vivo*, *J. Reprod. Fertil.*, 72, 67, 1984.
89. **Edirisinghe, W. R. and Wales, R. G.**, Influence of environmental factors on the metabolism of glucose by preimplantation mouse embryos *in vitro*, *J. Reprod. Fertil.*, 38, 411, 1985.
90. **Khurana, N. K. and Wales, R. G.**, Effects of prostaglandins E-2 and F-2α on the metabolism of [U-^{14}C] glucose by mouse morulae-early blastocysts *in vitro*, *J. Reprod. Fertil.*, 79, 275, 1987.
91. **Khurana, N. K. and Wales, R. G.**, Effects of oestradiol and progesterone on the metabolism of [U-^{14}C] glucose by mouse morulae and early blastocysts *in vitro*, *J. Reprod. Fertil.*, 79, 267, 1987.
92. **Yohkaichiya, T., Fukaya, T., Hoshiai, H., and Yajima, A.**, Improvement of mouse embryo development *in vitro* by prolactin, *Tohoku J. Exp. Med.*, 155, 241, 1988.
93. **Lavranos, T. C. and Seamark, R. F.**, Addition of steroids to embryo-uterine monolayer co-culture enhances embryo survival and implantation *in vitro*, *Reprod. Fertil. Dev.*, 1, 41, 1989.
94. **Harvey, M. B. and Kaye, P. L.**, IGF-2 receptors are first expressed at the 2-cell stage of mouse development, *Development*, 111, 1057, 1991.
95. **Rosenblum, I. Y., Mattson, B. A., and Heyner, S.**, Stage-specific insulin binding in mouse preimplantation embryos, *Dev. Biol.*, 116, 261, 1986.
96. **Harvey, M. B. and Kaye, P. L.**, Insulin increases the cell number of the inner cell mass and stimulates morphological development of mouse blastocysts *in vitro*, *Development*, 110, 963, 1990.
97. **Pritchard, M. L., Haydock, S. W., Wikarczuk, M. L., Farber, M., and Heyner, S.**, Effect of insulin on RNA synthesis in the preimplantation mouse embryo, *Biol. Reprod.*, 36, (Suppl. 1), 77, 1987.
98. **Harvey, M. B. and Kaye, P. L.**, Insulin stimulates protein synthesis in compacted mouse embryos, *Endocrinology*, 122, 1182, 1988.
99. **Wood, S. A. and Kaye, P. L.**, Effects of epidermal growth factor on preimplantation mouse embryos, *J. Reprod. Fertil.*, 85, 575, 1989.

100. Quinn, P. and Wales, R. G., Growth and metabolism of preimplantation mouse embryos cultured in phosphate-buffered medium, *J. Reprod. Fertil.*, 35, 289, 1973.
101. Minhas, B. S., Randall, G. W., Dodson, M. G., and Robertson, J. L., A limited exposure of murine oocytes and zygotes to phosphate buffered saline retards development *in vitro*, *Theriogenology*, 31, 229, 1989.
102. Mahadevan, M. M., Fleetham, J., Church, R. B., and Taylor, P. J., Growth of mouse embryos in bicarbonate media buffered by carbon dioxide, HEPES, or phosphate, *JIVET*, 3, 304, 1986.
103. Good, N. E., Winget, G. D., Winter, W., Connolly, T. N., Izawa, S., and Singh, R. M. M., Hydrogen ion buffers for biological research, *Biochemistry*, 5, 467, 1966.
104. Quinn, P., Barros, C., and Whittingham, D. G., Preservation of hamster oocytes to assay the fertilizing capacity of human spermatozoa, *J. Reprod. Fertil.*, 66, 161, 1982.
105. Behr, B. R., Stratton, C. J., Foote, W. D., Knutzen, V., and Sher, G., *In vitro* fertilization (IVF) of mouse ova in HEPES-buffered culture media, *JIVET*, 7, 9, 1990.
106. Quinn, P. and Harlow, G. H., The effect of oxygen on the development of preimplantation mouse embryos *in vitro*, *J. Exp. Zool.*, 206, 73, 1978.
107. Umaoka, Y., Noda, Y., Narimoto, K., and Mori, T., Effects of oxygen toxicity on early development of mouse embryos, *Mol. Reprod. Dev.*, 31, 28, 1992.
108. Thompson, J. G. E., Simpson, A. C., Pugh, P. A., Donnelly, P. E., and Tervit, H. R., Effect of oxygen concentration on *in vitro* development of preimplantation sheep and cattle embryos, *J. Reprod. Fertil.* 89, 573, 1990.
109. Noda, Y., Matsumoto, H., Umaoka, Y., Tatsumi, J., and Mori, T., Involvement of superoxide radicals in the mouse two-cell block, *Mol. Reprod. Dev.*, 28, 356, 1991.
110. Legge, M. and Sellens, M. H., Free radical scavengers ameliorate the 2-cell block in mouse embryo culture, *Hum. Reprod.*, 6, 867, 1991.
111. Pabon, J. E., Findley, W. E., and Gibbons, W. E., The toxic effect of short exposures to the atmospheric oxygen concentration on early mouse embryonic development, *Fertil. Steril.*, 51, 896, 1989.
112. Graves, C. N. and Biggers, J. D., Carbon dioxide fixation by mouse embryos prior to implantation, *Science*, 167, 1506, 1970.
113. May, J. V. and Hanshew, K., Organization of the *in vitro* fertilization/embryo transfer laboratory, in *Handbook of the Laboratory Diagnosis and Treatment of Infertility*, Keel, B. A. and Webster, B. W., Eds., CRC Press, Boca Raton, FL, 1990, 219.
114. Weiss, T. J., Warnes, G. M., and Gardner, D. K., Mouse embryos and quality control in human IVF, *Reprod. Fertil. Dev.*, 4, 105, 1992.
115. Gerrity, M., Mouse embryo culture bioassay, in *In Vitro Fertilization and Embryo Transfer*, Wolf, D. P., Ed., Plenum Press, New York, 1988, 57.
116. Fukuda, A., Noda, Y., Tsukui, S., Matsumoto, H., Yano, J., and Mori, T., Influence of water quality on *in vitro* fertilization and embryo development for the mouse, *JIVET*, 4, 40, 1987.
117. Silverman, I. H., Cook, C. L., Sanfilippo, J. S., Yussman, M. A., Schultz, G. S., and Hilton, F. H., Ham's F-10 constituted with tap water supports mouse conceptus development *in vitro*, *JIVET*, 4, 185, 1987.
118. Davidson, A., Vermesh, M. V., Lobo, R. A., and Paulson, R. J., Mouse embryo culture as quality control for human *in vitro* fertilization: the one-cell versus the two-cell model, *Fertil. Steril.*, 49, 516, 1988.
119. Fleming, T. P., Pratt, H. P. M., and Braude, P. R., The use of mouse preimplantation embryos for quality control of culture reagents in human in vitro fertilization programs: a cautionary note, *Fertil. Steril.*, 47, 858, 1987.
120. Parinaud, J., Reme, J.-M., Monrozies, X., Favrin, S., Sarramon, M.-F., and Pontonnier, G., Mouse system quality control is necessary before the use of new material for *in vitro* fertilization and embryo transfer, *JIVET*, 4, 56, 1987.

121. **Rinehart, J. S., Bavister, B. D., and Gerrity, M.,** Quality control in the *in vitro* fertilization laboratory: comparison of bioassay systems for water quality, *JIVET*, 5, 335, 1988.
122. **Whittingham, D. G. and Biggers, J. D.,** Fallopian tube and early cleavage in the mouse, *Nature*, 213, 942, 1967.
123. **Minami, N., Bavister, B. D., and Iritani, A.,** Development of hamster two-cell embryos in the isolated mouse oviduct in organ culture system, *Gamete Res.*, 19, 235, 1988.
124. **Krisher, R. L., Petters, R. M., Johnson, B. H., Bavister, B. D., and Archibong, A. E.,** Development of porcine embryos from the one-cell stage to blastocyst in mouse oviducts maintained in organ culture, *J. Exp. Zool.*, 249, 235, 1989.
125. **Sakkas, D., Batt, P. A., and Cameron, A. W. N.,** Development of preimplantation goat (*Capra hircus*) embryos *in vivo* and *in vitro*, *J. Reprod. Fertil.*, 87, 359, 1989.
126. **Gandolfi, F. and Moor, R. M.,** Stimulation of early embryonic development in the sheep by co-culture with oviduct epithelial cells, *J. Reprod. Fertil.*, 81, 23, 1987.
127. **Rexroad, C. E.,** Co-culture of domestic animal embryos, *Theriogenology*, 31, 105, 1989.
128. **Wiemer, K. E. and Cohen, J.,** Co-culture of mammalian embryos, in *From Ovulation to Implantation*, Evers, J. H. L. and Heineman, M. J., Eds., Elsevier, Amsterdam, 1990, 297.
129. **Wiemer, K. E., Cohen, J., Amborski, G. F., Wright, G., Wiker, S., Munyakazi, L., and Godke, R. A.,** *In vitro* development and implantation of human embryos following culture on fetal bovine uterine fibroblast cells, *Hum. Reprod.*, 4, 595, 1989.
130. **Wiemer, K. E., Malter, H. E., Cohen, J., Wright, G., Wiker, S. R., and Godke, R. A.,** Coculture of human zygotes on fetal bovine uterine fibroblasts: embryonic morphology and implantation, *Fertil. Steril.*, 52, 503, 1989.
131. **Bongso, A., Ng, S.-C., Fong, C.-Y., and Ratnam, S.,** Cocultures: a new lead in embryo quality improvement for assisted reproduction, *Fertil. Steril.*, 56, 179, 1991.
132. **Bongso, A., Ng, S.-C., and Ratnam, S.,** Co-cultures: their relevance to assisted reproduction, *Hum. Reprod.*, 5, 893, 1990.
133. **Bongso, A., Ng, S.-C., Sathananthan, H., Lian, N. P., Rauff, M. R., and Ratnam, S.,** Improved quality of human embryos when co-cultured with ampullary cells, *Hum. Reprod.*, 4, 706, 1989.
134. **Bongso, A., Ng, S.-C., Fong, C.-Y., and Ratnam, S.,** Improved fertilization rates of human oocytes in coculture, *JIVET*, 8, 216, 1991.
135. **Menezo, Y. J. R., Guerin, J. F., and Czyba, J. C.,** Improvement of human early embryo development *in vitro* by coculture on monolayers of vero cells, *Biol. Reprod.*, 42, 301, 1990.
136. **Takeuchi, K., Kaufmann, R. A., and Sandow, B. A.,** Enhanced mouse embryo development in oviductal and non-oviductal cell co-cultures is associated with reduced oxygen concentration in culture medium, *Proc. Am. Fertil. Soc.*, (Abstr.) O-019, 47th Annual Meeting, Orlando, Florida, 1991.
137. **Nasr-Esfahani, M., Johnson, M. H., and Aitken, R. J.,** The effect of iron and iron chelators on the *in-vitro* block to development of the mouse preimplantation embryo: BAT6 a new medium for improved culture of mouse embryos *in vitro*, *Hum. Reprod.*, 5, 997, 1990.
138. **Van Winkle, L. J., Haghighat, N., and Campione, A. L.,** Glycine protects preimplantation mouse conceptuses from a detrimental effect on development of the inorganic ions in oviductal fluid, *J. Exp. Zool.*, 253, 215, 1990.

Chapter 6

EMBRYO BIOPSY FOR PREIMPLANTATION DIAGNOSIS

Juan J. Tarín and Alan Trounson

TABLE OF CONTENTS

I. Introduction 116

II. Optimal Embryo Stage for Biopsy 117
    A. Biopsy of the First Polar Body 117
    B. Biopsy at Blastocyst Stage 117
    C. Biopsy at Cleavage Stages 118

III. Maximum Reduction of Cellular Mass 119

IV. Methods of Embryo Biopsy 120
    A. Comparative Studies of Different Biopsy Methods 124
        1. Oocytes in Metaphase II 124
        2. Cleavage Stages 125
        3. Blastocyst Stage 125

V. Conclusions 126

References 127

I. INTRODUCTION

Although it may be possible in the near future to diagnose some inherited diseases in early human embryos by noninvasive methods[1], in general, the diagnosis of genetic diseases, especially by DNA analysis, requires that one or more cells be biopsied from each embryo. Clearly, the greater the number of biopsied cells available for analysis, the more reliable any diagnosis is likely to be. However, there is a limitation on the cell number and/or cellular mass that can be removed without affecting the viability of the embryos. This limitation could be overcome either by allowing the biopsied cells to divide in culture before diagnosis or by removing larger numbers of nonessential cells from later stages of embryo development, e.g., the blastocyst stage. Nevertheless, biopsy presently involves the micromanipulation of fragile early stage embryos, extended culture *in vitro,* and delayed replacement *in vivo* or embryo cryopreservation. These additional manipulations may affect embryo development *in vitro* and/or embryo transfer results. For instance, it would be possible that the removal of even a single cell at the 2- or 4-cell stage may compromise the embryo's ability to form a normal blastocyst with an adequate number of inner cell mass (ICM) cells for normal development *in vivo*. In fact, in the mouse, biopsy of one-half of the blastomeres is correlated with a decrease in the proportion of ICM cells at the blastocyst stage[2] and with later *in vivo* development.[3,4] In addition, recently it has been suggested that mouse,[5] bovine,[6] and human[7] embryos at early cleavage stages may be more sensitive to micromanipulation than at later stages of development. A low[8] or even a complete failure to establish pregnancy[9] has been reported after transfer of either human morula and early blastocysts on day 5 or blastocysts on days 6 and 7 postinsemination, respectively. Finally, although it has been shown that biopsied mouse embryos can be successfully cryopreserved by ultrarapid freezing even though they have a punctured zona pellucida,[10] there is an increased risk that freezing-thawing may damage or destroy embryos.

A variety of embryo biopsy methods have been reported, including "blastomere aspiration," "blastomere extrusion," "mechanical division," and "trophectoderm (TE) herniation." This diversity in methodology is accompanied by a wide variation in the resulting embryo viability and in the acquisition of viable blastomeres suitable for genetic analysis. It is therefore essential to determine the optimal conditions for biopsy, avoiding as far as possible any damage to the embryos or blastomeres biopsied, so that the efficiency of the genetic diagnosis is maximized and pregnancy rates are maintained.

The present chapter analyzes the different approaches to embryo biopsy reported to date for preimplantation diagnosis for genetic defects. We have attempted to determine if conclusive information exists on the optimal embryo stage for biopsy and the maximum reduction of cellular mass that can be removed without compromising later embryo development *in vitro* and/or *in vivo*. Furthermore, special attention has been given to assess the different methods of embryo biopsy reported to date.

II. OPTIMAL EMBRYO STAGE FOR BIOPSY

A. BIOPSY OF THE FIRST POLAR BODY

Preimplantation diagnosis by removal and genetic analysis of the first polar body was reported by Verlinsky et al.[11] This approach is based on several principles which may appear attractive for its clinical application. For instance, the first polar body is not required for fertilization and normal embryonic development. Therefore, its removal should have no deleterious effect on the developing embryo. Furthermore, this strategy allows embryo transfer in the same *in vitro* fertilization (IVF) cycle, eliminating the need for cryopreservation. Nevertheless, there are several problems which may inhibit the clinical application of this approach. First, the procedure only allows the detection of maternal genetic defects. Second, there would be a considerable reduction in the number of embryos available for a transfer as a result of the possible crossing over between homologous chromosomes. For instance, in telomeric genes, half of the polar bodies analyzed will be heterozygous as a result of crossing over. In these cases, it will be impossible to predict the eventual haploid genotype after fertilization. One quarter will be homozygous for the normal gene, and only one quarter will be suitable for transfer (polar body homozygous for the mutant gene). Third, the genetic analysis that can be made after removal of the first polar body has a relatively low reliability because only a single nucleus can be used for genetic analysis.

In order to overcome these disadvantages, Verlinsky et al.[11] proposed that a second biopsy and analysis be undertaken in embryos resulting from later insemination and fertilization. The increased manipulation seemed to have no significant effect on embryo development to the blastocyst stage *in vitro* or on implantation rates.[12] However, if a second biopsy and analysis is needed for an accurate diagnosis and to confirm previous results, the polar body biopsy is redundant, since biopsy at cleavage stages can provide the minimal number of blastomeres ($n = 2$) to diagnose a genetic defect with acceptable reliability.

B. BIOPSY AT BLASTOCYST STAGE

Since the first successful preimplantation diagnosis was carried out in rabbit blastocysts,[13] the biopsy of TE cells at the blastocyst stage has been considered as the approach that offers more advantages in preimplantation diagnosis.[8,14-20] Biopsy of the blastocyst can provide the maximum number of cells for genetic analysis, and, clearly, the greater the number of biopsied cells available for analysis, the more reliable any diagnosis is likely to be. Another important advantage is that the TE cells removed are strictly extraembryonic, contributing only to placental tissues after implantation. In this sense, TE biopsy is an approach homologous to chorion villus biopsy, and, when the use of such a technique on human embryos is considered, there should be no ethical objections to its clinical application. Finally, by the blastocyst stage, especially in the TE, embryonic gene expression is more advanced than in cells of cleavage stage embryos, so it is possible to diagnose more inherited diseases by sensitive biochemical microassays.[21] However, the low pregnancy rate following IVF and transfer at blastocyst stage,[8,9] together with the relatively low proportion (between 14.5% and 42.0% according to Dokras et al.[17] and Hardy et al.,[22] respectively) of embryos that develop to the blastocyst stage *in vitro*, do not make this an attractive technique at the present time. In addition, there is heterogeneity in the rate of development of embryos to the blastocyst stage by day 5 and day 6.[7,22,23] These problems may prevent this approach being developed at the present time as a practical procedure in preimplantation diagnosis.

C. BIOPSY AT CLEAVAGE STAGES

The removal of one or more cells from embryos between the 2-cell and morula stages is the only feasible alternative to first polar body and blastocyst biopsies. However, not all of the cleavage stages have the same potential for success. For example, morulae are difficult to biopsy once compaction occurs, and the removal of one or more cells can affect their later postimplantation development.[5] Furthermore, it appears that early cleavage stage mouse[3,5] and cow[6] embryos may be more sensitive to micromanipulation than later stages. The optimum stage for biopsy in the mouse is the 8-cell stage, where the removal of one or two cells has minimal effect on the development to the blastocyst stage *in vitro*,[5] and in the cow, removal of up to half the cells of the 16-cell embryo prior to compaction.[6] Biopsy of embryos in these species at early cleavage stages results in retarded cleavage and development. Lawitts and Graves[3] reported that the development of half embryos of the mouse *in vitro* to the blastocyst stage was higher after mechanical division at the 8-cell stage than at 2-cell, 4-cell or morula stages. However, the highest survival rate of bisected embryos to live fetuses on days 15 to 18 of pregnancy was obtained with micromanipulated 4-cell embryos. According to the authors, the development of 2/4 embryos *in vitro* may have been more closely synchronized with the stage of pseudopregnancy of the recipients than embryos divided at the other cell stages because of their different rates of development *in vitro*. On the morning of day 4 prior to transfer, they observed that the majority of 1/2 embryos were at the morula stage, while the majority of 2/4 and 4/8 embryos were blastocysts. Virtually all half morulae developed to blastocyst during the same period. In the cow, Loskutoff et al.[6] found a lower total number of cells in blastocysts derived from half-embryos biopsied at the 2-cell stage than at the 4-cell stage, and both were lower than embryos biopsied at the 8- and 16-cell stages. However, untreated control embryos of the 2- and 4-cell stages showed retarded development in culture when compared with untreated 8- and 16-cell embryos. In the cow, early cleavage stages are more difficult to culture than later stage embryos and therefore less amenable to micromanipulation.

Recently, it has been suggested that this may also apply to human embryos.[7] Two types of 4- or 5-cell human embryos were found after biopsy of a quarter of their cells on day 2 after insemination. About half developed to the morula stage on day 4 (56%, 14/25) and the other half after day 4 (44%, 11/25). In both groups, the cleavage rate was retarded, although the retardation was more marked in embryos which reached the morula stage after day 4. This resulted in a smaller number of cells at the blastocyst stage on day 6 (40.8 ± 4.3 and 22.1 ± 1.5 for embryos which reached the morula stage on or after day 4, respectively) when compared to the expected cell numbers (47.7 ± 3.8). These results contrast with the proportional reduction in the total number of cells at the blastocyt stage found in 7/8 and 6/8 human embryos biopsied in the morning of day 3 after insemination.[23] Hence, it appears that human embryos are more sensitive to micromanipulation at 4- or 5-cells than at the 8-cell stage. In the same study,[7] only 8.7% (2/23) of the untreated control embryos which developed to blastocyst reached the morula stage after day 4, and the total number of cells of these blastocysts on day 6 (62.4 ± 4.7) was lower than that reported by Hardy et al.[23] in blastocysts derived from 8-cell embryos (78.5 ± 8.8).

III. MAXIMUM REDUCTION OF CELLULAR MASS

In the mouse and human, the timing of blastulation is constant and independent of cell number.[7,24] Hence, a reduction of cellular mass during cleavage results in blastocysts with reduced total cell numbers.[7,23,25-27] This reduction in the total number of cells at the blastocyst stage significantly reduces their capacity to form fetuses[28] and demonstrates that there is a lower limit to the cellular mass of the embryo compatible with normal development *in vivo*. In fact, in the mouse, development *in vitro* and *in vivo* is always affected after removal of half the embryo,[3,4,26,28] and may[29] or may not[10] be affected by removal of a quarter of cells, depending on subsequent cleavage rate.[5] In addition, several reviews on embryo manipulation in eutherian mammals[30-33] observe that the development of single blastomeres of 2-, 4-, and 8-cell embryos is lower in the mouse than in the cow, horse, rabbit, and sheep. Half-embryos produced by bisection of the embryo with either needles or with a microscalpel may also have a lower capacity for complete development in the mouse compared to the other species. This species difference may be explained by blastulation in the mouse at an earlier cleavage stage than other species.[33]

Similar to the pig,[34] untreated human embryos initiate blastulation after the fourth cleavage division.[22] This is earlier than in the mouse, where blastulation coincides with completion of the fifth cleavage division.[25,35] Hence, if embryo tolerance to a decrease in cellular mass is dependent on the cleavage stage at the time of cavitation, a cellular mass reduction innocuous to mouse embryos could be detrimental for human embryos.

In humans, little is known about the capacity for implantation and later development of embryos with a reduced cell mass. While there are reports of successful implantation and normal development of cryopreserved embryos with 5/8[36] or 1/4 intact blastomeres,[37] a systematic study by Handyside et al.[38] showed the effect of reducing embryonic cell mass by biopsy during cleavage on later implantation and development *in vivo*. According to this study, it appears that the developmental capacity of embryos of patients who were carriers of

X-linked recessive diseases was not decreased by the biopsy of 1/8 or 2/8 blastomeres of 6- to 8-cell embryos on day 3 after insemination. However, embryos biopsied at the 4- or 5-cell stages resulted in a reduction in the ratio of ICM:TE cells in blastocysts.[7] This may have negative consequences for postimplantation development because the fetus is derived from the ICM. In fact, in the mouse an insufficient number of ICM cells at the time of implantation may seriously affect later development *in vivo*.[26,39] Therefore, while biopsy of one quarter of the cells of human embryos on day 3 does not have a detrimental effect on implantation and development *in vivo*, development may be adversely affected if embryo biopsy is performed on day 2.

IV. METHODS OF EMBRYO BIOPSY

Different methods of embryo biopsy have been reported to date, including "aspiration," "extrusion," "mechanical division," and "herniation." Although some of these techniques can be used in all stages from the oocyte to the blastocyst (e.g., "aspiration" and "extrusion"), others are specific for a particular embryo stage (e.g., "mechanical division" and "herniation" for cleavage and blastocyst stages, respectively).

In the "aspiration" method, the first polar body or cells are removed by suction with a micropipette. The biopsy micropipette either can be forced through the zona pellucida as a needle[5,10,11,29,40,41] (Figure 1a) or be inserted through a hole or slit made in the zona pellucida by acid Tyrode's solution[7,23,42] or a sharpened dissection pipette[43] (Figure 1b).

For blastocyst biopsy, the zona pellucida is cut with a needle and the blastocyst can be induced[15,18,19] by micromanipulation to herniate through the cut. Thereafter, a biopsy micropipette aspirates a number of cells of the TE, and a microneedle or scissors cut off the sample (Figure 2a).

The "extrusion" method can be performed in three different ways:

1. "Displacement:" In this approach, an opening is made in the zona pellucida with a bevelled pipette; the bevelled pipette is then inserted at a second point and a gentle flow of medium injected through the pipette is used to dislodge, displace and protrude one or more blastomeres through the first puncture site in the zona pellucida[40,41] (Figure 3a); recently, Roudebush and Dukelow[44] have reported a modification of the "displacement" method where a pressure on the blastomeres together with a change in angulation of a micropipette are used to extrude one or more blastomeres through the zona pellucida;
2. "Stitch and pull:" This method was introduced by Schmutzler et al.[45] for biopsy of the first polar body and cells of cleavage stage embryos; the biopsy is carried out by drilling a hole through the zona with acid Tyrode's solution; the single cells are then pulled out by using stitching movements with a microneedle (Figure 3b). Recently, this technique has been used also at blastocyst stage;[46] several TE cells can be removed

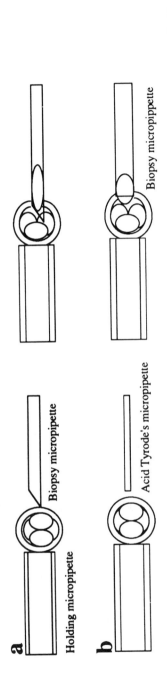

FIGURE 1. Biopsy of a single blastomere from a 4-cell embryo following two different methods of "aspiration": (a) the biopsy micropipette punctures the zona pellucida like a needle; (b) a hole is drilled in the zona pellcida with acid Tyrode's solution before a blastomere is removed by suction with a biopsy micropipette.

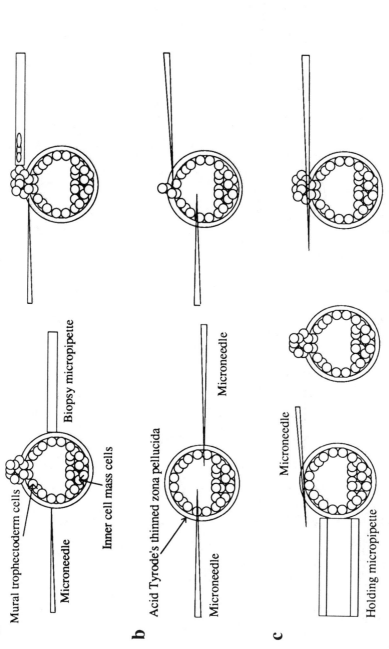

FIGURE 2. Biopsy of mural trophectoderm cells at the blastocyst stage following three different methods: (a) "Aspiration." The blastocyst is manipulated by the microinstruments to extrude a number of cells through the zona pellucida. The micropipette sucks a number of cells away from the trophectoderm cell layer while the microneedle cuts the cell contacts; (b) "Stitch and pull." After zona thinning with acid Tyrode's solution, the blastocyst is held at the abembryonic pole by two glass microneedles. The cells are removed through the zona pellucida by using stitching movements with a microneedle; (c) "Herniation." A slit is made in the zona pellucida opposite the inner cell mass using a microneedle. The embryos are then left in culture for several hours until a definite herniation of trophectoderm cells is visualized. The herniating cells are cut off by rubbing the end of a microneedle across the herniation against the bottom of a dish.

Embryo Biopsy for Preimplantation Diagnosis

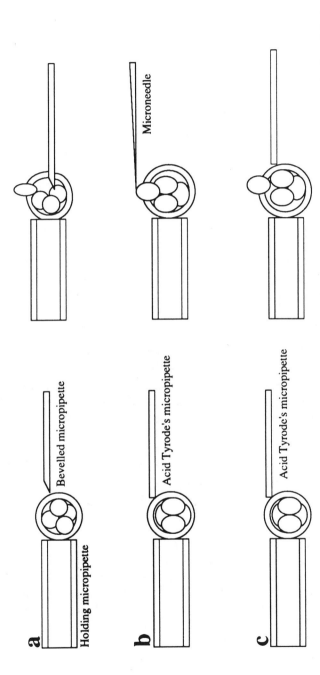

FIGURE 3. Biopsy of a single blastomere from a 4-cell embryo following three different methods of "extrusion": (a) "Displacement." An opening is made in the zona pellucida with a bevelled micropipette. One blastomere is displaced through the first puncture site using a gentle flow of medium injected through a second puncture site; (b) "Stitch and pull." A hole is drilled in the zona pellicida with acid Tyrode's solution. One blastomere is removed using stitching movements with a microneedle; (c) "Push." A hole is drilled in the zona pellucida with acid Tyrode's solution. One blastomere is squeezed through the zona opening by pushing against the zona with a micropipette at some distance from the hole.

through the zona pellucida, which is only partially dissolved with acid Tyrode's solution (Figure 2b);

3. "Push:" In this approach, described by Gordon and Gang,[47] after drilling the zona with acid Tyrode's solution or by mechanical dissection, the first polar body or the blastomeres are extruded through the hole by pushing against the zona with a micropipette at some distance from the hole (Figure 3c).

The "mechanical division" method involves the removal of the zona pellucida by digestion with pronase,[4,48] acid Tyrode's solution,[4,27,48] or by mechanical force (cutting the zona pellucida with a microblade).[3,4,28,48] The blastomeres are separated by aspirating the embryos into a finely drawn pipette. However, unlike the mouse, human embryos without a zona pellucida may divide in culture in a disorganized manner until the late 8-cell stage.[20] Hence, biopsy by "mechanical division" before the 8-cell stage could only be used in humans if the zona-free embryos were replaced in a recipient zona pellucida.

Finally, the "herniation" method is only used for embryo biopsy at the blastocyst stage.[16,17,49] A tear or slit is made in the zona pellucida opposite the ICM (Figure 2c). The embryos are then left in culture for several hours until a definite herniation of TE cells is visualized. The herniating TE cells are cut off with either a scalpel blade[16] or by rubbing the end of a siliconized glass needle across the waist of the herniation against the bottom of a dish.[17,49]

A. COMPARATIVE STUDIES OF DIFFERENT BIOPSY METHODS

A method of embryo biopsy used for preimplantation diagnosis must not have deleterious effects on embryo development *in vitro* and *in vivo*, or on blastomere viability after removal from the zona pellucida. Unfortunately, the majority of papers reporting embryo biopsy are concerned with the capacity of biopsied embryos to develop *in vitro* and/or *in vivo*.[5,7,10,23,29,38,41-43] The efficiency of the biopsy technique in the acquisition of intact viable blastomeres for chromosomal genetic analysis is only reported in a few studies.[40,44,50] Comparative studies between different biopsy methods are also scarce,[4,40,41,48] allowing only tentative conclusions to be made about an optimal method of embryo biopsy.

1. Oocytes in Metaphase II

Biopsy of the first polar body can be performed following the "aspiration," "push," or "stitch and pull" methods. Among these methods, the "stitch and pull" technique offers the lowest prospect of success because of the relatively low rate of embryonic development *in vitro* to the blastocyst stage (50%) reported in the mouse.[45] Although Gordon and Gang[47] did not report on the subsequent development of embryos *in vitro* or *in vivo* after first polar body biopsy using the "push" technique, they showed that this method is safe, rapid, and effective and did not interfere with subsequent *in vitro* fertilization.

In humans "aspiration" of the first polar body after puncturing the zona pellucida with a simple micropipette seems to have no major detrimental effect on fertilization and embryo development.[11]

2. Cleavage Stages

All of the comparative studies between different methods of embryo biopsy have been carried out at cleavage stages.[4,40,41,48]

In the mouse, no significant differences in embryo development *in vitro*[40,41] and *in vivo*[41] was observed after biopsy using the "displacement" and "aspiration" (puncturing the zona pellucida) methods. However, the number of blastomeres that remain viable and intact after biopsy is significantly higher using the "displacement" technique compared with "aspiration," irrespective of the embryo cleavage stage at the time of embryo biopsy.[40] Although confirmation of these results is needed, it seems that, at least in the mouse, the "displacement" approach is a less traumatic technique and is therefore likely to be more appropriate than the "aspiration" (puncturing the zona pellucida) procedure for preimplantation diagnosis.

No comparative study has been reported using the "stitch and pull," "push," and "aspiration" techniques after zona drilling with acid Tyrode's solution. However, it appears that the "stitch and pull" and "push" methods are not detrimental to embryo development to the blastocyst stage *in vitro* in the mouse.[45,47] While Gordon and Gang[47] reported 100% success rate in obtaining at least one intact blastomere for analysis, Schmutzler[51] observed that the "stitch and pull" technique may cause damage to the biopsied cells. Although, cellular lysis may not be a problem for genetic analysis using polymerase chain reaction (PCR),[51] it can be a serious handicap for *in situ* hybridization[43,52] or blastomere karyotyping.[53] Hence, the "stitch and pull" method may have limited value for preimplantation diagnosis.

In humans, exposure of oocytes to acid Tyrode's solution has been shown to be detrimental to oocyte viability[54] and to later preimplantation development.[55] Human embryos at the 4-cell stage also appear to be sensitive to this solution.[7] However, at the 8-cell stage, this technique does not appear to have any significant effects on embryo development to the blastocyst stage *in vitro*[23,42] or on implantation rate *in vivo*.[38] Although these authors[38,42] did not report the percentage of intact viable cells obtained after biopsy, it seems that in humans the "aspiration" technique after zona drilling with acid Tyrode's solution is a relatively innocuous approach for embryo biopsy at the 8-cell stage.

3. Blastocyst Stage

Although no comparative studies between the different methods of blastocyst biopsy have been reported and the implantation rate after biopsy following the "aspiration" method is still less than that of untreated embryos,[15,18] there are several reasons why the "aspiration" and "stitch and pull" techniques may result in a higher success rate than the "herniation" method. First, embryos can be biopsied as soon as the blastocele cavity appears because it is not necessary to wait until a herniation of TE cells occurs spontaneously. This increases the chance of transfer of the embryos without the additional need for embryo cryopreservation. Second, the number of TE cells sampled in human blastocysts following the "herniation" method depends on the time interval between slitting the zona and the biopsy of the herniation. A time interval of 18 to 24 h[17] or 12 to 18 h[56] could be excessive and result in the removal of too many cells. This may reduce embryo viability (as judged by recovery of blastocele),[18] human chorionic gonadotrophin (hCG) production,[56] and the potential for normal implantation and development.[16] Treatment with exogenous gonadotrophin may be required to maintain early pregnancy as reported for biopsied blastocysts of the marmoset monkey.[16] Third, in the mouse,[49] marmoset monkey,[16] and human,[17] only 42 to 59, 20 to 50, and 42 to 76% of the blastocysts herniate in culture after the time of culture established in each study (4, 24 to 48 and 18 to 24 h, respectively). This may limit the number of embryos which may be analyzed, reducing the number of embryos identified as suitable for transfer and the chance of establishing pregnancy.

V. CONCLUSIONS

Animal and human experiments have shown that removal of cells for preimplantation diagnosis of genetic diseases can be performed at various stages between the oocyte in metaphase II and blastocyst. However, biopsy of embryos at the 8-cell stage on day 3 after insemination can be regarded as the most practical at the present time because

1. In contrast to biopsy of the first polar body, a second biopsy analysis is not required for accurate genetic diagnosis and confirmation of previous results;
2. Human embryos on day 2 may be more sensitive than embryos on day 3 after insemination to micromanipulation;
3. Transfer of blastocyst stage human embryos results in a low pregnancy rate.

The limit of cellular mass that can be biopsied without affecting embryo development *in vitro* or *in vivo* in different species appears to be related to the time of blastulation, which is constant within each species and independent of cell number. In humans, this limit may be close to one quarter of the total cellular mass because this removal has no effect on development *in vitro* and *in vivo* if the cleavage rate of biopsied embryos is preserved.

Although only tentative conclusions can be made about an optimal method of embryo biopsy because of the lack of comparative studies, it appears that the "stitch and pull," "aspiration" (puncturing the zona pellucida), "mechanical division," and "herniation" techniques may have a limited value in preimplantation diagnosis because:

1. The "stitch and pull" method may reduce embryo development *in vitro* and damage the biopsied cells;
2. The "aspiration" method (puncturing the zona pellucida) may destroy a relatively large number of blastomeres;
3. The "mechanical division" method requires the removal of the zona pellucida, and in the absence of a zona pellucida human embryos divide in culture in a disorganized manner until late 8-cell stage;
4. The use of the "herniation" approach for TE biopsy at the blastocyst stage may limit the number of embryos for analysis, reducing the number of embryos which are suitable for transfer and the chance of establishing pregnancy.

REFERENCES

1. **Edwards, R. G. and Hollands, P.**, New advances in human embryology: implications of the preimplantation diagnosis of genetic disease, *Hum. Reprod.*, 3, 549, 1988.
2. **Rands, G. F.**, Cell allocation in half- and quadruple-sized preimplantation mouse embryos, *J. Embryol. Exp. Zool.*, 236, 67, 1985.
3. **Lawitts, J. A. and Graves, C. N.**, Viability of mouse half-embryos in vitro and in vivo, *Gamete Res.*, 20, 421, 1988.
4. **Nijs, M., Camus, M., and Van Sterteghem, A. C.**, Evaluation of different biopsy methods of blastomeres from 2-cell mouse embryos, *Hum. Reprod.*, 3, 999, 1988.
5. **Krzyminska, U. B., Lutjen, J., and O'Neill, C.**, Assessment of the viability and pregnancy potential of mouse embryos biopsied at different preimplantation stages of development, *Hum. Reprod.*, 5, 203, 1990.
6. **Loskutoff, N. M., Xu, K. P., and Betteridge, K. J.**, Effect of biopsy on the development of cleavage stage bovine embryos generated in vitro, *J. Reprod. Fertil.*, 7 (Abstr.), 35, 1991.
7. **Tarín, J. J., Conaghan, J., Winston, R. M. L., and Handyside, A. H.**, Human embryo biopsy on the second day post insemination for preimplantation diagnosis: removed of a quarter of embryo retards cleavage, *Fertil. Steril.*, 58, 970, 1992.
8. **Bolton, V. N., Wren, M. E., and Parsons, J. H.**, Pregnancies after in vitro fertilization and transfer of human blastocysts, *Fertil. Steril.*, 55, 830, 1991.
9. **Dawson, K. J., Rutherford, A. J., Winston, N. J., Subak-Sharpe, R., and Winston, R. M. L.**, Human blastocyst transfer, is it a feasible proposition?, *Hum. Reprod.*, 145 (Suppl.), 44, 1988.
10. **Wilton, L. J., Shaw, J. M., and Trounson, A. O.**, Successful single-cell biopsy and cryopreservation of preimplantation mouse embryos, *Fertil. Steril.*, 51, 513, 1989.
11. **Verlinsky, Y., Ginsberg, N., Lifchez, A., Valle, J., Moise, J., and Strom, C. M.**, Analysis of the first polar body: preconception genetic diagnosis, *Hum. Reprod.*, 5, 826, 1990.
12. **Verlinsky, Y., Cieslak, J., Evsikov, S., Milayeva, S., Strom, C., White, M., Lifchez, A., Moise, J., Ginsberg, N., and Applebaum, M.**, Effect of subsequent oocyte and blastomere biopsy on preimplantation development, 7th World Congress on IVF and Assisted Procreations, *Hum. Reprod.*, (Abstr.), 136, 1991.
13. **Gardner, R. L. and Edwards, R. G.**, Control of the sex ratio at full term in the rabbit by transferring sexed blastocysts, *Nature*, 218, 346, 1968.

14. **Whittingham, D. G. and Penketh, R.,** Prenatal diagnosis in the human preimplantation period, *Hum. Reprod.*, 2, 267, 1987.
15. **Monk, M., Muggleton-Harris, A. L., Rawlings, E., and Whittingham, D. G.,** Preimplantation diagnosis of HPRT-deficient male and carrier female mouse embryos by trophectoderm biopsy, *Hum. Reprod.*, 3, 377, 1988.
16. **Summers, P. M., Campbell, J. M., and Miller, M. W.,** Normal in-vivo development of marmoset monkey embryos after trophectoderm biopsy, *Hum. Reprod.*, 3, 389, 1988.
17. **Dokras, A., Sargent, I. L., Ross, C., Gardner, R. L., and Barlow, D. H.,** Trophectoderm biopsy in human blastocysts, *Hum. Reprod.*, 5, 821, 1990.
18. **Gomez, C. M., Muggleton-Harris, A. L., Whittingham, D. G., Hood, L. E., and Readhead, C.,** Rapid preimplantation detection of mutant (shiverer) and normal alleles of the mouse myelin basic protein gene allowing selective implantation and birth of live young, *Proc. Natl. Acad. Sci. U.S.A.*, 87, 4481, 1990.
19. **Monk, M., Handyside, A., Muggleton-Harris, A., and Whittingham, D.,** Preimplantation sexing and diagnosis of hypoxanthine phosphoribosyl transferase deficiency in mice by biochemical microassay, *Am. J. Med. Genet.*, 35, 201, 1990.
20. **Bolton, V. N.,** Embryo biopsy, in *The Embryo. Normal and Abnormal Development and Growth*, Capman, M., Grudzinskas, G., and Chard, T., Eds., Springer-Verlag, London, 1991, 63.
21. **Handyside, A. H. and Delhanty, D. A.,** Cleavage stage biopsy of human embryos and diagnosis of X-linked recessive disease, in *Preimplantation Diagnosis of Human Genetic Disease*, Edwards, R.G., Ed., Cambridge University Press, Cambridge, in press.
22. **Hardy, K., Handyside, A. H., and Winston, R. M. L.,** The human blastocyst: cell number, death and allocation during late preimplantation development in vitro, *Development*, 107, 597, 1989.
23. **Hardy, K., Martin, K. L., Leese, H. J., Winston, R. M. L., and Handyside, A. H.,** Human preimplantation development in vitro is not adversely affected by biopsy at the 8-cell stage, *Hum. Reprod.*, 5, 708, 1990.
24. **Pedersen, R. A.,** Potency, lineage, and allocation in preimplantation mouse embryos, in *Experimental Approaches to Mammalian Embryonic Development*, Rossant, J. and Pederson, R. A., Eds., Cambridge University Press, Cambridge, 1986, 3.
25. **Smith, R. and McLaren, A.,** Factors affecting the time of formation of the mouse blastocoele, *J. Embryol. Exp. Morphol.*, 41, 79, 1977.
26. **Nakagawa, A., Takahashi, Y., and Kanagawa, H.,** Studies on developmental potentials of bisected mouse embryos in vitro and in vivo, *Jpn. J. Vet. Res.*, 33, 121, 1985.
27. **Somers, G. R., Trounson, A. O., and Wilton, L. J.,** Allocation of cells to the inner cell mass and trophectoderm of 3/4 mouse embryos, *Reprod. Fertil. Dev.*, 2, 51, 1990.
28. **Zhouji, W., Trounson, A., and Dziadek, M.,** Developmental capacity of mechanically bisected mouse morulae and blastocysts, *Reprod. Fertil. Dev.*, 2, 683, 1990.
29. **Wilton, L. J. and Trounson, A. O.,** Biopsy of preimplantation mouse embryos: development of micromanipulated embryos and proliferation of single blastomeres in vitro, *Biol. Reprod.*, 40, 145, 1989.
30. **Anderson, G. B.,** Manipulation of the mammalian embryo, *J. Anim. Sci.*, 61 (Suppl. 3), 1, 1985.
31. **McLaren, A.,** Prenatal diagnosis before implantation: opportunities and problems, *Prenatal Diag.*, 5, 85, 1985.
32. **Fehilly, C. and Willadsen, S. M.,** Embryo manipulation in farm animals, *Oxford Rev. Reprod. Biol.*, 8, 379, 1986.
33. **Papaioannou, V. E. and Ebert, K. M.,** Comparative aspects of embryo manipulation in mammals, in *Experimental Approaches to Mammalian Embryonic Development*, Rossant, J. and Pedersen, R. A., Eds., Cambridge University Press, Cambridge, 1986, 67.
34. **Papaioannou, V. E. and Ebert, K. M.,** The preimplantation pig embryo: cell number and allocation to trophectoderm and inner cell mass of the blastocyst in vivo and in vitro, *Development*, 102, 793, 1988.
35. **Handyside, A. H. and Hunter, S.,** Cell division and death in the mouse blastocyst before implantation, *Roux's Arch. Dev. Biol.*, 195, 519, 1986.

36. **Trounson, A. and Mohr, L.,** Human pregnancy following cryopreservation, thawing and transfer of an eight-cell embryo, *Nature,* 305, 707, 1983.
37. **Veiga, A., Calderón, G., Barri, P. N., and Coroleu, B.,** Pregnancy after the replacement of a frozen-thawed embryo with less than 50% intact blastomeres, *Hum. Reprod.,* 2, 321, 1987.
38. **Handyside, A. H., Kontogianni, E. H., Hardy, K., and Winston, R. M. L.,** Pregnancies from biopsied human preimplantation embryos sexed by Y-specific DNA amplification, *Nature,* 344, 768, 1990.
39. **Rossant, J.,** Postimplantation development of blastomeres isolated from 4- and 8-cell mouse eggs, *J. Embryol. Exp. Morphol.,* 36, 283, 1976.
40. **Roudebush, W. E., Kim, J. G., Minhas, B. S., and Dodson, M. G.,** Survival and cell acquisition rates after preimplantation embryo biopsy: use of two mechanical techniques and two mouse strains, *Am. J. Obstet. Gynecol.,* 162, 1084, 1990.
41. **Takeuchi, K., Sandow, B. A., Morsy, M., Kaufmann, R. A., Beebe, S. J., and Hodgen, G. D.,** Pre-clinical models for human pre-embryo biopsy and genetic diagnosis: I. Efficiency and normalcy of mouse pre-embryo development after different biopsy techniques, *Fertil. Steril.,* 57, 425, 1992.
42. **Handyside, A. H., Penketh, R. J. A., Winston, R. M. L., Pattinson, J. K., Delhanty, J. D. A., and Tuddenham, E. G. D.,** Biopsy of human preimplantation embryos and sexing by DNA amplification, *Lancet,* i, 347, 1989.
43. **Grifo, J. A., Boyle, A., Fisher, E., Lavy, G., DeCherney, A. H., Ward, D. C., and Sanyal, M. K.,** Preembryo biopsy and analysis of blastomeres by in situ hybridization, *Am. J. Obstet. Gynecol.,* 163, 2013, 1990.
44. **Roudebush, W. E. and Dukelow, W. R.,** Embryonic biopsy by cell displacement maintains an intact isolated blastomere without disrupting development, *Zool. Sci.,* 8, 323, 1991.
45. **Schmutzler, A. G., Schmutzler, R. K., Krebs, D., and Gordon, J. W.,** Polar body and blastomere biopsy in the mouse, Abstract, 2nd Joint ESCO-ESHRE Meeting, *Hum. Reprod.,* (Abstr.), 1990, 7.
46. **Muggleton-Harris, A. L. and Findlay, I.,** In-vitro studies on "spare" human preimplantation embryos in culture, *Hum. Reprod.,* 6, 85, 1991.
47. **Gordon, J. W. and Gang, I.,** Use of zona drilling for safe and effective biopsy of murine oocytes and embryos, *Biol. Reprod.,* 42, 869, 1990.
48. **Nijs, M. and Van Steirteghem, A. C.,** Assessment of different isolation procedures for blastomeres from two-cell mouse embryos, *Hum. Reprod.,* 2, 421, 1987.
49. **Nijs, M. and Van Steirteghem, A. C.,** Developmental potential of biopsied mouse blastocysts, *J. Exp. Zool.,* 256, 232, 1990.
50. **Kola, I. and Wilton, L.,** Preimplantation embryo biopsy: detection of trisomy in a single cell biopsied from a four-cell mouse embryo, *Mol. Reprod. Dev.,* 29, 16, 1991.
51. **Schmutzler, R. K.,** Current developments in preimplantation genetic analysis, *Foc. Reprod.,* 1, 14, 1991.
52. **Griffin, D. K., Handyside, A. H., Penketh, R. J. A., Winston, R. M. L., and Delhanty, J. D. A.,** Fluorescent in-situ hybridization to interphase nuclei of human preimplantation embryos with X and Y chromosome specific probes, *Hum. Reprod.,* 6, 101, 1991.
53. **Roberts, C., Lutjen, J., Krzyminska, U., and O'Neill, C.,** Cytogenetic analysis of biopsied preimplatantion mouse embryos: implications for prenatal diagnosis, *Hum. Reprod.,* 5, 197, 1990.
54. **Garrisi, G. J., Talansky, B. E., Grunfeld, I., Sapira, V., Navot, D., and Gordon, J. W.,** Clinical evaluation of three approaches to micromanipulation-assisted fertilization, *Fertil. Steril.,* 54, 671, 1990.
55. **Malter, H. E. and Cohen, J.,** Partial zona dissection of the human oocyte: a nontraumatic method using micromanipulation to assist zona pellucida penetration, *Fertil. Steril.,* 51, 139, 1989.
56. **Dokras, A., Sargent, I. L., Gardner, R. L., and Barlow, D. H.,** Human trophectoderm biopsy—morphology and hCG secretion of biopsied blastocysts, *J. Reprod. Fertil.,* 7 (Abstr.), 20, 1991.

Chapter 7

FERTILIZATION USING MICROMANIPULATION TECHNIQUES

Alan Trounson and A. Henry Sathananthan

TABLE OF CONTENTS

I. Introduction 132

II. Techniques Which Disrupt the Zona Pellucida 132

III. Injection of Sperm into the Perivitelline Space 133
    A. The Technique of Microinjecting Sperm into the Perivitelline Space 135
    B. Sperm Quality and Success of Microinjection 138
    C. The Acrosome Reaction of Sperm and Microinjection 139
    D. Fusion of the Sperm and Oocyte after Microinjection 140
    E. Is There an Effective Block to Polyspermy at the Vitelline Membrane? 142

IV. Direct Injection of Sperm into the Ooplasm 143
    A. Injection of Acrosome Defective Sperm into the Oocyte 143
    B. Injection of Immotile Sperm into the Perivitelline Space or Directly into the Oocyte 145

V. Conclusions 147

References 148

I. INTRODUCTION

The severely infertile male who is azoospermic or produces insufficient motile sperm for the insemination of oocytes, even in microdroplets of culture medium under oil, has few prospects for the resolution of his infertility. As semen quality reduces, the proportion of oocytes fertilized by insemination decreases, and in cases of multiple defects of sperm concentration, motility, and morphology, IVF success rates may be severely compromised.[1] Fertilization may also be difficult to achieve with sperm recovered from the epididymis.[1] These problems have raised interest in the possibility of using micromanipulation techniques which would enable the sperm direct access to the oocyte, without the need to pass through the natural glycoprotein barrier which surrounds the oocyte, known as the zona pellucida. The zona has an important function in preventing polyspermic fertilization in many species, including the human. When an acrosome-reacted spermatozoon digests its way through the zona and fuses with the oolemma, the cortical granules which lie close to the oocyte plasma membrane are released into the perivitelline space, hardening the zona and preventing any supernumerary sperm from passing through.[2] While there may be a secondary block to polyspermy operative at the vitelline membrane, this does not always prevent polyspermy, and the insemination of oocytes with perforated zonae can result in a dramatic increase in polyspermy.[3]

Micromanipulation techniques can be broadly classified as (1) those which involve opening the zona to enable direct access of sperm to the oocyte following insemination, (2) the introduction of sperm into the perivitelline space by microinjection techniques, and (3) the injection of a sperm directly into the cytoplasm of the oocyte. These techniques may enable the fertilization of oocytes with low quality sperm or, in the case of microinjection techniques, with very few sperm. In the case of direct cytoplasmic injection of sperm, only a single spermatozoon is required for each oocyte. These new methods are evolving rapidly and represent major advances in the treatment of severe male factor infertility.

II. TECHNIQUES WHICH DISRUPT THE ZONA PELLUCIDA

Gordon and Talansky[4] reported a method for digesting a hole in the zona pellucida of the mouse using acidified culture medium, which enabled the reduction of sperm concentrations for achieving fertilization *in vitro* by a factor of about 100. Despite the disruption of the integrity of the zona, polyspermy was not increased when oocytes were inseminated with diluted sperm. This technique was termed zona drilling. Further use of this technique in human IVF,[3] produced fertilized oocytes (10 of 47 drilled oocytes = 25%), but five oocytes were polyspermic (50%). When compared to zona-intact control oocytes inseminated with sperm from the same patients (25% fertilized), the results were disappointing. Malter and Cohen[5] compared the zona drilling technique with mechanical tearing of the zona using a sharp microneedle inserted through the zona. The mechanical tearing method was termed partial zona dissection (PZD), and the rupture in the zona was achieved by manipulation of the oocyte impaled on a microneedle, against the stationary suction pipette.[5] Polyspermy exceeded 50% in both the PZD and zona drilled oocytes, but more oocytes were monospermic after PZD (24%) than after zona drilling (13%). Blastocysts developed from PZD oocytes, but cleavage did not occur in zona drilled oocytes, raising doubts about the viability of human oocytes exposed to acidified Tyrode's medium. The fertilization rate achieved increased from 33% in control (conventional insemination) oocytes to 68% in PZD oocytes. In a further report by the same group,[6] fertilization rate in control oocytes was 47% and in PZD treated oocytes was 68%. The high rate of fertilization in control oocytes makes it difficult to conclude that severe male factor patients were being treated in these studies. However, pregnancies were obtained after transfer of a mixture of PZD and control oocytes that were fertilized in these studies. It was impossible to determine if the pregnancies were a result of PZD treated oocytes.

It is surprising that zona drilled human oocytes should be so dramatically affected by acid Tyrode's medium, because development of mouse oocytes fertilized after zona drilling appears to be unaffected.[7,8] Garrisi et al.[9] compared zona drilling of human oocytes with acid Tyrode's medium with PZD and a mechanical method of zona perforation after treatment with chymotrypsin. Their patients were genuine male factor cases in which only 4% of oocytes fertilized in the control group. While embryos cleaved after zona drilling with acid Tyrode's medium, their development included a high rate of fragmentation, granulation, and uneven cleavage. Similar problems occurred after treatment of oocytes with chymotrypsin but not with PZD. Interestingly, the fertilization rates for the micromanipulated oocytes were not significantly different among the three methods (18 to 25%). Zona drilling and PZD were also compared by Payne et al.[10] While both techniques appeared to increase fertilization rates (around 30%) from those achieved in previous insemination cycles or those for control oocytes, 24% of zona drilled and 12% of PZD oocytes degenerated after 42 h culture, and no pregnancies were obtained using either technique.

These observations may indicate that PZD is the preferred method of zona perforation for human oocytes and that insemination of oocytes with mechanically torn zonae with sperm from severely infertile male factor patients should improve the prospect of fertilization. It is also possible that the treatment of patients with methylprednisolone (16 mg/d) for four d after oocyte recovery and with another two d of tetracycline (250 mg, four times daily) may improve implantation and development of embryos arising from PZD,[11] although the physiological basis for this remains obscure.

III. INJECTION OF SPERM INTO THE PERIVITELLINE SPACE

The technique for microinjection of sperm into the perivitelline space of the oocyte to achieve fertilization was developed by Metka et al.[12] and Laws-King et al.[13] They showed that human oocytes could be fertilized by bypassing the zona pellucida and that the fertilized oocytes would cleave normally *in vitro*.[13]

TABLE 1
Summary of Results for Sperm Microinjection for 1991 at the Infertility Medical Centre, Melbourne, Involving Patients with Severe Male Factor Infertility

Number of cycles of treatment (number of patients)	111	(83)
Number of mature oocytes microinjected	910	
Number of monospermic fertilized oocytes	187	(21%)
Number of polyspermic fertilized oocytes	61	(7%)
Total fertilized oocytes	248	(27%)
Number of monospermic fertilized which cleaved normally	164	(88%)
Number of embryos transferred (number frozen)	142	(10)
Number of cycles resulting in embryo transfer	66	(60%)
Number of preclinical pregnancies	1	(1.5%)
Number of clinical pregnancies	7	(11%)
Total pregnancies	8	(12%)

Note: Patients who had previously failed conventional IVF on at least two occasions or those with too few sperm for insemination of oocytes in microdroplets.

Data provided by Lacham, O., Fuscaldo, G., and D. Sobieszczuk.

In the mouse, it was shown that oocytes fertilized after microinjection of a spermatozoon into the perivitelline space developed normally to term.[14] These results raised interest in the possibility of using the microinjection technique to improve the prospect of fertilization in severely infertile men.[15] Pregnancy was first reported using this technique for the injection of seven to ten sperm from a severely oligiospermic patient into the perivitelline space of his wife's oocytes.[16] Concerns were raised about the possible increase in chromosomal abnormalities which may result from using low quality sperm from severely infertile men, particularly if the sperm are selected and microinjected into the perivitelline space. In an analysis of karyotypes of oocytes fertilized with low quality sperm using this procedure, Kola et al.[17] were unable to detect any increase in aneuploidy or chromosomal rearrangements.

The microinjection of multiple sperm into the perivitelline space was used by Fishel et al.[18] to achieve fertilization in IVF patients who had failed to fertilize oocytes in previous attempts at IVF. Using a mean of 3.4 sperm for each oocyte, 15% of the microinjected oocytes fertilized, and three pregnancies initiated when the resulting embryos were transferred. The rate of detectable polyspermy was low (4%). When it compared with PZD, Cohen et al.[19] reported that sperm microinjection resulted in a significantly higher fertilization rate (30% compared to 13% for PZD) when 1 to 12 sperm were injected into the perivitelline space. Pregnancies in this study were obtained with a mixture of techniques including conventional insemination, PZD, and microinjection of sperm into the perivitelline space.

Pregnancies have also been reported by ourselves[20,21] and others[22] using sperm microinjection, and the technique is now in routine clinical use in our own IVF program (Table 1). The microinjection technique is a very useful addition to the new reproductive technologies which aid the treatment of severe male factor infertility.

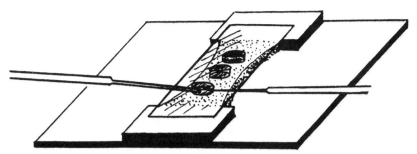

FIGURE 1. Micromanipulation chamber with three droplets of medium containing oocytes, sperm, and a wash drop, surrounded by lightweight paraffin oil. A suction pipette and a microinjection pipette attached to micromanipulators are introduced from opposite directions.

A. THE TECHNIQUE OF MICROINJECTING SPERM INTO THE PERIVITELLINE SPACE

The technique involves a laboratory-made coverslip micromanipulation chamber[14] with dimensions under the coverslip of 30 × 23 × 2 mm. Two or three column drops of about 5 mm diameter are placed in line and surrounded by lightweight paraffin oil (Figure 1). One of the drops contains the sperm preparation, and another contains the oocytes. A wash drop of culture medium (Hepes buffered M2 medium) is sometimes included to ensure that the desired number of sperm are placed in the perivitelline space. The entire chamber is maintained at 37°C on a warming stage. For micromanipulation, oocytes are held stationary on a suction pipette polished by the heated filament of a microforge (de Fonbrune, Beaudouin, Paris, France), leaving an opening of about 15 µm (Figure 2). Pipettes used for injecting sperm are made from thin walled capillaries, reduced by a micropipette puller (David Kopf Instruments, Tujunga, CA, USA) and ground to 45° with an 8 to 12 µm opening using a micropipette grinder (Groschopp Co., Viersen, Germany). The suction and injection pipettes are attached to micromanipulators (Ernst Leitz, Wetzlar, Germany), and manipulation is carried out under inverted microscopy.

Sperm are drawn into the micropipette with a minimum amount of culture medium. When available, motile sperm with apparently normal morphology are chosen for microinjection, and care is taken not to damage the sperm during aspiration into the pipette. Normally one to ten sperm are injected into the perivitelline space,[20] and the number may be titrated against the severity of patients' sperm quality. Larger numbers of sperm have been microinjected into the perivitelline space to increase fertilization rates, but this will also result in increased rates of polyspermy.[20,22] The number of sperm used can be determined in a particular IVF program by the maximum number of two pronucleate oocytes obtained using a range of sperm numbers. Increasing sperm numbers in excess of ten would be akin to using PZD where access to the oocyte cell is only restricted to those which are able to enter the perforated zona. The microinjected sperm frequently move around in the perivitelline space but may also attach to the oocyte vitelline membrane or the inner surface of the zona pellucida. Microinjected oocytes are returned to culture and examined 16 to 20

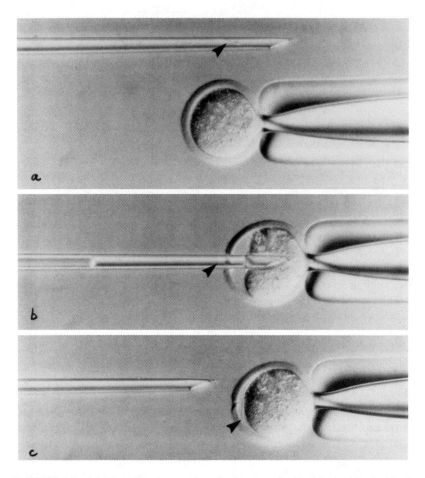

FIGURE 2. Microinjection of a spermatozoon under the zona pellucida: (a) microinjection pipette containing a spermatozoon (indicated by arrow), and an egg to be injected; (b) with the pipette pushing a considerable distance into the egg and with the intact plasma membrane folded around the end of the pipette, the head of the spermatozoon is ejected onto the surface of the plasma membrane. The pipette is then partially retracted while still discharging medium until the sperm tail is ejected; (c) the pipette is then fully retracted, usually leaving the entire sperm under the zona. In some cases, the tail escapes through the hole made in the zona. This probably does not influence whether or not the egg will be fertilized, since 9 out of 20 eggs have been fertilized by a spermatozoon injected with the tail intentionally protruding. Four of these eggs developed to term upon transfer to recipients. Photographs were taken using an immotile sperm and differential interference-contrast optics. The shank of the pipette was bent with a microforge so that the end of the pipette could be raised to touch the under-surface of the coverslip. The end of the injection pipette (o.d. 15 μm) was bevelled and sharpened to facilitate puncture of the zona. Lysis of the plasma membrane after puncture of the zona was infrequent — about 1 in 15 eggs. (From Mann, J. R., *Biol. Reprod.*, 38, 1077–1083, 1988. With permission.)

h later for the formation of pronuclei. Those with multiple pronuclei should be discarded.

Sperm may be treated with a number of capacitation and acrosome reacting agents, and stimulants of motility, prior to microinjection. We have used

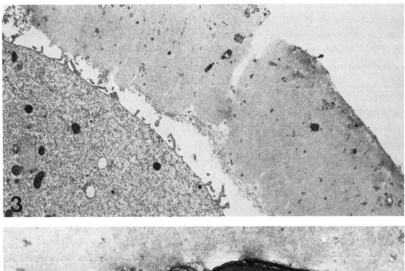

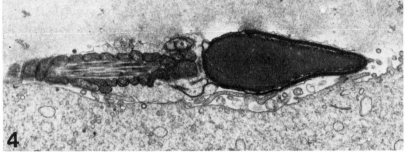

FIGURE 3. Perforation slit through the zona pellucida made by the needle (48 h after microinjection). Egg structure is well preserved. (Original magnification × 9100.) (From Sathananthan, A. H., Ng, S. C., Trounson, A. O., Bongso, A., Laws-King, A., and Ratnam, S. S., *Hum. Reprod.*, 4, 574–583. 1989. With permission.) **FIGURE 4.** Acrosome intact sperm in the perivitelline space of an oocyte after microinjection. Sperm structure is well preserved.(Original magnification × 21,000.) (From Ng, S. C., Bongso, T. A., Sathananthan, A. H., and Ratnam, S. S., *Fertil. Steril.*, 53, 203–219, 1990. With permission.)

follicular fluid, phospholipid (PC12), and incubation with cyclic nucleotides without markedly improving fertilization rates. Treatment of sperm with the motility stimulants 2-deoxyadenosine and pentoxyfilline may improve fertilization rates, but it is very important to remove 2-deoxyadenosine before sperm are microinjected into the perivitelline space. The presence of this drug can induce a block to embryo cleavage. We have shown that the fertilization rate of microinjected oocytes co-incubated with a dilute solution of the sperm used for microinjection is increased when compared with microinjected oocytes cultured without sperm.[20,21] However, definitive methods for sperm treatment which guarantee elevated fertilization rates need to be developed and demonstrated in large-scale clinical studies.

The perforation in the zona pellucida made by the fine microinjection needle (Figure 3) is much finer than that made by PZD or zona drilling. The perforation remains open in unfertilized oocytes examined 72 h after microinjection, but it is unlikely to compromise early embryonic development. Sperm and oocyte structure is normally well preserved after microinjection (Figures 3 and 4), and cortical granules are not released at the time of microinjection.[13,23] Parthenogenetic activation (formation of a single pronucleus) is also a rare occurrence after microinjection.[23]

B. SPERM QUALITY AND SUCCESS OF MICROINJECTION

The initial sperm concentration, motility, and morphology in semen samples have had no major effect on the fertilization rate of microinjected oocytes in our own studies[20] and similar observations have been made by others,[18,24] although in patients with severe teratozoospermia, embryos derived by PZD may have reduced viability.[19] Sperm remaining after microinjection, those in the perivitelline space and in the ooplasm, have been examined for ultrastructural defects.[23] Abnormalities of the sperm head have included bizarre shapes and forms (Figure 5) which affect the acrosome, nucleus, and postacrosomal region. Viable sperm with apparently normal head structure are also found among totally immotile sperm (Figure 6).

Poor quality or immotile sperm invariably have midpiece and tail defects,[25,26] and our recent investigations even show centriolar aberrations in the neck region as well, which might have implications in sperm motility (see below), since the functional proximal centriolar complex is regarded as the kinetic center for flagella motility. However, such defects are also encountered in some sperm from normal semen samples. Nuclear or chromatin aberrations in poor quality sperm also are prevalent in some normal sperm samples; these may cause genetic defects or abnormal development after microinjection, though this has yet to be experimentally confirmed. Indeed, sperm with nuclear defects have been incorporated into ooplasm after microinjection.[23] Further, many abnormal sperm have been located in the perivitelline space[23] (Figure 5), and a few have been observed fusing with the oocyte after microinjection.[27] Fertilization of oocytes by abnormal sperm remains a concern in microinjection because it is not possible to select a "normal" spermatozoon with the light microscope. Nor is it feasible to distinguish between dead and living sperm when the sperm are immotile (Figure 6).[25] Dead sperm often have been seen in the perivitelline space of oocytes after microinjection. Having examined sperm from patients with a high incidence of dead sperm in their semen,[25] it is easy to identify these by electron microscopy after microinjection. Dead or moribund sperm have complex surface membranes, leached acrosomes, and, occasionally, degeneration of the midpiece and tail. Centrioles and axonemal microtubules may also be disorganized. The low rates of fertilization reported for microinjection is usually attributed to the poor quality of sperm, and this usually involves three or more defects of sperm quality.[28] Multiple sperm injection into the perivitelline space has an added advantage in that there could be some natural selection of sperm at the oolemma.

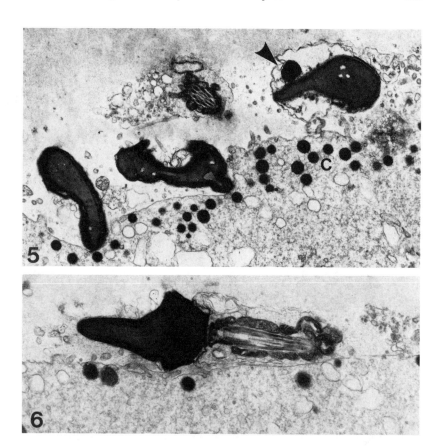

FIGURE 5. Three abnormal sperm microinjected into the perivitelline space of an oocyte. One sperm is undergoing the acrosome reaction (arrow), and the oocyte has not fertilized (C = cortical granules) (Original magnification × 15,400.) (From Ng, S. C., Bongso, T. A., Sathananthan, A. H., and Ratnam, S. S., *Fertil. Steril.*, 53, 203–219, 1990. With permission.)
FIGURE 6. Immotile sperm in the PVS of an oocyte after microinjection. The acrosome is intact and the sperm head looks normal in structure. (Original magnification × 19,600.) (Reproduced from Sathananthan, A. H., Ng, S. C., Bongso, A., and Ratnam, S. S., in *Micromanipulation in Human Reproduction*, Fishel, S. and Symonds, E. M., Eds., Edward Arnold, London, in press. With permission.)

C. THE ACROSOME REACTION OF SPERM AND MICROINJECTION

It is well established that sperm capacitation and the acrosome reaction are important prerequisites for gamete membrane fusion for IVF (see Chapter 13) and for sperm microinjection.[23,29] Human sperm need to be capacitated for 1 to 2 h during sperm preparation to induce the acrosome reaction. Ng et al.[28] have used the Ficoll method for isolating sperm from poor quality semen and a 4 to 6 h capacitation time was used successfully for immotile sperm.[30] Laws-King et al.[13] used Percoll separation combined with a strontium-substituted medium

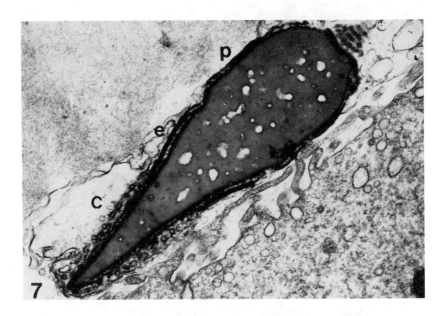

FIGURE 7. Acrosome reacting sperm in the perivitelline space of an oocyte 4 h after microinjection. The acrosome (C) has vesiculated while the equatorial segment (e) is still intact. P = postacrosomal region. (Original magnification × 35,700.) (From Ng, S. C., Bongso, T. A., Sathananthan, A. H., and Ratnam, S. S., *Fertil. Steril.*, 53, 203–219, 1990. With permission.)

to synchronize sperm capacitation for microinjection of single sperm. Although it is desirable to use acrosome-reacted sperm for microinjection, we have shown that the sperm-acrosome reaction can occur in the perivitelline space of oocytes (Figure 7) after microinjection. Such sperm completed the acrosome reaction at the surface of the zona pellucida, which is the usual site where sperm binding and the acrosome reaction occur. Induction of a physiological acrosome reaction with solubilized zonae or the glycoprotein ZP3 needs to be investigated in the human (see Chapter 13). Since the acrosome reaction can also occur in the perivitelline space of microinjected oocytes both in the human[23] and mouse,[31] the inner region of the zona pellucida may be as good a site as its outer surface in the induction of the acrosome reaction.

D. FUSION OF THE SPERM AND OOCYTE AFTER MICROINJECTION

The process of gamete membrane fusion has been observed in two oocytes, but the sperm were grossly abnormal.[27] Evidently, the postacrosomal region of the sperm plasma membrane had fused with the oolemma, as during normal fertilization *in vitro*. This event has been well documented in the mouse.[32] Sperm incorporated into the ooplasm show decondensation of chromatin and vesiculation of the nuclear envelope (Figure 8), while the midpiece remains attached to the spermhead. Even a fertilization cone with superficial

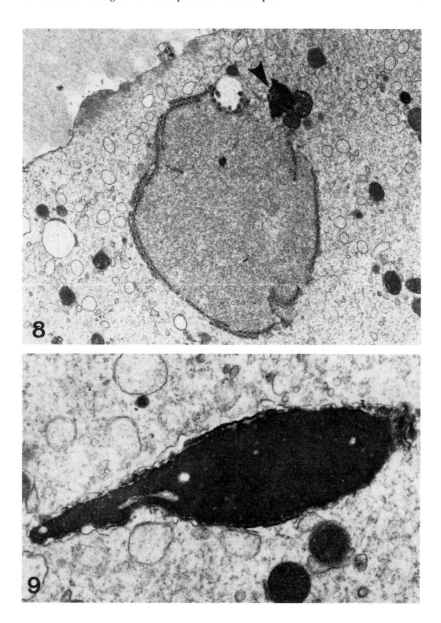

FIGURE 8. Spermhead decondensing chromatin in a fertilized ovum four h after microinjection soon after its incorporation. The centriolar complex (arrow) is evident at the base of the head. (Original magnification × 17,500.) (From Sathananthan, A. H., Ng, S. C., Trounson, A. O., Bongso, A., Laws-King, A., and Ratnam, S. S., *Hum. Reprod.,* 4, 574–583, 1989. With permission.)

FIGURE 9. Sperm incorporated into the ooplasm of a tripronuclear ovum after microinjection. Note partially reacted acrosome and a membrane bound vacuole around spermhead. The chromatin has not decondensed. (Original magnification × 35,700.) (From Sathananthan, A. H., Ng, S. C., Bongso, A., and Ratnam, S. S., in *Micromanipulation in Human Reproduction,* Fishel, S. and Symonds, E. M., Eds., Edward Arnold, London, in press. With permission.)

microfilaments is formed during sperm incorporation, which is a phagocytic response elicited by the oocyte. However, when sperm are microinjected into immature germinal vesicle oocytes or early human embryos,[33] sperm are incorporated into the ooplasm but do not decondense their chromatin (Figure 9). Hence, it is necessary that the oocyte should be mature before microinjection is carried out. However, the majority of microinjected oocytes remain unfertilized. Karyotypes of unfertilized oocytes show that most of them are haploid.[34] Many of these oocytes, examined by electron microscopy 24 to 48 h after microinjection, were aging and showed spindle defects, large conglomerations of cortical granules, and progressive vacuolation of the ooplasm. Poor fertilization results have been reported in postmature or aging oocytes.[13]

E. IS THERE AN EFFECTIVE BLOCK TO POLYSPERMY AT THE VITELLINE MEMBRANE?

Although multiple sperm are commonly injected into the perivitelline space, the majority of oocytes fertilized after microinjection with sperm from genuine male factor patients are monospermic.[18,20,23,27] Monospermic oocytes show two distinct pronuclei (Figure 10), while polyspermic oocytes often have three (Figure 11) or more pronuclei, indicating simultaneous penetration by two or more sperm. Fertilized oocytes also have acrosome-reacted sperm in their perivitelline space, suggesting there may be a vitelline block to polyspermy at the level of the oolemma.

It is clear that cortical granule exocytosis occurs during fertilization by sperm placed in the perivitelline space, and there is incorporation of the cortical granule membrane as well as sperm plasm, a membrane at the moment the sperm fuses with the oocyte, changing the overall nature of the oolemma. A vitelline block to polyspermy also exists in the mouse after microinjection of multiple sperm into the perivitelline space, which seems to be stronger than that observed in the human.[15] In the mouse, polyspermy is a rare occurrence, even when there is a high incidence of acrosome-reacted sperm in the perivitelline space of oocytes after microinjection. Further capacitated sperm injected into the perivitelline space of pronuclear stage oocytes and 2- to 8-cell human embryos do not result in refertilization, although sperm are incorporated into membrane-bound vacuoles within the ooplasm and their spermheads remain unexpanded (Figure 12).[33] A similar situation exists in the mouse. Hence, there is little doubt that a secondary block to polyspermy exists in mouse oocytes, and a weaker block also exists in human oocytes. Microinjection of multiple sperm into the perivitelline space should increase the proportion of normally fertilized human oocytes, as long as the number of sperm is carefully titrated against sperm quality. Simply increasing sperm numbers irrespective of sperm quality will increase the proportion of polyspermic oocytes and may have little effect on the number of normally fertilized oocytes for transfer.[20]

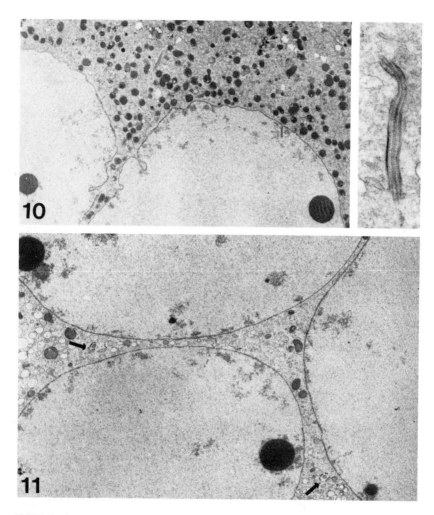

FIGURE 10. Normal bipronuclear ovum obtained after single sperm microinjected into the perivitelline space. × 7000. The sperm tail axoneme (arrow) is enlarged on the side (serial section). (Original magnification × 44,100.) (From Sathananthan, A. H., Ng, S. C., Trounson, A. O., Bongso, A., Laws-King, A., and Ratnam, S. S., *Hum. Reprod.*, 4, 574–583, 1989. With permission.) **FIGURE 11.** Tripronuclear ovum obtained after microinjection of multiple sperm into the perivitelline space. Two sperm tails are found in two different locations (arrows). (Original magnification × 15,400.)

IV. DIRECT INJECTION OF SPERM INTO THE OOPLASM

Mammalian sperm inserted directly into the cytoplasm of oocytes can result in decondensation of the sperm head and formation of pronuclei[35,36] and normal preimplantation embryo development.[37] Acrosome defective human sperm form pronuclei at high rates (90%) when microinjected into hamster oocytes.[38]

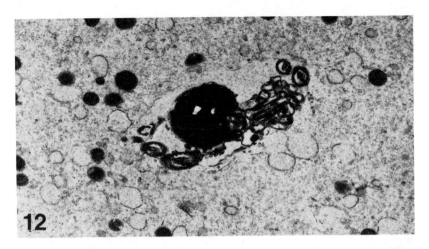

FIGURE 12. Abnormal sperm microinjected directly into the cytoplasm of an oocyte. (Original magnification × 17,500.)

One of the major problems has been a high rate of degeneration of oocytes when pierced by the microinjection pipette, but Lazendorf et al. achieved a high rate of oocyte survival when injecting human sperm into hamster[38] and human oocytes.[39] In their study examining the direct injection of sperm into human oocytes, 6 of 20 oocytes (30%) formed pronuclei and 4 of the 20 oocytes (20%) degenerated.[39] These data have encouraged researchers to reexamine this procedure for the treatment of severe male infertility, and pregnancies have been obtained using the technique.[40]

The cytoplasmic sperm injection technique entails the drawing of very fine pipettes, just large enough to draw in a sperm head and sharp enough to perforate both the zona and the oocyte plasma membrane. Sperm may be immobilized by freezing and thawing in buffered culture medium.[39] This will also damage the sperm head membranes, which may aid decondensation of the injected sperm head in the ooplasm. Sonication has also been used to prepare human sperm for microinjection, but this has resulted in increased structural abnormalities of chromosomes (27%) and multiple breaks and rearrangements (64%) when karyotypes were examined in oocytes directly injected with these sperm.[41] There were fewer chromosomal abnormalities (15%) and multiple breaks and rearrangements (24%) when sperm were stored at 4°C for 1 to 3 d in TEST-yolk buffer, but in zona-denuded oocytes fertilized by freshly collected human sperm, only 11 to 12% structural and numerical abnormalities were observed.[41] These observtions have raised concerns about the direct injection of sperm into oocytes, particularly when sonicated or stored at 4°C.

Not all sperm injected into the cytoplasm decondense and form pronuclei. Some sperm are enclosed in membrane-bound vacuoles (Figure 12). The membrane may be an invagination of the oolemma, and sperm-oocyte membrane fusion may occur in these vacuoles.[23] A few sperm heads may remain unexpanded within the ooplasm even 24 h after injection, and some of these may show stages of acrosome reaction. Abnormal sperm forms (Figure 12) are more prevalent within the ooplasm, since selection of normal sperm is not always possible with light microscopy. Separation of the sperm head and tail may also prejudice embryo development, because the sperm centriole-centrosome complex is inherited by the fertilized ovum and could play a role in early cleavage (see Chapter 13).

Formation of pronuclei and early embryo cleavage have been obtained by direct injection of sperm from severely infertile patients in our own clinical studies,[42] but further work is required to confirm the viability of embryos transferred.

A. INJECTION OF ACROSOME DEFECTIVE SPERM INTO THE OOCYTE

Globozoospermia, or the round-headed sperm syndrome, is a rare condition characterized by sperm lacking acrosomes and post-acrosomal sheaths.[43,44] Such sperm are not able to penetrate the zona pellucida nor to fuse with the oocyte and need to be injected into the ooplasm. However, round-headed sperm have motility characteristics within the normal range.[43] Although they have no acrosomes (Figure 13), an occasional sperm shows a feeble attempt to produce an acrosome within Golgi membranes.[25] Rarely, these sperm have attenuated heads like normal sperm. Round-headed sperm have proximal centrioles and midpieces with mitochondria and axonemes. When injected into the perivitelline space, they do not fuse with the oocyte (Figure 14). Those injected directly into the ooplasm, after demembranation by plunging into liquid nitrogen, also remain unexpanded (Figure 15). This experiment needs to be repeated without demembranation of sperm, since the technique damages sperm surface membranes. Round-headed sperm fail to bind or penetrate the oocyte in the hamster egg-penetration test.[44]

B. INJECTION OF IMMOTILE SPERM INTO THE PERIVITELLINE SPACE OR DIRECTLY INTO THE OOCYTE

Men with Kartegener's Syndrome, a rare clinical condition, produce immotile sperm which will fertilize oocytes after microinjection, resulting in embryonic development.[23,28,30] It was shown in previous studies of fertilization *in vitro* that sperm motility was not essential for sperm-oocyte fusion and sperm incorporation (see Chapter 13), since sperm could be incorporated into the oocyte tail first. Examination by transmission electron microscopy of washed immotile sperm pellets from five patients revealed a population of sperm with normal head structure undergoing various stages of the acrosome reaction.[25] Those examined after microinjection may also complete the acrosome reaction in the perivitelline space. Immotile sperm, however, have a variety of head, midpiece, and tail abnormalities,[25] and some lack dynein arms in their axonemes[26,30] that contribute to their immotility. Since the sperm are merely washed and centrifuged before microinjection, the chance

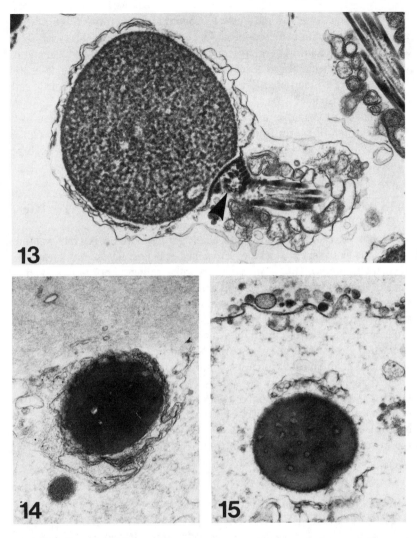

FIGURE 13. Round-headed sperm without an acrosome and postacrosomal segment. The proximal centriole is visible in the neck region (arrow). (Original magnification × 26,250.) **FIGURE 14.** A round-headed sperm microinjected into the PVS of an oocyte. The oocyte was not fertilized. (Original magnification × 25,400.) **FIGURE 15.** Demembranated round-headed sperm injected directly into the ooplasm. The nucleus has not decondensed and the egg has also degenerated. (Original magnification × 23,400.)

of injecting dead or moribund sperm is high. Recent studies have shown that immotile sperm, especially those with stumpy midpieces lacking tails, have a variety of proximal centriolar defects in addition to axonemal tail aberrations.[27] Others lack centrioles, while a few have normal proximal centrioles similar to those of motile sperm. We have to look now at testicular biopsies to determine the development of centriolar derivatives from the two centrioles during spermiogenesis, since the distal centriole is not functional. Surrounding the proximal centriole is an electron-dense centrosomal substance which anchors the two central microtubules of the axoneme; this complex is regarded as the kinetic center of flagellar motility. A few of the immotile sperm from two patients showed wriggling movements with no forward progression. There are ethical concerns regarding the treatment of patients with Kartegener's syndrome, since it is an autosomal recessive genetic condition. No pregnancies have been reported after microinjection of immotile sperm.

V. CONCLUSIONS

Micromanipulation techniques are now providing a new therapy for the treatment of male factor infertility. There has been an evolution of techniques used to treat infertile men from conventional insemination *in vitro* to insemination of oocytes in microvolumes and disruption of the zona pellucida to microinjection techniques. It seems likely that these various options will all be used in the future, depending on the severity of the abnormalities identified in the patient's semen quality and sperm. It is very likely that direct injection of sperm into the ooplasm will be used extensively for patients where very few sperm are available, and probably for patients requiring surgical recovery of epididymal or testicular sperm. It is essential that embryologists working in IVF develop micromanipulation skills as a normal component of their technical capacity.

Pregnancies are being obtained by many IVF clinics using the micromanipulation techniques described in this chapter, and research is continuing to improve the capacity of sperm to fertilize the ooycte. The preferred procedure would be to microinject a single spermatozoon either directly into the ooplasm or into the perivitelline space, in order to control the wastage of oocytes which are polyspermic after micromanipulation. This will require new techniques to ensure that the microinjected spermatazoon is capable of completing the fertilization process. This may mean that that physiological capacitation and acrosome reaction processes need to be bypassed in preparing sperm for microinjection.

The mechanical micromanipulation techniques are likely to be supplemented with or replaced by laser microbeam technology.[46] The laser optical trap can be used to move cells around in a micromanipulation chamber without causing physical damage to the cells. Laser beams can also be used to make small perforations in the zona pellucida and to destroy supernumerary pronuclei. Ultimately, this technology may allow embryo biopsy and DNA amplification using the polymerase chain reaction (PCR) in sealed micromanipulation chambers, and may be used for sperm fertilization techniques considered to be beyond the scope of present mechanical manipulation techniques.

REFERENCES

1. **Trounson, A., Yates, C., Temple-Smith, P., Southwick, G., and Lacham, O.,** The value of IVF for male infertility management, in *Perspectives in Andrology*, Vol. 53, Serio, M., Ed., Serono Symposia Publications, Raven Press, New York, 1989, 421–429.
2. **Sathananthan, A.H. and Trounson, A.O.,** Ultrastructure of cortical granule release and zona interaction in monospermic and polyspermic human ova fertilized *in vitro*, *Gamete Res.*, 6; 225–234, 1982.
3. **Gordon, J. W., Talansky, B. E., Grunfeld, L., Richards, C., Garrisi, G. J., and Laufer, N.,** Fertilization of human oocytes by sperm from infertile males after zona pellucida drilling, *Fertil. Steril.*, 50, 68–73, 1988.
4. **Gordon, J. W. and Talansky, B. E.,** Assisted fertilization by zona drilling: a model for correction of oligospermia, *J. Exp. Zool.*, 239, 347–354, 1986.
5. **Malter, H. E. and Cohen, J.,** Partial zona dissection of the human oocyte: a nontraumatic method using micromanipulation to assist zona pellucida penetration, *Fertil. Steril.*, 51, 139–148, 1989.
6. **Cohen, J., Malter, H., Wright, G., Kort, H., Massey, J., and Mitchell, D.,** Partial zona dissection of human oocytes when failure of zona pellucida penetration is anticipated, *Hum. Reprod.*, 4, 435–442, 1989.
7. **Talansky, B. E. and Gordon, J. W.,** Cleavage characteristics of mouse embryos inseminated and cultured after zona pellucida drilling, *Gamete Res.*, 21, 277–287, 1988.
8. **Depypere, H. T., McLaughlin, K. J., Seamark, R. F., Warnes, G. M., and Matthews, C. D.,** Comparison of zona cutting and zona drilling as techniques for assisted fertilization in the mouse, *J. Reprod. Fertil.*, 84, 204–211, 1988.
9. **Garrisi, G. J., Sapira, V., Talansky, B. E., Navot, D., Grunfeld, L., and Gordon, J. W.,** Clinical evaluation of three approaches to micromanipulation-assisted fertilization, *Fertil. Steril.*, 54, 671–677, 1990.
10. **Payne, D., McLaughlin, K. J., Depypere, H. T., Kirby, C. A., Warnes, G. M., and Matthews, C. D.,** Experience with zona drilling and zona cutting to improve fertilization rates of human oocytes *in vitro*, *Hum. Reprod.*, 6, 423–431, 1991.
11. **Cohen, J., Kort, H., Malter, H., Massey, J., Elsner, C., and Mayer, R. N.,** Immunosuppression supports implantation of zona pellucida dissected human embryos, *Fertil. Steril.*, 53, 622–665, 1990.
12. **Metka, M., Haromy, T., Huber, J., and Schurz, B.,** Artificial insemination using a micromanipulator, *Fertiltät*, 1, 41–44, 1985.
13. **Laws-King, A., Trounson, A., Sathananthan, A. H., and Kola, I.,** Fertilization of human oocytes by microinjection of a single spermatozoon under the zona pellucida, *Fertil. Steril.*, 48, 637–642, 1987.
14. **Mann, J. R.,** Full term development of mouse eggs fertilized by a spermatozoon microinjected under the zona pellucida, *Biol. Reprod.*, 38, 1077–1083, 1988.
15. **Trounson, A., Peura, A., and Lacham, O.,** Fertilization of mouse and human eggs by microinjection of single spermatozoa under the zona pellucida, *J. Reprod. Fertil.*, Suppl. 38, 145–152, 1989.
16. **Ng, S. C., Bongso, A., Sathananthan, A. H., Chan C. L. K., Wong, P. C., Hagglund, L., Anandakumar, C., Wong, Y. C., and Goh, V. H. H.,** Pregnancy after transfer of multiple sperm under the zona, *Lancet*, 2, 790, 1988.
17. **Kola, I., Lacham, O., Jansen, R. P. S., Turner, M., and Trounson, A.,** Chromosomal analysis of human oocytes fertilized by microinjection of spermatozoa into the perivitelline space, *Hum. Reprod.*, 5, 575–577, 1990.
18. **Fishel, S., Johnson, J., Jackson, P., Grossi, S., Antinori, S., and Versaci, C.,** Subzonal insemination for the alleviation of infertility, *Fertil. Steril.*, 54, 828–835, 1990.

19. Cohen, J., Adler, A., Alikani, M., Talansky, B. E., Malter, H. E., and Rosenwaks, Z., Partial zona dissection or subzonal sperm insertion: microsurgical fertilisation alternatives based on evaluation on sperm and embryo morphology, *Fertil. Steril.*, 56, 696–706, 1991.
20. Sakkas, D., Lacham, O., Gianaroli, L., and Trounson, A., Sub-zonal microinjection (SUSM) in cases of severe male factor infertility and repeated IVF failure, *Fertil. Steril.*, 57, 1279, 1992.
21. Lacham, O. and Trounson, A., The need for microinjection in human reproduction, in *Micromanipulation in Human Reproduction,* Fishel, S. and Symonds, E.M., Eds., Edward Arnold, London, in press.
22. Lippi, J., Turner, M., and Jansen, R. P. S., Pregnancies after *in vitro* fertilization by sperm microinjection into the perivitelline space, *Proc. 46th Annu. Meet. Am. Fertil. Soc.,* (Abstr) 529, 1990.
23. Sathananthan, A. H., Ng, S. C., Trounson, A. O., Bongso, A., Laws-King, A., and Ratnam, S. S., Human microinsemination by injection of single or multiple sperm: ultrastructure, *Hum. Reprod.*, 4, 574–583, 1989.
24. Cohen, J., Talansky, B. E., Malter, H. M., Alikani, M., Adler, A., Reing, A., Berkeley, A., Graf, M., Davis, O., Liu, H., Bedford, J. M., and Rosenwaks, Z., Microsurgical fertilization and teratozoospermia, *Hum. Reprod.*, 6, 118–123, 1991.
25. Sathananthan, A. H., Ng, S. C., Ho, J., Tok, V., and Ratnam, S. S., Ultrastructural assessment of human sperm for techniques in assisted reproductive technology, unpublished data.
26. Palmblad, J., Mossberg, B., and Afzelius, B. A., Ultrastructural cellular and clinical features of the immotile cilia syndrome, *Annu. Rev. Med.*, 35, 481–485, 1984.
27. Sathananthan, A. H., Ng., S. C., Bongso, A., and Ratnam, S. S., Sperm microinjection and microfertilization, in *Micromanipulation in Human Reproduction,* Fishel, S. and Symonds, E.M., Eds., Edward Arnold, London, in press.
28. Ng, S. C., Bongso, T. A., Sathananthan, A. H., and Ratnam, S. S., Fertilization by micro-insemination, in *Progress in Obstetrics and Gynaecology,* Studd, J., Ed., 9, 227–244, 1991.
29. Ng, S. C., Bongso, T. A., Sathananthan, A. H., and Ratnam, S. S., Micromanipulation: its relevance to human IVF, *Fertil. Steril.*, 53, 203–219, 1990.
30. Bongso, T. A., Sathananthan, A. H., Wong, P. C., Ratnam, S. S., Anandakumar, C., and Ganatra, S., Human fertilization by microinjection of immotile spermatozoa, *Hum. Reprod.*, 4, 175–179, 1989.
31. Lacham, O., Trounson, A., Holden, C., Mann, J., and Sathananthan, A. H., Fertilization and development of mouse eggs injected under the zona pellucida with single spermatozoa treated to induce the acrosome reaction, *Gamete Res.*, 23, 1–11, 1989.
32. Sathananthan, A. H., Trounson, A., Peura, A., and Lacham, O., Fertilization in the mouse by single or multiple sperm injection: ultrastructure, *Asst. Reprod. Technol./ Androl.*, (Suppl. 3,1–14), 1992.
33. Ng, S. C., Sathananthan, A. H., Bongso, T. A., Ratnam, S. S., Tok, V. C. N., and Ho, J. K. C. Subzonal transfer of multiple sperm (MIST) into early human embryos, *Mol. Reprod. Dev.*, 26, 253–260, 1990.
34. Ng, S. C., Bongso, T. A., and Ratnam, S. S., Microinsemination: genetic aspects, *Arch. Androl.*, 25, 261–270, 1990.
35. Uehara, T. and Yanagimachi, R., Microsurgical injection of spermatozoa into hamster eggs with subsequent transformation of sperm nuclei into male pronuclei, *Biol. Reprod.*, 15, 467–470, 1976.
36. Thadani, V. M., A study of hetero-specific sperm-egg interactions in the rat, mouse and deer mouse using *in vitro* fertilization and sperm injection, *J. Exp. Zool.*, 212, 435–453, 1980.
37. Markert, C. L., Fertilizaion of mammalian eggs by sperm injection, *J. Exp. Zool.*, 228, 195–201, 1983.

38. **Lazendorf, S., Maloney, M., Ackerman, S., Acosta, A., and Hodgen, G. D.**, Fertilizing potential of acrosome-defective sperm following microsurgical injection into eggs, *Gamete Res.*, 19, 329–337, 1988.
39. **Lazendorf, S. E., Slussor, M. S., Maloney, M. K., Hodgen, G. D., Veek, L. L., and Rosenwaks, Z.**, A pre-clinical evaluation of pronuclear formation by microinjection of human spermatozoa into human oocytes, *Fertil. Steril.*, 49, 835–842, 1988.
40. **Van Steirtegham, A.**, personal communication.
41. **Martin, R. H., Ko, E., and Rademaker, A.**, Human sperm chromosome complements after microinjection of hamster eggs, *J. Reprod. Fertil.*, 84, 179–186, 1988.
42. **Lacham, O. and Trounson, A.**, unpublished data.
43. **Aitken, R. J., Kerr, L., Bolton, V., and Hargreave, T.**, Analysis of sperm function in globozoospermia: implications for mechanism of sperm-zona interaction, *Fertil. Steril.*, 54, 701–707, 1990.
44. **La Londe, L., Langlais, J., Antaki, P., Chapdelaine, A., Robers, K.D., and Blean, G.**, Male infertility associated with round-head acrosomeless spermatozoa, *Fertil. Steril.*, 49, 316–321, 1988.
45. **Sathananthan, A. H.**, Inheritance of paternal centrioles and male infertility, *Proc. XIIIth World Cong. Gyn. Obstet.*, Singapore, 1629 (Abstr.), 209, 1991.
46. **Tadir, Y., Wright, W. H., Vafa, O., Liaw, L. H., Asch, R., and Berns, M. W.**, Micromanipulation of gametes using laser microbeams, *Hum. Reprod.*, 6, 1011–1016, 1991.

Chapter 8

GENETIC ANALYSIS OF THE PREIMPLANTATION EMBRYO

Marie Dziadek and Marilyn Bakker

TABLE OF CONTENTS

I. Background 152
   A. Principles of the Polymerase Chain Reaction 152

II. Methods 155
   A. Preparation of Cell Lysates 155
   B. PCR Reaction Mixture 155
   C. Controls 155
   D. Automated PCR 158
   E. Visualization of PCR Products 158

III. One-Step PCR Assay 159
   A. Embryo Sexing 159
   B. Single Gene Detection 161

IV. Two-Step PCR Assay 162
   A. Procedure 162
   B. Sensitivity 162

V. Problem Solving 164
   A. Sample Contamination 164
      1. Preventative Measures 164
   B. Absence of Amplification Product 165
      1. Considerations 165

VI. Diagnostic Assays Using PCR 166
   A. Analysis of Deletions 166
   B. Restriction Digestion of PCR Products 167
   C. Allele-Specific Oligonucleotide Probing 167
   D. Analysis by ARMS 167
   E. Heteroduplex Analysis 168
   F. Direct Sequencing 168
   G. Multiplex Analysis 168

VII. Clinical Application of Preimplantation Genetic Diagnosis 168

References 169

I. BACKGROUND

Approximately 1% of all newborn babies are affected with a severe genetic disease. Advances in recombinant DNA techniques over recent decades have provided a better understanding of the molecular basis of many of these inherited disorders. Prenatal diagnosis of inherited genetic diseases by DNA diagnosis is now available for a large number of human disorders and is increasing annually.[1] Analyses by restriction fragment length polymorphisms (RFLPs) using Southern blotting are now being replaced by diagnostic techniques using the polymerase chain reaction (PCR), due to the greater speed and relative simplicity of this procedure.[2] Prenatal diagnosis by RFLP analysis is not routinely feasible with less than 10^5 to 10^6 cells and can take 10 d to complete, while PCR techniques can be done on much smaller samples and, as shown in this chapter, are feasible with one or a few cells removed from preimplantation embryos. Genetic diagnosis using PCR can be done on blastomeres isolated from 4- or 8-cell embryos, or from trophoblast cells biopsied at the blastocyst stage of development (see Chapter 6). Diagnostic techniques using PCR for gene amplification can be achieved in 5 to 8 h, making this procedure particularly applicable to analysis of preimplantation embryos.

Genetic diagnosis of preimplantation embryos is potentially feasible for all disorders where a PCR assay can be developed. The number of human genetic diseases that can be diagnosed by PCR-based analyses is now close to 50 (Table 1). However, modification of the existing techniques to allow analysis of a single diploid genome presents problems which are not encountered when higher cell numbers are used (e.g., after chorionic villus sampling). Extremely stringent sterile laboratory conditions are required to prevent sample contamination, and specific controls are necessary to demonstrate the accuracy of the gene amplification reaction.

The major application of this technique is for the diagnosis of single gene defects. However, diagnosis of embryo sex is also possible using these procedures; this application can aid in identification of male embryos affected by an X-linked disorder for which no DNA diagnostic tests are yet available (e.g., X-linked mental retardation syndromes).

A. PRINCIPLES OF THE POLYMERASE CHAIN REACTION

The polymerase chain reaction is based on the enzymatic amplification of a DNA sequence flanked by two primers which hybridize to opposite strands

TABLE 1
List of Human Genetic Diseases for Which a PCR-Based Diagnosis Has Been Developed

Acute intermittent porphyria (AIP)	Hereditary fructose intolerance
Adenosine deaminase (ADA) deficiency	Hereditary persistence of fetal hemoglobin (HPFH)
Amyloidotic polyneuropathy	
Antithrombin III (ATIII) deficiency	Hypoxanthine phosphoribosyl-transferase (HPRT) deficiency
ApoC deficiency	
ApoB deficiency	Hypophosphatasia
ApoE deficiency	Insulin resistance type A
Becker muscular dystrophy (BMD)	Laron dwarfism
C1 inhibitor deficiency	Lesch-Nyhan syndrome
Cystic fibrosis (CF)	Leukocyte adhesion deficiency
Duchenne muscular dystrophy (DMD)	Maple syrup urine disease
Dysfibrinogenemia	Non-insulin-dependent diabetes mellitus (type II diabetes)
Ehlers-Danlos syndrome IV	
Ehlers-Danlos syndrome VII	Osteogenesis imperfecta
Elliptocytosis	Ornithine transcarbamylase (OTC) deficiency
Encephalomyopathy, mitochondrial	
Fabry disease	Phenylketonuria (PKU)
Familial hypercholesterolemia	Protolipid protein deficiency
Glucose-6-phosphate dehydrogenase (G6PD) deficiency	Retinoblastoma
	Sandhoff disease
Gaucher's disease	Sickle cell anemia
Gerstmann-Straussler syndrome	Spondyloepiphyseal dysplasia
Gyrate atrophy	Tay-Sachs disease
Hemophilia A (F8C deficiency)	Thalassemia beta (HBB)
Hemophilia B (F9 deficiency)	Thalassemia delta (HBD)
Heparin cofactor II deficiency	von Villebrand disease type IIA

From Reiss, J. and Cooper, D. N., *Hum. Genet.*, 85, 1, 1990.

of the target sequence. The most important requirement for the establishment of a PCR diagnostic assay is knowledge of the nucleotide sequence which distinguishes the specific mutation from the normal DNA sequence. Oligonucleotide primers (usually 20 base pairs in length) are synthesized; these are complementary to sequences on either side of the mutation and usually separated by 150 to 600 bp (Figure 1a). Primer sequences similar in their AT/GC ratio are chosen for the PCR reaction, since annealing conditions are likely to be the same. The simple formula $(n_{A/T} \times 2°C) + (n_{G/C} \times 4°C)$ gives a reasonable estimate of the melting temperature of oligonucleotide primers which are 20 bp in length. However, the melting temperature of primer:DNA hybrids is also affected by the actual nucleotide sequence, and a specific formula has been developed to give a more accurate estimate of the annealing temperature than the nucleotide composition alone.[3] Our own experience suggests that these formulae are only useful in providing a rough guide in the choice of primers, and that the actual melting temperatures can only be determined empirically.

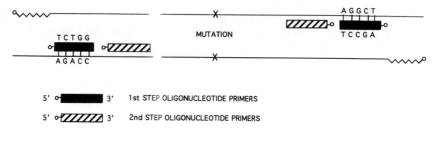

FIGURE 1. (A) Diagram showing the position of oligonucleotide primers designed to bind to each DNA strand on either side of the mutation site. "Nested" primers used in the second step are designed to bind internally to the first step oligonucleotide primers.

Each PCR cycle involves three phases which operate at different temperatures (Figure 1b):

1. Separation of the double-stranded DNA template by denaturation at 95°C;
2. Annealing of oligonucleotide primers to complementary sequences on the DNA template at a temperature between 50 and 65°C, depending on the melting temperature of the primer:DNA hybrid;
3. Replication of a new DNA strand in a 5' to 3' direction from the bound primers takes place at a temperature optimal for the DNA polymerase (about 72°C).

Repeated cycles result in the amplification of the DNA segment defined by the 5' ends of the PCR primers. The extension product of each primer in a given cycle serves as the template for the second primer in the next cycle, resulting in an exponential accumulation of the specific target fragment. Theoretically, each PCR cycle results in the duplication of existing sequence copies, and thus, after 20 cycles, 10^6 copies are expected from a single genome. However, the PCR reaction is not necessarily 100% efficient in each cycle, and some studies indicate efficiencies of around 70% in particular reactions.[4,5]

In initial studies, enzymatic DNA synthesis was performed using the Klenow fragment of *Escherichia coli* DNA polymerase I.[5] The thermal instability of the Klenow fragment required the addition of fresh enzyme after each denaturation cycle. The discovery of a heat-stable DNA polymerase from the *Thermus aquaticus* thermophilic bacterium (Taq polymerase) allowed the development of automated PCR with no addition of enzyme in each cycle.[6] The higher optimal temperature for the Taq polymerase (72°C) compared to the Klenow fragment (37°C) significantly improved the specificity of amplification, since only genomic sequences precisely complementary to the oligonucleotide primers form stable complexes at the higher temperature.

II. METHODS

A. PREPARATION OF CELL LYSATES

All handling of cells is done in a UV sterilized biohazard cabinet. After biopsy of preimplantation embryos, cells are collected by mouth pipette and rinsed in phosphate buffered saline (PBS) (1 drop) containing 25 ng/µl salmon sperm DNA. Cells are then placed in 1 µl of 200 µg/ml proteinase K in 1× PCR buffer which is overlaid with approximately 30 µl light paraffin oil to prevent evaporation. After incubation at 58°C for 1 h the enzyme is inactivated by denaturation at 93.5°C for 10 min. The PCR reaction mix can then be added directly to each tube.

B. PCR REACTION MIXTURE

The reaction mixture is made up as a stock solution which is aliquoted and frozen at −20°C. This solution appears to be unaffected by two to three cycles of freeze-thawing. The stock solution is tested for possible DNA contamination during preparation before use in diagnostic assays by running PCR cycles without addition of cell lysates or DNA. Stock solutions which generate a PCR product are immediately discarded. The reaction mixture contains the following ingredients (allowing for 10% dilution by DNA sample):

67 mM Tris-HCl pH 8.8 (at 25°C)
16.6 mM $(NH_4)_2SO_4$
0.45% Triton X-100
200 µg/ml gelatin
2.5 mM $MgCl_2$
200 µM each of dATP, dCTP, dGTP, dTTP
3 µg/ml of each oligonucleotide primer (20 mer)
50 units/ml Taq polymerase

The reaction mixture is added to the tubes containing DNA or cell samples (usually 2 µl cell lysate or DNA preparation), by pipetting 18 µl under the layer of paraffin oil. The activity of the Taq polymerase may vary somewhat between batches, and so it is useful to titrate the enzyme against a minimal amount of DNA template (e.g., 5 ng) to determine the optimal amount to be used for maximal amplification. While 2.5 mM $MgCl_2$ is optimal for most reactions, the $MgCl_2$ should be titrated for each primer pair. The concentration required can be affected by the method of template preparation, as, for example, if the DNA sample is redissolved in buffer containing EDTA.

C. CONTROLS

Three negative solution controls are included in each PCR assay performed to eliminate the possibility of false diagnosis due to sample contamination. These include:

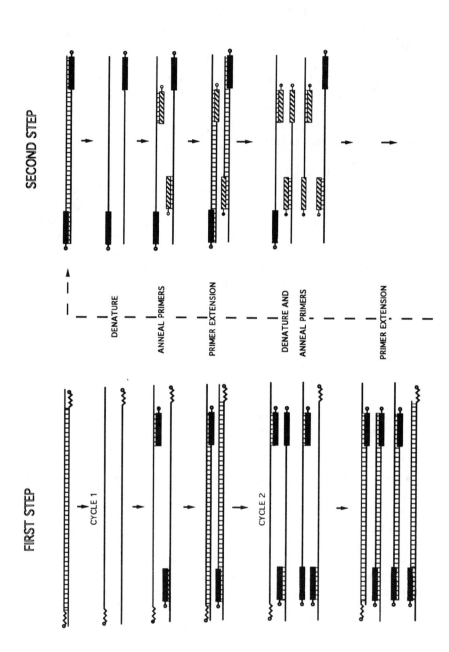

Genetic Analysis of the Preimplantation Embryo

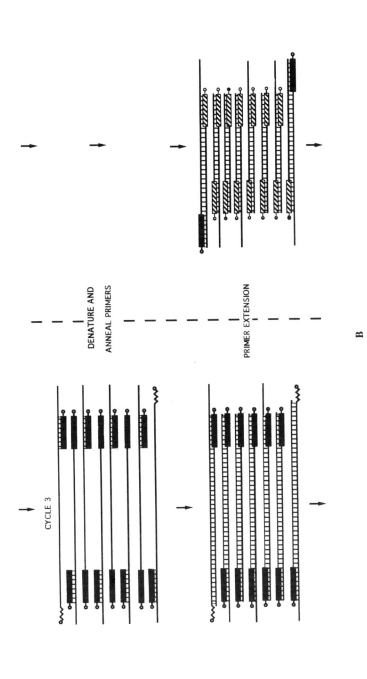

FIGURE 1. (B) Diagram showing the sequence of DNA denaturation, annealing of primers, and primer extension during successive cycles of the polymerase chain reaction. In the second step or "nested" reaction, the amplification product is smaller than in the first.

1. an aliquot of embryo culture medium used during embryo biopsy, which is added to the Proteinase K under oil
2. an aliquot of PBS + salmon sperm DNA, which is used for cell collection
3. a sterile H_2O sample to control for aerosol contamination during sample preparation

A positive control is also included in each assay (50 ng purified DNA) to ensure that all components necessary for the reaction were indeed present and active.

D. AUTOMATED PCR

The PCR machine used in our laboratory is one of Australian design and manufacture (Innovonics, Melbourne, Australia), which consists of three water baths through which the samples are transferred by means of a robotic arm. This system provides an extremely rapid temperature change and enables 48 samples to be completed in less than 2 h. An analysis of the performance of various different thermocycling machines has recently been published.[7] We have optimized the PCR cycle on our machine to be

1. 60 sec denaturation at 93.5°C
2. 60 sec annealing at 55 to 66°C (depending on primers)
3. 60 sec extension at 72°C (depending on the product length; $\leq$ 500 bp for 60 sec and 1.0 kb for 90 sec)

The actual annealing temperature used in a particular assay is optimized by trial and error. The approximate melting temperature is calculated from the AT/GC content of the primers (see above) or from the formula from Rychlik et al.[3] and the optimal annealing temperature is usually 3 to 4°C below the calculated melting temperature. However, it is generally useful to test a range of temperatures around the theoretical melting temperature for each set of oligonucleotide primers used. Non-specific fragments which are sometimes amplified can be eliminated by increasing the annealing temperature by a few degrees without affecting the amplification of specific fragments.

Our analyses have indicated that 35 cycles of PCR are optimal in a one-step assay, and an additional 35 cycles are optimal for the two-step assay. Increasing the number of cycles beyond this does not appear to increase the amount of specific product, but increases non-specific amplification signals which can interfere with visualization of specific products (Figure 4).

E. VISUALIZATION OF PCR PRODUCTS

An aliquot (usually 15 μl) of the PCR product is analyzed by gel electrophoresis using Nusieve (FMC) Agarose. Amplified products larger than 400 bp are optimally separated on 1% gels, while 2% gels are used for products less than 400 bp. Ethidium bromide (0.3 μg/ml) is added to the agarose prior to casting the gel. After electrophoresis in TAE buffer for 1 h at 70 volts, the separated bands are visualized under UV illumination for an immediate diagnosis.

The amplified products can also be transferred to membrane filters for analysis by Southern blotting. In this case, either a 1:1 mixture of Nusieve agarose and conventional molecular biology grade agarose or a straight conventional agarose gel should be used for electrophoresis, since, in our experience, DNA does not transfer efficiently from Nusieve Agarose. Oligonucleotide primers used for PCR amplification cannot be used for probing the filters, as these will hybridize to all PCR products generated, including non-specific products. Oligonucleotide probes which bind to an internal sequence are 5' end-labeled for hybridization. The specific techniques used for diagnosis after or during PCR amplification are described in a later section of this chapter.

III. ONE-STEP PCR ASSAY

A. EMBRYO SEXING

Male cells can be identified by the presence of a highly repetitive sequence (DYZ1) on the long arm of the Y chromosome (500 to 8,000 copies).[8] Amplification of this repeated sequence is equivalent to amplification of a single gene from at least 500 cells, and is readily visualized after a single-step PCR assay. Amplification of a 149 bp fragment from this repeated Y chromosome sequence has already been used successfully for determining the sex of preimplantation human embryos after IVF.[9] We have used oligonucleotide primers, which amplify sequences within each repeated unit (Table 2), rather than those used by Handyside et al.[9] which amplify across adjacent units. Our PCR assay amplifies a fragment of 395 bp and appears to produce a higher intensity signal than observed in previous reports. An amplified product is readily visualized after 35 cycles of PCR using 10 pg of template DNA (Figure 2), and assays using dilutions of male and female DNA have been 100% accurate in determining sex. However, for clinical application, it is important to be absolutely certain that absence of amplification is diagnostic of a female embryo rather than due to a technical failure of the reaction, since non-amplified embryos are selected for transfer. When an alpha-satellite repetitive sequence on the X chromosome[10] (Table 2) is included as a positive control, there is a significant loss in sensitivity of the positive control amplification when the two pairs of primers are used simultaneously in the reaction (Figure 2). Primers used to amplify the DYZ1 repeated sequence also interfered with amplification of several other control sequences. An alternative assay using primers to amplify centromeric alpha-satellite repeated sequences on the Y chromosome[10] was less sensitive than the DYZ1 amplification, but only minimally affected X chromosome control primers in the same reaction (Figure 2).

Female patients who choose preimplantation embryo sexing should be tested for the absence of Y chromosome sequences in their own DNA. In very rare cases, translocation of the long arm of the Y chromosome onto the X or other chromosomes is seen in women, which will obviously interfere with the sexing assay. In these cases, amplification of centromeric alpha-satellite repeated sequences on the Y chromosome[10] should be used for embryo sexing, since these sequences are not translocated.

TABLE 2
Oligonucleotide Primers and Conditions Used for PCR Assays Described in This Chapter

Gene/Chromosome	Reference	Oligonucleotide primer sequence (5'-3')	Optimal annealing temperature	Optimal ($MgCl_2$)	Size of amplified product
Human Y-chromosome (DYZ1 locus)	8	HY1: CTCTATCTGAGTGATTTTATTGCA HY2: TGTACTGGAAAGGACTCGAATTTCA	52–64°C	2.5 mM	395 bp
Human Y-chromosome (DYZ3 locus)	10	Y-A: TGAAAACTACACAGAAGCTG Y-B: ACACATCACAAAGAACTATG	56°C	3.75 mM	1.0 kb
Human X alpha satellite (DXY1 locus)	10	X-3A: ATAATTTTCCCATAACTAAACACA X-4A: TGTGAAGATAAAGGAAAAGGCTT	55°C	3.75 mM	500 bp
Human 18s ribosomal	35	R1: AATACATGCCACGGGCGCT R2: CCCGCTCCCAAGATCCAACT	66°C	3.75 mM	528 bp
Mouse Mov-13 locus:	36	coll A: TCAGCTTTGTGGACCTCCGG coll B: GACCCCTCTATACAGAACGC	58°C	5 mM	A-B: 135 bp A-M: 283 bp
	37	MMuLV: CTTCTGCTCCCCGAGCTCAA	58°C	2.5 mM	367 bp
Mouse adult α-globin:	38	Hbα1A: AAGAAGGTCGCCGATGCGCT Hbα1B: AGGTCAGCACGGTGCTCACA			
nested:		Hbα2A: CGGTGCCTTGTCTGCTGA Hbα2B: TCCAGAGAGGCATGTACCGC	58°C	2.5 mM	280 bp
Mouse β-actin:	39	βAc1A: GCAAGAGAGGTATCCTGACC βAc1B: CTCCTGCTCGAAGTCTAGAG	58°C	2.5 mM	499 bp
nested:		βAc2A: CACGCACGATTTCCCTCTCA βAc2B: CTACAATGAGCTGCGTGTGG	58°C	2.5 mM	361 bp

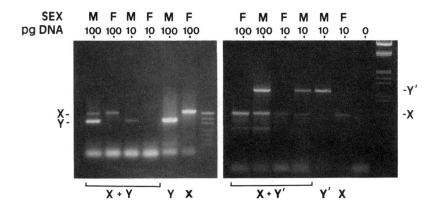

FIGURE 2. Amplification of human Y-chromosome specific sequences using primers to amplify a 395 bp fragment of the DYZ1 locus (Y) or a 1.0 kb fragment of the DYZ3 locus (Y'). Amplification of a 500 bp fragment of the DXZ1 centromeric locus on the X chromosome (X) is included as a positive control. The signal obtained after amplification of 100 pg of male (M) or female (F) DNA is much stronger when the DYZ1 and DXZ1 primers are used individually than when combined in the same reaction (compare lanes 1 and 2 with lanes 5 and 6 in the first panel). When 10 pg of DNA is used, no X-chromosome signal is visualized. In contrast, the DYZ3 primers do not significantly interfere with amplification of the DXZ1 locus, and both X and Y' signals are seen when 10 pg of DNA is used as the template (shown in the second panel). A no DNA control is shown in the last lane. Molecular weight markers are HpaII digested pUC19 in panel 1 and EcoRI/HindIII digested lambda phage in panel 2.

B. SINGLE GENE DETECTION

Our initial studies were done with the Mov-13 mouse mutation, in which a single copy of the murine Moloney leukemia virus has inserted into the collagen α1(I) gene.[11] A PCR assay using three primers was set up to distinguish the three genotypes (Table 2) in cultured cell lines[12] and to determine the minimum cell numbers required for accurate diagnosis using a one-step PCR assay. Our results showed that 100% accuracy in diagnosis could be achieved with 50-cell aliquots, which reduced slightly to 92% when 10-cell aliquots were used (Figure 3). The sensitivity was not improved by either increasing the number of PCR cycles beyond 40, or by adding additional enzyme. A similar result was obtained when primers were used to amplify the α-globin genes, indicating that a one-step PCR assay is only applicable for diagnosis of single gene disorders when DNA from 50 or more cells is available for amplification. In contrast to these studies, Li et al.[4] have shown that the β-globin gene can be amplified from single human cells in 84% of samples, and the low density lipoprotein receptor gene in 55% of samples containing single sperm, using 50 cycles of PCR. In these studies, the amplified products were visualized after dot blotting onto nylon membranes and hybridization with radioactively labelled allele-specific oligonucleotide probes. A simpler and faster alternative to this hybridization step is the two-step PCR assay.

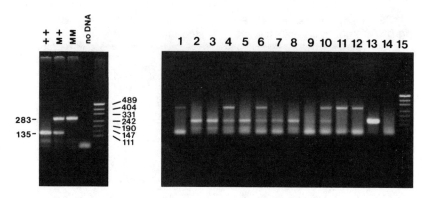

FIGURE 3. Amplification of 0.5 µg DNA from wild type (++), heterozygous (M+) and homozygous (MM) Mov13 cell lines using three oligonucleotide primers (Table 2) in a one-step PCR assay to amplify fragments of 135 and 283 bp. Size markers from HpaII digested pUC19 are indicated. One-step amplification of 12 randomly selected, coded 10-cell aliquots from the three cell lines are shown in the second panel. Actual genotypes are: (++) in lanes 2,3,5,7; (M+) in lanes 4,6,9,10; (MM) in lanes 1,11,12. Only the sample in lane 9 could not be diagnosed. Lanes 13 and 14 show amplification of a positive wild type control, and a no DNA control, respectively. pUC19 molecular weight markers are shown in lane 15.

IV. TWO-STEP PCR ASSAY

A. PROCEDURE

In a two-step PCR assay, the amplified product from the first step is used as a template for another round of PCR using a second pair of oligonucleotide primers internal to the first pair (frequently called "nested" primers) (Figure 1a). Thus, a slightly smaller PCR product is produced after the second round (Figures 1b, and 4). An aliquot from the first reaction (2 µl) is added to a new reaction mix, and another 35 cycles of PCR are performed exactly as for the first step. This second step increases the time of the total assay by up to two h but need not affect the type of diagnostic procedure which is used for a particular gene disorder.

B. SENSITIVITY

We have used the mouse α-thalassemia mutation to establish the two-step PCR reaction on single mouse embryos and biopsied blastomeres, using one set of four primers to amplify the adult α-globin genes and another set of four primers to amplify a control gene, in this case the β-actin gene (Figure 4). Initial studies were done on embryos from a normal mouse strain to determine the sensitivity of the two-step amplification. We observed an amplification signal in only 75 to 90% of samples and found that both the α-globin and β-actin genes did not always amplify in these control embryonic cells. In the majority of cases (20 to 40%) this was due to lack of amplification of the β-actin gene rather than the α-globin gene (1 to 2%), possibly due to the presence of two adult α-globin genes. Absence of amplification may be

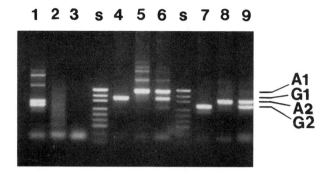

FIGURE 4. Amplification of sequences from the mouse adult α-globin gene (G) and mouse β-actin gene (A) using one-step or two-step reactions. Lane 1 shows amplification signals (A2, G2) from 100 pg mouse DNA after 35 cycles of PCR in each step of a two-step reaction. 70 cycles of PCR in a one-step reaction produced a smear of non-specific bands (lane 2), while no signal was detected after 35 cycles (lane 3). The amplification products from each step of a two-step reaction are shown for each primer pair used individually (lanes 4, 5 and 7, 8) or in combination (lanes 6 and 9). The amplification products from the second step (A2, G2) are clearly smaller than those from the first step (A1, G1). Molecular weight markers (HpaII digested pUC19) are shown (lanes s).

partly due to interference between two different primer pairs in one reaction mix, as was observed in PCR assay to sex embryos (see section above). However, in assays where primers for β-actin amplification were omitted, the α-globin gene was still not amplified in about 25% of cases when control embryos were used. A similar proportion (17%) of unamplified samples was also found in a study to detect the β-globin gene using a two-step PCR assay.[13] The reason for failure of amplification is not clear, but the data indicate some differences in the accessibility or stability of different DNA sequences in the original sample.

Our analysis of embryos from matings of heterozygous α-thalassemic mice has shown the expected 20 to 30% homozygous embryos in which the β-globin genes are deleted (negative for α-globin and positive for β-actin) (Hendrey and Bakker, unpublished). Thus, several studies including our own have demonstrated that an accurate genetic analysis of single cells biopsied from preimplantation embryos is feasible in the majority of cases. Further work is required to modify the procedures to achieve a 100% success rate in amplification and thus to allow diagnosis of all embryos which are biopsied. Since it may be impossible to achieve 100% accuracy using single cells for diagnosis, the preferred approach is to do a duplicate analysis from each embryo after the removal of two separate blastomeres at the 8-cell stage, and, in addition, to increase the amount of DNA for the PCR assay by allowing the blastomeres to undergo a few cell divisions in culture (see Chapter 6). An additional cell culture step would require embryo freezing prior to transfer. To apply these techniques to genetic diagnosis of human preimplantation embryos as a clinical procedure, the following criteria need to be met in each laboratory planning to offer this service:

1. Sensitivity: amplification of DNA must occur in close to 100% of samples;
2. Reliability: amplification of contaminating DNA must be excluded, and appropriate controls for contamination need to be included in each assay;
3. Accuracy: accuracy of the diagnosis must be controlled for by positive and negative control reactions in each assay.

V. PROBLEM SOLVING

A. SAMPLE CONTAMINATION

The potential for contamination of samples is of major concern in genetic diagnosis from single cells, since these techniques have been established specifically to amplify sequences from single gene copies. Contamination has been found to occur in most laboratories where PCR work is done, including our own. Sources of contamination can include deposition of human cells on tubes and pipettes used for sample preparation through handling or by aerosols, as well as transfer of DNA fragments amplified in previous reactions.

1. Preventative Measures

a. Separate pipettors should be kept solely for pre-PCR use and must be decontaminated by treatment with 0.25 M HCl and then 0.25 M NaOH prior to use;
b. The pre-PCR equipment and work area (including freezers) should be kept physically separate from the equipment and area used to amplify DNA and analyze PCR products;
c. All pre-PCR sample handling should be done in a biohazard hood with sterile gloves and using sterilized plasticware;
d. A stock PCR reaction mix should be pretested for contamination and then aliquoted for use;
e. Three negative solution controls should always be included in each PCR assay, as described in the Methods section;
f. Treatment of reaction mixtures with UV-irradiation,[14] DNase I or restriction enzymes[15] or other decontamination tricks are not useful when single cells are being analyzed unless 100% effectiveness can be guaranteed. The additional handling of reagents may increase the risk of contamination rather than be effective in decontamination.

The only effective way to prevent contamination is to use strictly sterile laboratory procedures at all stages prior to amplification. The ideal situation is to have two quite separate laboratories which are dedicated to single cell gene amplification, one for all pre-PCR sample preparation and the second for PCR amplification, electrophoresis, and analysis.

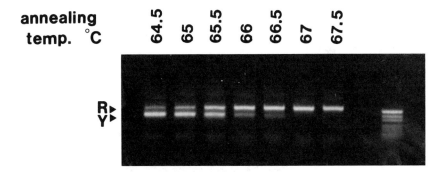

FIGURE 5. Effect of the annealing temperature on the amplification signal when two pairs of primers are used in the same reaction to amplify human 18s ribosomal sequences (R) and the human Y chromosome DYZ1 locus sequences (Y). 10 ng of human male DNA were amplified in each reaction, using a $MgCl_2$ concentration of 2.5 mM. In this experiment 65.5°C was the best compromise when these two pairs of primers were used in combination.

B. ABSENCE OF AMPLIFICATION PRODUCT

Absence of PCR amplification can be due to suboptimal reaction conditions or to deterioration of template DNA before the reaction is initiated. Optimal conditions for the particular assay (i.e., each primer pair used) should be established in the first instance since optimal PCR conditions vary considerably for different primer pairs.

1. Considerations

a. The amount of enzyme in the reaction may not be sufficient. Each new batch of Taq polymerase should be pretested for its activity and the amount used in each reaction altered accordingly;

b. Our studies have shown that the annealing temperature used is critical in determining the sensitivity of the reaction, and that different primer pairs behave quite differently at different temperatures irrespective of their estimated melting temperatures. A temperature difference of 0.5°C can have a significant effect on the degree of amplification depending on the primers used (Figure 5). It is probably important to choose primer pairs which have similar annealing temperatures determined empirically by trial and error rather than elucidation from the sequence. This is particularly important when two sets of primers are used in one reaction;

c. The denaturation temperature may be too high and the time held at this temperature too long, causing damage to the DNA template. We have observed significant differences between 93.5 and 95°C;

d. The PCR machine may not hold the set temperatures accurately, and this should be checked if significant day-to-day variations are seen in the degree of amplification. Automated apparatus consisting of three set temperature baths may be more stable than those utilizing thermostatically controlled changes in a heating block;

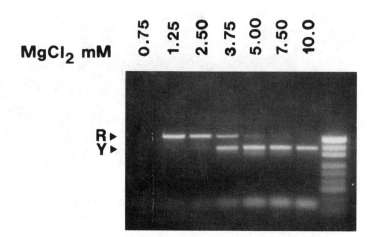

FIGURE 6. Effect of MgCl$_2$ concentration on the amplification signal when the two pairs of primers described in Figure 5 are used in combination. A constant annealing temperature of 64.5°C was used in this experiment, with 1 ng human male DNA as the template in each reaction. The MgCl$_2$ concentration affects the two amplification signals independently and appears optimal at 3.75 mM in this particular reaction.

e. The magnesium concentration is an important variable and should be optimized for each new set of primers (Figure 6);
f. A number of different primer pairs should be tried and the best selected;
g. Carrier DNA should be used when the starting template is minimal (e.g., 1 cell) to prevent damage to template DNA by either mechanical shearing or enzymic degradation from cellular DNAses, and to prevent the sample sticking to the tube.

VI. DIAGNOSTIC ASSAYS USING PCR

The molecular basis for single gene disorders is very heterogeneous. For example, at least 90 different mutations are known to produce the β-thalassemia phenotype.[16] A variety of different methods have been developed which allow the potential diagnosis of all mutations. Several possible methods can be used to diagnose a specific mutation, depending on whether the mutation is: (1) an insertion or deletion, (2) a single nucleotide substitution that affects an enzyme restriction site, or (3) a single substitution that does not affect a restriction site.

A. ANALYSIS OF DELETIONS

For disorders caused by large genetic deletions such as in α-thalassemia and Duchenne muscular dystrophy (DMD), diagnosis can be made by observing the presence or absence of the sequences in the amplified samples (Figure 4). The DMD locus is extremely large (>2 megabases), and partial deletions (several hundred kilobases) occur in 50 to 60% of patients and account for most of the mutations thus far characterized.[17] Deletions of the α-globin genes in α-thalassemia are smaller than for DMD but nevertheless involve regions of DNA ranging from less than a kilobase to several kilobases in size.[16]

Small deletions or insertions within the sequence spanned by the oligonucleotide primers can be detected by a change in the size of the amplified product.

B. RESTRICTION DIGESTION OF PCR PRODUCTS

If the mutation results in the loss or gain of a restriction site, restriction fragments produced after digestion of the amplified product can be used to diagnose the mutation. DNA from heterozygous individuals will show three bands, while affected homozygotes will show either one band (if the restriction site is lost) or two bands (if a new restriction site has appeared). Restriction digestion of PCR products has been used for the diagnosis of hemophilia A,[18,19] cystic fibrosis,[20] and many other genetic disorders.

It is also possible to introduce artificial fragment length polymorphisms (A-RFLPs) into the amplification products when the mutation does not affect a restriction site. Ward et al.[21] introduced a single nucleotide mismatch into the 3' end of the oligonucleotide primer positioned immediately adjacent to the polymorphic base in a β-thalassemia mutation.

C. ALLELE-SPECIFIC OLIGONUCLEOTIDE PROBING

Radioactive or biotinylated oligonucleotide probes can be used to analyze amplified DNA after dot-blotting onto a solid support such as nitrocellulose or nylon. The analysis is conducted at high stringency to eliminate partially mismatched hybridization of probes to target DNA. This procedure is frequently used to distinguish amplified fragments which do not differ in size, as are seen for diagnosis of sickle cell anemia, β-thalassemia[22] and cystic fibrosis.[23] Analysis of β-thalassemia can be simplified by amplification of the entire β-globin gene in each case, with subsequent hybridization using oligonucleotide probes specific for each mutation to screen the products.[24]

D. ANALYSIS BY ARMS

In addition to their use for screening PCR products after amplification, allele-specific oligonucleotides can be used to discriminate between alleles during the PCR reaction.[25] This amplification refractory mutation system (ARMS) is a relatively simple and reliable technique which allows genotype diagnosis solely by inspection of the PCR reaction products after gel electrophoresis. The procedure is based on the observation that oligonucleotides with a mismatched 3' residue will not function as primers in PCR under the appropriate conditions.[25] Oligonucleotide primers are made so that the 3'-nucleotide of one primer is allele-specific. However, in some cases this mismatch is not sufficient to be completely refractory to extension, and further deliberate mismatches can be introduced near the 3' end to prevent enzymic extension. The specificity of mismatch extension can also be controlled by increasing the specificity of the PCR reaction. Thus, increasing the annealing temperature can prevent the generation of mismatched products. Old et al.[26] increased the length of primers to 30 base pairs, which permitted them to use a 65°C annealing temperature and prevent the amplification of nonspecific bands.

The F508 cystic fibrosis mutation is responsible for 70% of all cystic fibrosis mutations and involves a specific 3 bp deletion.[23] Ballabio et al.[27] designed allele-specific oligonucleotide primers corresponding to the wild type and F508 alleles and demonstrated the specific amplification of the two alleles using two separate reactions for each individual. The three primers could also be used in a competitive oligonucleotide priming reaction when one of the allele-specific primers was radioactively labelled at its 5′ end. Radioactivity was predominantly incorporated only when the perfectly matched primer was present.

E. HETERODUPLEX ANALYSIS

Nagamine et al.[28] have shown that heterozygote individuals carrying deletions or insertions of 18 bp could be identified by spurious migration of heteroduplex DNA in gel electrophoresis using PCR products. More recently, Keen et al.[29] report that single base mismatches can be detected using this technique. Electrophoretic analysis of heteroduplex formation has been used to detect the 3 bp deletion in the F508 cystic fibrosis mutation.[30]

F. DIRECT SEQUENCING

Sequencing of PCR products provides an absolutely specifc diagnosis of mutations and has been used in diagnosis of alpha-1 antitrypsin deficiency.[31] However, this is a time consuming technique and probably not appropriate if the techniques described above can be applied to the particular genetic disorder being diagnosed. Sequencing of PCR fragments can always be used to confirm a diagnosis when time permits.

G. MULTIPLEX ANALYSIS

Multiplex DNA amplification involves the simultaneous amplification of widely separated sequences in the one reaction. This procedure has been developed for screening hemizygous genetic loci which are susceptible to deletions, such as the DMD and steroid sulfatase genes.[17,32] Chamberlain et al.[17] were able to simultaneously amplify six deletion prone exons in one PCR reaction and readily identify regions which fail to amplify, by gel electrophoresis. Although this technique has greatest application in mutation screening, it may also be important in prenatal diagnosis of relatively frequently occurring disorders such as DMD, where one third of all cases result from a new mutation.[33,34]

VII. CLINICAL APPLICATION OF PREIMPLANTATION GENETIC DIAGNOSIS

Couples at risk of transmitting a genetic disease to their offspring may prefer preimplantation embryo diagnosis to later methods of prenatal diagnosis (chorionic villus sampling, amniocentesis), which rely on a therapeutic abortion to prevent the birth of a baby affected with the disease. Couples will know whether they are at risk because of a previously affected child or a family history of a particular genetic disease. Appropriate genetic and IVF counselling and development of a single-cell PCR assay to diagnose the specific mutation in the couple are essential requirements before the couple is admitted to an IVF program for preimplantation embryo genetic diagnosis.

REFERENCES

1. **Cooper, D. N. and Schmidtke, J.,** Diagnosis of genetic disease using recombinant DNA, *Hum. Genet.,* 77, 66, 1987.
2. **Reiss, J. and Cooper, D. N.,** Application of the polymerase chain reaction to the diagnosis of human genetic disease, *Hum. Genet.,* 85, 1, 1990.
3. **Rychlik, W., Spencer, W. J., and Rhoads, R. E.,** Optimization of the annealing temperature for DNA amplification in vitro, *Nucl. Acids Res.,* 18, 6404, 1990.
4. **Li, H., Gyllensten, U. B., Ciu, X., Saiki, R. K., Erlich, H. A., and Arnheim, N.,** Amplification and analysis of DNA sequences in single human sperm and diploid cells, *Nature,* 335, 414, 1988.
5. **Saiki, R. K., Scharf, S., Faloona, F., Mullis, K. B., Horn, G. T., Erlich, H. A., and Arnheim, N.,** Enzymatic amplification of β-globin genomic sequence and restriction site analysis for diagnosis of sickle cell anemia, *Science,* 230, 1350, 1985.
6. **Saiki, R. K., Gelfand, D. H., Stoffel, S., Scharf, S. J., Higuchi, R. G., Horn, T. T., Mullis, K. B., and Erlich, H. A.,** Primer-directed enzymatic amplification of DNA with a thermostable DNA polymerase, *Science,* 239, 487, 1988.
7. **Hoelzel, R.,** The trouble with PCR machines, *TIG,* 6, 237, 1990.
8. **Nakahori, Y., Mitani, K., Yamada, M., and Nakagome, Y.,** A human Y-chromosome specific repeated DNA family (DYZ1) consists of a tandem array of pentanucleotides, *Nucl. Acids Res.,* 14, 7569, 1986.
9. **Handyside, A. H., Kontogianni, E. H., Hardy, K., and Winston, R. M. L.,** Pregnancies from biopsied human preimplantation embryos sexed by Y-specific DNA amplification, *Nature,* 344, 768, 1990.
10. **Warburton, P. E., Greig, G. M., Haaf, T., and Willard, H. F.,** PCR amplification of chromosome-specific alpha satellite DNA: definition of centromeric STS markers and polymorphic analysis, *Genomics,* 11, 324, 1991.
11. **Schnieke, A., Harbers, K., and Jaenisch, R.,** Embryonic lethal mutation in mice induced by retrovirus insertion into the alpha 1(I) collagen gene, *Nature,* 304, 315, 1983.
12. **Dziadek, M., Timpl, R., and Jaenisch, R.,** Collagen synthesis by cell lines derived from Mov-13 mouse embryos which have a lethal mutation in the collagen I gene, *Biochem. J.,* 244, 375, 1987.
13. **Holding, C. and Monk, M.,** Diagnosis of beta-thalassemia by DNA amplification in single blastomeres from mouse preimplantation embryos, *Lancet,* ii, 532, 1989.
14. **Sarkar, G. and Sommer, S. S.,** Shedding light on PCR contamination, *Nature,* 343, 27, 1990.
15. **Furrer, B., Candrian, U., Wieland, P., and Luthy, J.,** Improving PCR efficiency, *Nature,* 346, 324, 1990.
16. **Kazazian, H. H.,** The thalassemia syndromes: molecular basis and prenatal diagnosis in 1990, *Semin. Haematol.,* 27, 209, 1990.
17. **Chamberlain, J. S., Gibbs, R. A., Ranier, J. E., Nguyen, P.N., and Caskey, C. T.,** Deletion screening of the Duchenne muscular dystrophy locus via multiplex DNA amplification, *Nucl. Acids Res.,* 16, 11141, 1988.

18. **Kogan, S. C., Doherty, M., and Gitschier, J.,** An improved method for prenatal diagnosis of genetic diseases by analysis of amplified DNA sequences. Application to hemophilia A, *N. Engl. J. Med.,* 317, 985, 1987.
19. **Wehnert, M., Shukova, E. L., Surin, V. L., Schroeder, W., Solovjev, G.Ya., and Herrmann, F. H.,** Prenatal diagnosis of haemophilia A by the polymerase chain reaction using the intragenic HindIII polymorphism, *Prenatal Diagn.,* 10, 529, 1990.
20. **Feldman, G. L., Williamson, R., Beaudet, A., and O'Brien, W. E.,** Prenatal diagnosis of cystic fibrosis by DNA amplification for detection of KM-19 polymorphism, *Lancet,* ii, 102, 1988.
21. **Ward, M. A., Olivieri, N. F., Ng, J., and Roeder, J. C.,** Detection of β-thalassemia using an artificial-restriction fragment length polymorphism generated by the polymerase chain reaction, *Nucl. Acids Res.,* 19, 959, 1990.
22. **Saiki, R. K., Chang, C. A., Levenson, C. H., Warren, T. C., Boehm, C. D., Kazazian, H. H., and Erlich, H. A.,** Diagnosis of sickle cell anemia and β-thalassemia with enzymatically amplified DNA and non-radioactive allele-specific oligonucleotide probes, *N. Engl. J. Med.,* 319, 537, 1988.
23. **Kerem, B. S., Rommens, J. M., Buchanan, J. A., Markiewicz, D., Cox, T. K., Chakravarti, A., Buchwald, M., and Tsui, L. C.,** Identification of the cystic fibrosis gene: genetic analysis, *Science,* 245, 1073, 1989.
24. **Kazazian, H. H., Jr. and Boehm, C. D.,** Molecular basis and prenatal diagnosis of β-thalassemia, *Blood,* 72, 1107, 1988.
25. **Newton, C. R., Graham, A., Heptinstall, L. E., Powell, S. J., Summers, C., Kalsheker, N., Smith, J. C., and Markham, A. F.,** Analysis of any point mutation in DNA. The amplification refractory mutation system (ARMS), *Nucl. Acids Res.,* 17, 2503, 1989.
26. **Old, J. M., Varawalla, N. Y., and Weatherall, D. J.,** Rapid detection and prenatal diagnosis of β-thalassemia: studies in Indian and Cypriot populations in the UK, *Lancet,* ii, 834, 1990.
27. **Ballabio, A., Gibbs, R. A., and Caskey, C. T.,** PCR test for cystic fibrosis deletion, *Nature,* 343, 220, 1990.
28. **Nagamine, C. M., Chan, K., and Lau, Y.-F.,** A PCR artifact: generation of heteroduplexes, *Am. J. Hum. Genet.,* 45, 337, 1989.
29. **Keen, J., Lester, D., Inglehearn, C., Curtis, A., and Bhattacharya, S.,** Rapid detection of single base mismatches as heteroduplexes on hydrolink gels, *TIG,* 7, 5, 1991.
30. **Rommens, J., Kerem, B- S., Greer, W., Chang, P., Tsui, L.-C., and Ray, P.,** Rapid nonradioactive detection of the major cystic fibrosis mutation, *Am. J. Hum. Genet.,* 46, 395, 1990.
31. **Newton, C. R., Kalsheker, N., Graham, A., Powell, S., Gammack, A., Riley, J., and Markham, A. F.,** Diagnosis of α1-antitrypsin deficiency by enzymatic amplification of human genomic DNA and direct sequencing of polymerase chain reaction products, *Nucl. Acids Res.,* 16, 8233, 1988.
32. **Ballabio, A., Ranier, J. E., Chamberlain, J. S., Zollo, M., and Caskey, C. T.,** Screening for steroid sulfatase (STS) gene deletions by multiplex DNA amplification, *Hum. Genet.,* 84, 571, 1990.
33. **Koenig, M., Hoffman, E. P., Bertelson, C. J., Monaco, A. P., Feener, C. C., and Kunkel, L. M.,** Complete cloning of the Duchenne muscular dystrophy (DMD) cDNA and preliminary genomic organization of the DMD gene in normal and affected individuals, *Cell,* 50, 509, 1987.
34. **Witkowski, J.,** The molecular genetics of Duchenne muscular dystrophy: the beginning of the end? *TIG,* 4, 27, 1988.
35. **Gonzales, I. L. and Scmickel, R. D.,** The human 18s ribosomal RNA gene: evolution and stability, *Am. J. Hum. Genet.,* 38, 419, 1986.
36. **Harbers, K., Kuehn, K., Delius, H., and Jaenisch, R.,** Insertion of retrovirus into the first intron of α1(I) collagen gene leads to embryonic lethal mutation in mice, *Proc. Natl. Acad. Sci. U.S.A.,* 81, 1504, 1984.

37. **Shinnick, T., Lerner, R., and Sutcliff, J.,** Nucleotide sequence of Moloney murine leukemia virus, *Nature,* 293, 543, 1981.
38. **Nishioka, Y. and Leder, P., T**he complete sequence of a chromosomal mouse α-globin gene reveals elements conserved throughout vertebrate evolution, *Cell,* 18, 875, 1979.
39. **Alonso, S., Minty, A., Bourlet, Y., and Buckingham, M.,** Comparison of three actin-coding sequences in the mouse; evolutionary relationships between the actin genes of warm-blooded vertebrates, *J. Mol. Evol.,* 23, 11, 1986.

Chapter 9

CHROMOSOMAL ANALYSIS OF PREIMPLANTATION MAMMALIAN EMBRYOS

Ismail Kola, A. Henry Sathananthan, and Lyn Gras

TABLE OF CONTENTS

I. Introduction 174

II. Techniques Used for Cytogenetic Analysis 175
    A. Metaphase Spreads and Karyotypes 175
    B. Analysis of Single Blastomeres Generated by Embryo Biopsy Procedures 178
    C. Sister Chromatid Exchanges 178

III. Analysis and Interpretation of Data 179

IV. Applications of Cytogenetic Analysis of Preimplantation Mammalian Embryos 183
    A. Studying the Developmental Biology of Human Embryos 183
    B. Evaluating the Safety of New Techniques Used in Human *In Vitro* Fertilization 185
    C. Analysis of Blastomeres Following Embryo Biopsy 188
    D. The Elucidation of the Mechanisms of Drug-Induced Perturbation of Development 189

V. Conclusion 191

References 192

I. INTRODUCTION

Reports of the culture, manipulation, and developmental biology of preimplantation mammalian embryos date back to the end of the last century and the turn of the current century. Schenk in 1880[1] first reported an attempt to culture mammalian embryos *in vitro* when he observed the first cleavage-division in the rabbit and guinea pig after inseminating ovarian ova of these species. Several years later in 1893, Onanoff,[2] claimed the *in vitro* fertilization of rabbit and guinea pig oocytes. Furthermore, it was claimed that these oocytes were cultured to the 8-cell stage *in vitro*, and that further development of these embryos was obtained by transfer into the abdominal cavity of males or females.

Indeed, some of the most profound and incisive observations in the fields of developmental biology and cytogenetics were made and proposed in the earlier part of this century, albeit that such observations were often made on invertebrate preimplantation embryos. Boveri[3,4] in the early 1900s proposed that unfertilized oocytes contain centrosomes from male gametes at the time of fertilization, and that centrioles associated with such centrosomes organize the first mitotic spindle. These observations were made on sea urchin oocytes and have subsequently been shown to be true for a wide variety of animal species. This theory of fertilization by Boveri[3,4] is a classic one, and it ranks alongside his other fundamental predictions of chromosomal instability and rearrangements being etiological in the development of tumors and cancers.

Similar to the far-sighted and profound theories by Boveri, O. Hertwig and F. Fol (see Wilson[5]) first reported that sea urchin oocytes fertilized by two spermatozoa form multipolar cleavage spindles, and the embryo cleaves directly to 3- or 4-cells. After the initial multipolar division, cleavage proceeds by regular bipolar divisions, and morphologically normal looking blastulae are produced. However, the majority of these normal looking blastulae produce a wide range of abnormal or "monstrous" larvae, which die later on. A minority of these normal looking blastulae do develop into normal larvae. These observations of Hertwig and Fol were interpreted by Wilson[5] as suggesting that chromosomes consisted of genes and that individual chromosomes contain different genes.

The astute observations of Hertwig and Fol and the interpretation of these observations by Wilson[5] have, however, only been proven conclusively after the elucidation of the structure of DNA, and the localization of genes. In an analogous manner, Schenk's[1] and Onanoff's[2] initial reported success of *in vitro* fertilization and culture of mammalian preimplantation embryos have only become routine techniques in other mammalian species in the last four decades. Furthermore, the extent to which Boveri's[4,5] theories of fertilization were applicable to mammalian species is only recently being appreciated. This appreciation has, in part, been catalyzed by cytogenetic and/or chromosomal analysis of human embryos.

In addition to generating useful information on mammalian developmental biology, cytogenetic analysis of preimplantation mammalian embryos has also proven to be extremely valuable for other purposes. Valuable insights into the cytogenetics of human gametes and preimplantation embryos have been gained by analyzing gametes or embryos obtained from human *in vitro* fertilization programs. Cytogenetic analysis of mammalian oocytes and embryos has also proven useful for establishing the safety of procedures used in human *in vitro* fertilization programs. Furthermore, cytogenetic analysis of mammalian preimplantation embryos is also being investigated for its potential use in preimplantation embryo biopsy procedures. In this chapter, the following will be discussed: (1) techniques used for cytogenetic analysis, (2) methods used to analyze the data, and (3) applications of these techniques.

II. TECHNIQUES USED FOR CYTOGENETIC ANALYSIS

The technique we have found to be most reproducible and efficient in our hands is based on that originally devised by Tarkowski.[6] Although numerous other techniques have been proposed, we have found that the Tarkowski[6] technique is simplest and most efficient. The biggest problem with this technique, however, is that artifactual results may be obtained by the overspreading of chromosomes. Nevertheless, with appropriate modifications and sufficient practice, it is possible, to reduce substantially the over-spreading of chromosomes. The following technique is the one routinely used in our laboratory to spread unfertilized oocytes and preimplantation mammalian embryos.

A. METAPHASE SPREADS AND KARYOTYPES

Embryos are cultured in the presence of colcemid (4 µg/ml of culture medium). Metaphase arresting agents such as colcemid interfere with the assembly of microtubules in spindle formation and thereby cause accumulation of metaphases in culture. The time of incubation in colcemid is dependent on the stage and species of embryos being studied. Generally with morula- and blastocyst-stage embryos, a 4 h incubation period is sufficient, since a number of cells will be blocked at metaphase over such a time period. This is so because the cells of these later-stage embryos are asynchronous, and at any given time a random number of cells will be at or about to enter metaphase. However, if a greater number of metaphase cells is required, or if you want to ensure that metaphase cells are obtained, then the time of incubation in colcemid should be increased. The time of incubation in colcemid may be increased up to a maximum of 12 h. However, we find that more than 6 h of incubation in colcemid adversely affects the morphology of chromosomes obtained in metaphase spreads. It is advisable to incubate earlier cleavage-stage embryos in colcemid for periods greater than 2 h, to ensure that metaphase cells are obtained for analysis. In our experience, it is also necessary to incubate human embryos in colcemid for longer periods of time to ensure that a sufficient number of metaphase cells are obtained. Oocytes are not cultured in colcemid since ovulated or mature oocytes block at metaphase of the second meiotic division. Oocytes can be spread for up to 48 h after retrieval. In some animal experiments, it may be desirable or necessary to evaluate the chromosomes directly after flushing from the oviduct or uterus (without culturing them *in vitro*). In such situations, colchicine (2 mg/kg body weight) can be injected intraperitoneally into the animals 2 h before the retrieval of embryos.[7,8]

Embryos are ready for spreading after incubation in colcemid. It is important to remember, however, that before oocytes are spread, the cumulus cells must be removed. The oocyte should be as naked as possible. The presence of cumulus cells may interfere with the quality of the spread. This will occur in the first instance by the cumulus cells sticking to the glass slide, and thus reducing the extent to which individual chromosomes will be visible. Second, the cumulus cells may also interfere with the visibility of the chromosomes since both will stain up with the Giemsa stain. Cumulus cells are removed by incubating oocytes in a small drop (approximately 20 to 50 µl) of prewarmed hyaluronidase (1 mg/ml, Sigma, U.S.A.) dissolved in phosphate-buffered-saline (PBS). After approximately 2 to 3 min of incubation at 37°C, the oocytes are rinsed in PBS and gently aspirated up and down a finely pulled pipette. This aspiration procedure is continued until the oocyte is entirely free from cumulus cells. It is also important to ensure that the pipette does not have any ragged edges since this will puncture the zona pellucida and lyse the oocyte.

Oocytes and embryos are spread onto glass slides. It is preferable that high quality clean glass slides are used. Slides should be free from grease. The presence of grease will retard or inhibit the free movement of oocytes and embryos on glass slides, and thus lead to poorly spread or ill-defined individual chromosomes. It is also important to make a small circle (approximately 3 to 5 mm in diameter) in the center of the bottom surface of the glass slide. The circle is made with a diamond pencil. This circle is used to mark the position where the embryo or oocyte should be placed. This process makes the localization of the embryo easier after staining. The circle should be made before the slides are cleaned. Fragments of glass which result from making the circle will interfere with the spreading of chromosomes. Ideally, glass slides are cleaned with a toothbrush and 7X detergent and thereafter thoroughly rinsed in water.

The first step in the spreading procedure is the incubation of the oocyte or embryo in hypotonic solution. The hypotonic solution employed in our laboratory is tri-sodium citrate constituted in Milli-Q water. The concentration of sodium citrate varies from 0.5% to 1.0%. Higher concentrations will be used with oocytes and earlier-stage embryos, whereas lower concentrations will be used with later-stage embryos (8-cell to blastocyst). The hypotonic solution is added in droplets of approximately 50 µl to 35 mm tissue-culture dishes. These small size droplets make it easier to find the oocytes/embryos. The transfer into hypotonic solution should occur with a minimal amount of PBS. The oocytes or embryos are left in the hypotonic solution for about 10 min at 37°C, depending on how they swell. The swelling of the oocytes or embryos is monitored by visual observation through a microscope. Generally, if a lower concentration of hypotonic solution is used, then the time of incubation should be lower since the embryo or oocyte will swell faster and vice versa. Human oocytes,[9] fertilized zygotes,[10,11] and early cleavage-stage embryos[12] are incubated in 1% trisodium citrate for up to 10 min. Blastocyst-stage embryos[13] are incubated in 0.5% tri-sodium citrate for 10 to 15 min. These hypotonic treatments result in excellent metaphase spreads. After incubation in hypotonic solution, the oocytes or embryos are transferred onto the center of the circle on the premarked cleaned glass slide. The volume of hypotonic solution used for the transfer of the embryo should be as small as possible, but it should not be so small that the embryo dries up during subsequent procedures. If too much hypotonic solution is transferred across, the excess can be drawn off using a finely pulled mouth-controlled pipette. Care should be taken, however, not to shift the oocyte or embryo out of the circle, or worse, pull it into the pipette.

Fixation of the embryo on the glass slide follows the hypotonic treatment. We routinely use freshly prepared methanol and glacial acetic acid for this purpose (made up in a ratio of 3:1, respectively). It is critical that the methanol and glacial acetic acid are high quality reagents and that the stock is not too old. We routinely dedicate methanol and glacial-acetic acid stocks for chromosomal analysis only. The glass pipette has a finely pulled end and a rubber bung attached to it. The fixative is added onto the embryo in a drop-wise fashion immediately after the excess hypotonic fluid is drawn off from around the embryo. The fixative is added by holding the pipette approximately 2 cm behind the embryo, and dropping one drop of fixative onto the embryo or oocyte while gently blowing onto the embryo. The embryo should swing around and stop not too far from its original position. The fixative quickly evaporates from the glass slide. The fixative around the embryo will usually be the last to evaporate. Thus, it will appear to the investigator that the fixative is contracting towards the embryo. The next drop of fixative should be dropped just before the previous drop of fixative around the embryo has evaporated. The process should be continued until approximately 4 to 5 drops of fixative have been added. If the volume of fixative per drop is too large or if the drops are added too quickly, the oocyte or embryo could be lost by being washed away. Alternatively, if the oocyte or embryo does not swing on addition of the first drop of fixative, or if the sample dries out, poorly defined chromosomes will be obtained. Thereafter, the slides are air dried at room temperature. It is preferable to fix one embryo or oocyte per glass slide. This prevents any possibility of chromosomes from one metaphase being washed to that of another and thereby confounding the data.

Staining can be carried out 10 to 15 min after the slides have been air dried at room temperature if G-banding of chromosomes is not required. Slides are stained with 10% Giemsa solution made up in PBS at a pH of 6.8. (This buffer is commercially available in tablet form and can be readily dissolved in water.) It is important to use a Giemsa solution that is relatively fresh (not more than a couple of days old). Furthermore, the Giemsa solution should be filtered through Whatman filter paper. If the Giemsa solution is not adequately filtered, debris can accumulate on the glass slides, and this will certainly interfere with the analysis of chromosomes.

If chromosomes are to be G-banded, then the slides should be allowed to air dry at room temperature for approximately one week. Slides should be stored in such a manner that they are protected from dust. For G-banding, the slides are individually immersed in a 0.1% trypsin solution in a coplin jar for 10 to 30 sec. The exact conditions of trypsin treatment may need to be titrated for each batch of trypsin and each set of experiments. Overexposure to trypsin will result in the swelling of chromosomes and a ghost-like appearance. Underexposure will result in the absence of bands. To determine the optimum time of exposure of slides to trypsin, it is advisable to test a series of metaphase slides of similar age by incubating for varying time intervals. It is recommended to start with 10 sec exposure to trypsin, and to increase the exposure if the chromosomes are unbanded. In any event, it is generally more difficult to obtain good G-banding with chromosomes from oocytes and preimplantation embryos as compared to that for other cells. The slides should be rinsed in two changes of PBS after trypsin treatment. Staining of slides is carried out in a 10% Giemsa solution for a period of 3 to 5 min. Metaphases with clear G-banding, good contrast between banded regions, and no chromosome scattering may be photographed using technical Pan high-contrast film. Karyotypes are then constructed from these G-banded photographs.

B. ANALYSIS OF SINGLE BLASTOMERES GENERATED BY EMBRYO BIOPSY PROCEDURES

Single biopsied blastomeres are cultured overnight under oil in a 5% CO_2-in-air incubator in microdrops of medium containing 4 mg/ml BSA and a final concentration of 0.1 µg/ml colcemid. The cells are spread by incubating individual cells in 0.5 to 0.6% trisodium citrate solution for 1 min.[14] The cells are then transferred onto glass slides as described before.

Fixative is quickly dropped onto the slides in a stepwise fashion as follows: the first drop is applied directly onto the cell and the next five drops individually washed onto the cell by dropping the fixative onto the sides of the cell, blowing after each drop to facilitate better chromosome spreading. The slides are then stained in 10% Giemsa solution as previously described.

C. SISTER CHROMATID EXCHANGES

The principal on which sister chromatid differentiation is based is shown in Figure 1. Embryos are cultured in dishes at 37°C for 48 h. Throughout the 48 h culture period, dishes are kept in the dark in the incubator by being placed in black boxes with loosely fitting tops. Embryos are cultured in the presence of $1 \times 10^{-7} M$ BrdU (Sigma, St. Louis, U.S.A.) for the first 24 h of the culture period, and $1 \times 10^{-7} M$ thymidine (Sigma, St. Louis, U.S.A.) for the next 24 h. For the last 3 h of the second 24 h culture period, colcemid is added to the cultures. At the end of the 48 h culture period, the embryos are incubated in hypotonic solution (trisodium citrate). Thereafter, the embryos are fixed onto

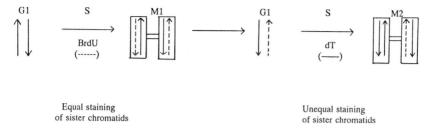

FIGURE 1. A diagrammatic representation of the differentiation of sister chromatids using BrdU in the first cycle and thymidine in the second cycle. (Adapted from Latt, S. A., *Annu. Rev. Genet.*, 15, 11, 1981. With permission.)

glass slides with methanol/glacial acetic acid as described before. The slides are then aged by being kept at 4°C for 2 to 3 d. After this period, the slides are exposed to a solution of Hoechst 33258 (5 µg/ml) for 20 min at room temperature. Thereafter, the slides are irradiated at 254 nm for 1 h, and then incubated at 60°C for 1 h.[15] The slides are then stained with a 10% Giemsa solution for approximately 10 min.

III. ANALYSIS AND INTERPRETATION OF DATA

The data derived from the cytogenetic evaluation of preimplantation mammalian embryos can be analyzed in several different ways. For the detection of the rate of aneuploidies, the number of chromosomes in each metaphase can be counted. For this purpose it is sufficient to stain the spreads with Giemsa only and not to G-band them. If, however, it is necessary (or desirable) to investigate the total number of chromosomes per metaphase and to identify which of the chromosomes have been lost or gained, then Giemsa staining only (without G-banding) will only facilitate (at best) the identification of the groups of chromosomes that are involved in the aneuploidy. G-banding is essential for the identification of the specific chromosome(s) involved in the aneuploidy. Furthermore, the G-banding of chromosomes is also necessary for the identification of structural chromosomal anomalies such as translocations. Sister chromatid exchanges are used for the detection of more subtle genotoxic and DNA-damaging events.

Regardless of the method of analysis, we always employ at least two investigators to carry out the microscopic evaluation of slides. It is also preferable that the slides be coded so that at least one (and if possible both) of the investigators carrying out the microscopic evaluation are blind to the identity of specific slides. Microscopic evaluation is carried out by locating embryos or oocytes on the glass-slide using either the 4× or 10× objective (40× and 100× magnification, respectively). Metaphases are then evaluated under the 100× objective (1000× magnification) using oil and an oil-immersion lens. Ideally, there should be minimum overlap of individual chromosomes, and yet all the chromosomes should be simultaneously viewed within the field of the 100× objective. The chromosomes can then be counted and the results recorded. The position of the metaphase spread should also be recorded alongside the results using an England-Finder. If the results are unclear or abnormal, the metaphase spread can be photographed using technical Pan high-contrast film. G-banded preparations should be photographed for karyotype construction.

The manner of handling the data which emanates from cytogenetic analysis of preimplantation mammalian embryos or oocytes also merits attention. One of the major problems with the Tarkowski[6] technique is that artifactual losses of chromosomes can occur because of overspreading. In essence, overspread metaphases can be (and should be) excluded from the data. However, even if there is no evidence of overspreading and a chromosomal loss (e.g., monosomy) is detected, the question of whether this is real or artifactual is important. Many workers in the field have approached this problem by excluding hypoploidies from their data and only taking into account those cells with the expected euploid chromosome number and hyperploid cells. They then double the number of hyperploid cells. It could be argued that if chromosome losses are a problem with the technique, then it is possible that some of the cells with the expected number of chromosomes could indeed be hyperploid cells with artifactual losses of chromosomes. For example, consider a hyperhaploid oocyte with 25 chromosomes, 2 of which are lost due to a technical artifact; on analysis this oocyte will appear to have 23 chromosomes. Thus, it will be considered to be normal, whereas in reality it is abnormal. This error (or underestimate) is then doubled because the aneuploidy figure is derived by doubling the hyperploidy rate. It can therefore be concluded that the incidence of aneuploidy is underestimated in cases where the artifactual losses of chromosomes are a problem and where the data are handled in the above manner. The degree of underestimation will be related to the extent to which overspreading of chromosomes occurs. If it is true that oocytes and embryonic cells fulfill a major correlate of the theory of nondisjunction, which states that the incidence of hyperploidies and hypoploidies is balanced (see[9,16]), then the difference between hypo- and hyperploidies will give an indication of the extent of artifactual losses. The hypoploidies in such a situation would be an overestimate, whereas the hyperploidies would be an underestimate. On the basis of a mathematical model, it could be argued that even if artifactual losses of chromosomes occur, the true incidence of chromosomal aneuploidy is the total of hyperploid (an example of a hyperhaploid metaphase spread and karyotype is shown in Figure 2(a) and (b), respectively) and hypoploid cells. This mathematical model is demonstrated below.

Assumptions:

1. That the incidence of hyperploidies and hypoploidies is the same in the cells being investigated. This is one of the important postulates of nondisjunction. Furthermore, this is acknowledged as such by workers who calculate the incidence of aneuploidy by doubling the hyperploidy rate.

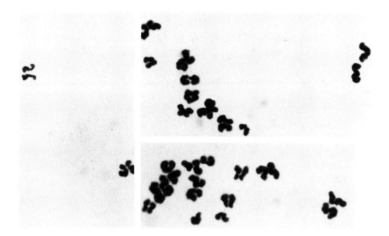

FIGURE 2(a). A metaphase spread from an uninseminated human oocyte, obtained using the technique described in this chapter. (Original magnification × 1000.) (From Gras, L., McBain, J., Trounson, A., and Kola, I., *Hum. Reprod.*, 7, 1396, 1992. With permission.)

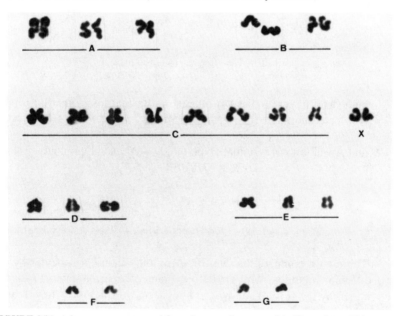

FIGURE 2(b). A karyotype constructed from the metaphase spread in Figure 2(a). This oocyte was hyperhaploid with an extra chromosome from the C group. (Original magnification × 1000.) (From Gras, L., McBain, J., Trounson, A., and Kola, I., *Hum. Reprod.*, 7, 1396, 1992. With permission.)

2. That the rate of technical, artifactual losses is constant throughout the experiment. Thus the actual number of hypoploidies (HYPO) is the observed number of hypoploidies (x) minus the artifactual losses (a), whereas the actual number of hyperploidies (HYPER) is the observed

TABLE 1
A Comparison of the Rates of Aneuploidy in Human Oocytes Using Two Different Formulae

Study	Ref.	Aneuploidy (HYPO + HYPER)	2 × HYPER
Wramsby and Liedholm	20	25%	0%
Martin et al.	21	30%	4%
Wramsby et al.	22	57%	19%
Tarin et al.	23	21%	0%
Gras et al.	9	31%	32%
Michelmann and Mettler	24	3%	6%
Wramsby and Fredga	25	56%	8%
Veiga et al.	26	11%	18%
Bongso et al.	27	21%	16%
Van Blerkom and Henry	28	8%	3%
Djalali et al.	29	27%	4%
Papadopoulos et al.	30	24%	16%
Ma et al.	31	26%	22%
Pieters et al.	32	21%	0%
Pellestor	16	27%	25%
Mean + S.D.		25.9 ± 14.8%	11.5 ± 10.3%

Note: The data used are those from the published literature.

number of hyperploidies (y) plus the artifactual losses that have been considered normal.

Actual Aneuploidy = Actual Hyperploidy + Actual Hypoploidy
 = HYPO + HYPER
 = $(x - a) + (y + a)$
 = $x - a + y + a$
 = $x + y$
 = Observed Hypoploidies + Observed Hyperploidies

In Table 1 we compare the rates of aneuploidy in human oocytes by the two different methods. The aneuploidy rate of approximately 26% (as determined by the formula above) in human oocytes is higher than that of human spermatozoa, which is approximately 10%.[7,18] This higher figure of aneuploidies in oocytes concurs with the data from aborted human conceptuses, which demonstrate that trisomes in embryos/fetuses are more frequently maternal in origin.[19] Furthermore, the use of the above formula also results in a lower percentage of variability between published reports as compared to the formula of doubling the hyperploidy rates (a standard deviation of 57% from the mean as compared to a 90% standard deviation, respectively).

IV. APPLICATIONS OF CYTOGENETIC ANALYSIS OF PREIMPLANTATION MAMMALIAN EMBRYOS

The relevance of cytogenetic evaluations of mammalian preimplantation embryos and gametes to human and mammalian genetics is obvious. However, it is still worthwhile to emphasize that our current perceptions of the incidences of chromosomal anomalies in humans is based on data derived from aborted conceptuses. Conceptuses with specific types of chromosomal abnormalities fail to develop to the stage of clinically recognized pregnancies. For instance, monosomic mammalian conceptuses die in the pre- or peri-implantation period of pregnancy.[14,33] Furthermore, trisomy 1 human conceptuses are hardly ever recognized in spontaneously aborted material (perhaps because this is the largest human autosome, and more genes are involved in the gene dosage perturbations that occur). Thus, our current data on incidences of cytogenetic abnormalities in mammalian conceptuses are based on a skewed population. The study of preimplantation human embryos overcomes these problems.

The cytogenetic analysis of preimplantation mammalian embryos has also been used for the following purposes in our laboratory:

A. STUDYING THE DEVELOPMENTAL BIOLOGY OF HUMAN EMBRYOS

Boveri's[3,4] theory of fertilization proposed that the inheritance of paternal centrosomes is important for the organization of the first mitotic spindle. These data are based on the sea urchin. However, data from Schatten et al.[34] demonstrated that, in the mouse, the mitotic spindle is organized by maternally inherited mitotic spindles. On the basis of the data on the mouse, it was presumed that this was true for mammals in general. In 1987 we[12,35] suggested that this generalization may not necessarily apply to humans. Our suggestion was based on a study of the cleavage patterns and karyotypic status of tripronuclear human oocytes and embryos.[12] It has been proposed[35] that paternal centrosomes may (partly, at least) be involved in the organization of the first mitotic spindle. This has recently been confirmed by transmission electron microscopy (TEM) of pronuclear oocytes.[36] Earlier TEM studies had demonstrated a centriole in an early human embryo closely associated with a developing male pronucleus 3 h after insemination.[37]

Our data[12] on the study of tripronuclear human oocytes (Figure 3(a)) demonstrated that these oocytes cleaved either to 2-cells (Figure 3(b)), or to 2-cells plus an extrusion (Figure 3(c)), or to 3-cells (Figure 3(d)) after the first division. The karyotypic status of the resulting embryos was either mosaic (a chromosome complement between triploidy and diploidy), or triploid (Figure 3(e)), or diploid (Figure 3(f)). On the basis of this data, a model has been proposed to explain the mechanisms whereby such cleavage patterns were occurring (Figure 4a).[35,38] Such cleavage patterns may be occurring through the

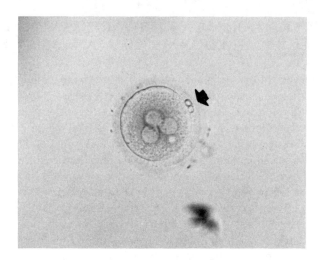

FIGURE 3(a). Photomicrograph of a tripronuclear human zygote. The photomicrograph shows three pronclei. The first and second polar bodies are shown by the arrow. The presence of two polar bodies demonstrates that the tripronuclear state is due to dispermic fertilization. (Original magnification × 200.) (From Kola, I., Trounson, A., Dawson, G., and Rogers, P., *Biol. Reprod.*, 37, 395, 1987. With permission.)

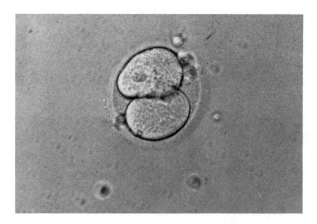

FIGURE 3(b). Photomicrograph of a 2-cell embryo resulting from cleavage of a tripronuclear human oocyte. (Original magnification × 200.) (From Kola, I., Trounson, A., Dawson, G., and Rogers, P., *Biol. Reprod.*, 37, 395, 1987. With permission.)

formation of either bipolar or tripolar spindles at the first mitotic division. Evidence has subsequently been obtained for both three-cornered (Figure 4(b)) and two-cornered spindles (Figure 4(c)) in tripronuclear human oocytes.[36] Transmission electron microscopy has also shown that tripronuclear oocytes could arise by the simultaneous penetration of two spermatozoa (Figure 4d),[39] confirming dispermy.

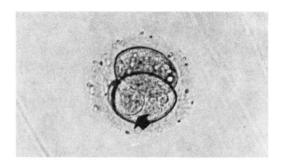

FIGURE 3(c). Photomicrograph of a 2-cell plus extrusion embryo derived from a tripronuclear human oocyte. The arrow shows the extrusion. (Original magnification × 200.) (From Kola, I., Trounson, A., Dawson, G., and Rogers, P., *Biol. Reprod.*, 37, 395, 1987. With permission.)

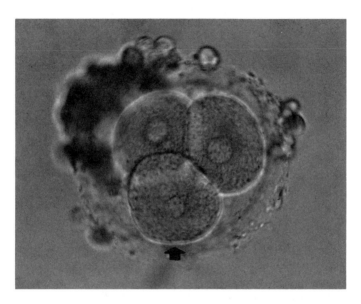

FIGURE 3(d). Photomicrograph of a 3-cell embryo that resulted from the direct and synchronous cleavage of a triponuclear human oocyte. One blastomere (arrowed) is binucleated. (From Kola, I. and Trounson, A. O., in *The Cell Biology of Fertilization*, Schatten, G. and Schatten, H., Eds., Academic Press, New York, 277, 1989. With permission.)

B. EVALUATING THE SAFETY OF NEW TECHNIQUES USED IN HUMAN *IN VITRO* FERTILIZATION

Using cytogenetic analysis of mammalian preimplantation embryos, the safety of new techniques used in human *in vitro* fertilization procedures has been investigated. For instance, we have tested the safety of procedures for vitrification of oocytes. The data[10] have demonstrated that vitrified oocytes and those that had been exposed to the VS1 vitrification solution developed into

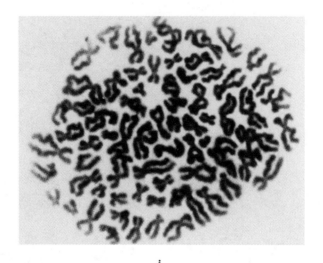

FIGURE 3(e). A triploid metaphase spread (3(e)(i)) derived from the embryo in Figure 3(b) and the construction of the karyotype from the metaphase spread (3(e)(ii)). (Original magnification × 1000.) (From Kola, I., Trounson, A., Dawson, G., and Rogers, P., *Biol. Reprod.*, 37, 395, 1987. With permission.)

viable fetuses at a rate much lower than corresponding controls. Furthermore, the data also demonstrated that a significantly higher number of oocytes that were vitrified had chromosomal aneuploidies. On the basis of such data, we had stopped the vitrification of mouse oocytes using VSI solution. Subsequently, we have investigated the effects on chromosomal integrity of different variables (such as straw handling and DMSO concentration) which occur in the freezing of mouse embryos[40] and the incidence of chromosomal abnormalities in oocytes fertilized by sperm microinjection procedures.[11] It has demonstrated that the incidence of aneuploidies is not significantly elevated in oocytes fertilized by sperm microinjection procedures as compared to oocytes fertilized by routine *in vitro* fertilization procedures.

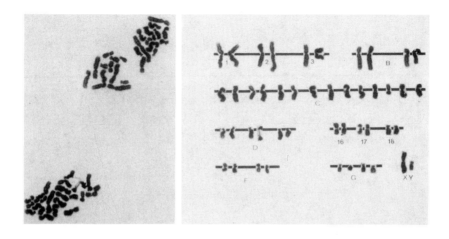

i ii

FIGURE 3(f). A diploid metaphase spread (3(f)(i)) derived from the embryo in Figure 3(c) and the construction of the karyotype from the metaphase spread (3(f)(ii)). (Original magnification × 1000.) (From Kola, I., Trounson, A., Dawson, G., and Rogers, P., *Biol. Reprod.*, 37, 395, 1987. With permission.)

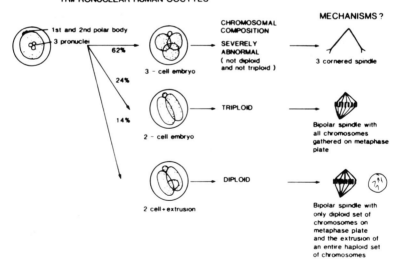

FIGURE 4(a). Diagram demonstrating the cleavage patterns and karyotypic analysis, chromosomal composition, and possible mechanisms of triponuclear human zygote development. (From Kola, I. and Trounson, A. O., in *The Cell Biology of Fertilization,* Schatten, G. and Schatten, H., Eds., Academic Press, New York, 277, 1989. With permission.)

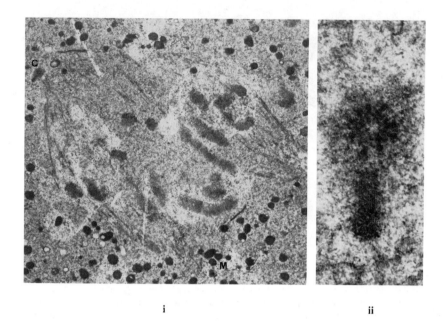

i ii

FIGURE 4(b). Section of a tripolar spindle of a 3PN embryo at syngamy. (i) Two centrioles masked by osmiophilic centrosomal material are seen at one of the three poles. MTs extend from each pole toward the chromosomes in the central region of spindle. M, mitochondria. (Original magnification × 6000.) (ii) The two centrioles at higher magnification, aligned at right angles to each other. Both centrioles are associated with dense centrosomal material, which obscures their structure. (Original magnification × 65,000.) (From Sathananthan, H., Kola, I., Osborn, J., Trounson, A., Ng. S. C., Bongso, A., and Ratnam, S. S., *Proc. Natl. Acad. Sci. U.S.A.*, 88, 4806, 1991. With permission.)

Another question that has been addressed using chromosomal analysis is whether superovulation procedures used in IVF significantly impacted on the incidence of chromosomal aneuploidies.[41] It has been shown that the incidence of chromosomal aneuploidies in superovulated oocytes is not significantly different statistically from oocytes retrieved from nonstimulated (natural) cycles.[9] These data suggest the possibility that the higher incidence of aneuploidies detected in human oocytes[16,42] relative to that in animal oocytes[43,44] is not attributable to the process of superovulation *per se*. It may be that human gametes in general have a higher aneuploidy rate, or that the higher aneuploidy rate may be related to the infertility status of the patients, especially since the data on nonstimulated oocytes in our study[9] is based on oocytes derived from IVF patients.

C. ANALYSIS OF BLASTOMERES FOLLOWING EMBRYO BIOPSY

Highly efficient procedures for obtaining quality metaphase spreads from single cells biopsied from preimplantation mouse embryos have been

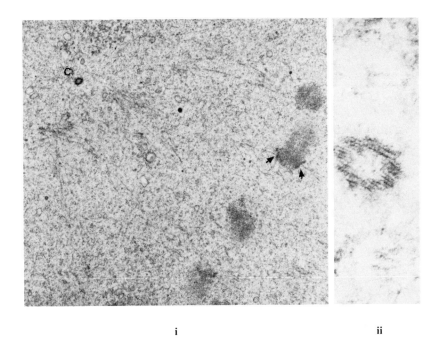

i   ii

FIGURE 4(c). Bipolar spindle developed from a 3PN embryo in syngamy. (i) A centriole (C) is visible at one pole of half a spindle depicted in this electron micrograph. Spindle MTs extend from the pole to chromosomes, connecting at kinetochores (arrowheads). The spindle zone is usually devoid of other organelles. (Original magnification × 13,200.) (ii) Centriole in oblique cross section at higher magnification. It presents the typical 9 + 0 structure, consisting of nine triplets of MTs arranged in a circle. (Original magnification × 65,000.) (From Sathananthan, H., Kola, I., Osborn, J., Trounson, A., Ng. S. C., Bongso, A., and Ratnam, S. S., *Proc. Natl. Acad. Sci. U.S.A.*, 88, 4806, 1991. With permission.)

developed. In our laboratory, approximately 80% of metaphase spreads were suitable for analysis[14] (Figure 5). Furthermore, biopsied cells were 100% predictive of the karyotype of the fetus and correlated absolutely with the morphology of the fetus. The limitations of applying this technique to humans for the detection of chromosomal anomalies is dependent on (1) achieving even higher rates of success with obtaining metaphase spreads, (2) determining the incidence of chromosomal mosaicism in human preimplantation embryos, (3) developing efficient and reproducible banding techniques for the detection of anomalies such as translocations, and (4) establishing that the biopsy procedure does not affect the subsequent viability of human embryos.

D. THE ELUCIDATION OF THE MECHANISMS OF DRUG-INDUCED PERTURBATION OF DEVELOPMENT

The mouse has been used as a model to study the mechanisms of drug-induced perturbation of preimplantation embryos. Our data[7,8,13,15] chal-

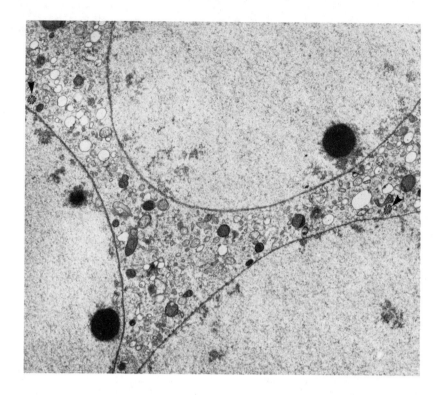

FIGURE 4(d). Tripronuclear embryo developed after multiple sperm injection into the perivitelline space of an oocyte. Two sperm tails (in cross section) are evident at two different locations between the pronuclei (arrows), indicating dispermic fertilization. (Original magnification × 15,400.) (From Sathananthan, A. H. and Chen, C., *Gamete Res.*, 15, 177, 1986. With permission.)

lenged the interpretation of the so-called "all or none" phenomenon proposed for the exposure of preimplantation mammalian embryos to teratogens. This phenomenon proposed that if exposure to a teratogen or embryotoxic agent occurred during the preimplantation period of development, then the embryo was either killed before implantation or it survived to be normal. Embryos exposed to drugs such as cyclophosphamide survived.[13] These surviving embryos had higher rates of chromosomal aberrations and sister chromatid exchanges.[8,15] The developmental consequences of these genotoxic events manifested only after implantation, in that a greater number of embryos were resorbed and fetuses had lower birth weights.[15] Cyclophosphamide-induced chromosomal aberrations in preimplantation embryos and subsequent resorptions in postimplantation embryos were induced (partly, at least) by the generation of reactive oxygen molecules. This conclusion is based on the finding that treatment with antioxidants reduced the frequency of these abnormalities.

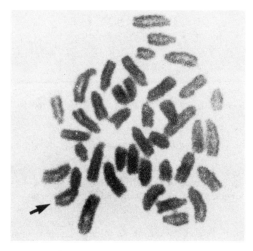

FIGURE 5. Photomicrograph of a metaphase spread of a single cell biopsied from a 4-cell embryo. The photomicrograph shows 38 chromosomes plus one Robertsonian translocation chromosome (arrow), giving the cell a euploid karyotype. (Original magnification × 1,250.) (From Kola, I. and Wilton, L., *Mol. Reprod. Dev.*, 29, 16, 1991. With permission.)

V. CONCLUSION

The techniques described in this chapter are those which we have found in our laboratory to be the most useful and efficient for the chromosomal analysis of preimplantation mammalian embryos. Clearly, relative to the cytogenetic analysis of somatic cells, these techniques still require further development. We do find, for instance, that even with the use of the same protocol, different investigators will achieve different rates of success. Furthermore, the technical difficulties of the technique are compounded by the limitation of material. Nevertheless, even with these limitations, the technique has been useful in addressing fundamental questions in mammalian biology and human medicine. The data that have emanated from studies carried out thus far have given new and important insights into the genetics of human embryos, the developmental biology of human embryos, and the potential uses and problems of novel techniques developed for human *in vitro* fertilization and other assisted reproductive technologies. In the future, these cytogenetic techniques will be developed even further and refined. These will then be even more useful than they currently are.

REFERENCES

1. **Schenk, S. L.,** Das Saugethierei Kunstlick befruchtet au ßerhalb des mutterthieres, *Mutt. Embr. Int. K.K. Univ. Wien.,* 1, 107, 1880.
2. **Onanoff, J.,** Recherches sur la fecondation et la gestation des mammifers, *C.R. Soc. Biol. (Paris),* 45, 719, 1893.
3. **Boveri, T.,** *Ueber mehrpolige Mitosen als Mittel zur Analyse des Zellkerus: V.P.M.G.* XXXV, 1902.
4. **Boveri, T.,** *Zellen-Studien VI,* Fischer, Jena, 1907.
5. **Wilson, E. B.,** *The Cell in Development and Heredit.,* MacMillan, New York, 1928, 916.
6. **Tarkwoski, A. K.,** An air-drying method for chromosome preparations from mouse eggs, *Cytogenetics,* 5, 394, 1966.
7. **Kola, I. and Folb, P.I.,** Chlorpromazine inhibits the mitotic index, cell number and formation of blastocysts and delays implantation of CBA mouse embryos, *J. Reprod. Fertil.,* 76, 527, 1986.
8. **Kola, I., Folb, P. I., and Parker, M. I.,** Maternal administration of cyclophoshamide induces chromosomal aberrations and inhibits cell number, histone- and DNA-synthesis in preimplantation mouse embryos, *Teratogenesis, Carcinogenesis and Mutagenesis,* 6, 115, 1986.
9. **Gras, L., McBain, J., Trounson, A., and Kola, I.,** The incidence of chromosomal aneuploidies in stimulated and unstimulated (natural) uninseminated human oocytes, *Hum. Reprod.,* 7, 1396, 1992.
10. **Kola, I., Kirby, C., Shaw, J. M., Davey, A., and Trounson, A. O.,** Vitrification of mouse oocytes results in aneuploid zygotes and malformed fetuses, *Teratology,* 38, 467, 1988.
11. **Kola, I., Lacham, O., Jansen, R. P. S., Turner, M., and Trounson, A.,** Chromosomal analysis of human oocytes fertilized by microinjection of spermatozoa into the perivitelline space, *Hum. Reprod.,* 5, 575, 1990.
12. **Kola, I., Trounson, A., Dawson, G., and Rogers, P.,** Tripronuclear human oocytes: altered cleavage patterns and subsequent karyotypic analysis of embryos, *Biol. Reprod.,* 37, 395, 1987.
13. **Kola, I. and Folb, P. I.,** The effects of cyclophosphamide on alkaline phosphatase activity and on *in vitro* post-implantation murine blastocyst development, *Dev. Growth and Differ.,* 27, 125, 1985.
14. **Kola, I. and Wilton, L.,** Preimplantation embryo biopsy: detection of trisomy in a single cell biopsied from a four-cell mouse embryo, *Mol. Reprod. Dev.,* 29, 16, 1991.
15. **Kola, I., Vogel, R., and Spielmann, H.,** Co-administration of ascorbic acid with cyclophosphamide (CPA) to pregnant mice inhibits the clastogenic activity of CPA in preimplantation murine blastocysts, *Mutagenesis,* 4, 297, 1989.
16. **Pellestor, F.,** Frequency and distribution of aneuploidy in human female gametes, *Hum. Genet.,* 86, 283, 1991.
17. **Martin, R. H., Rademaker, A. W., Hildebrand, K., Long-Simpson, L., Peterson, D., and Yamamoto, J.,** Variation in the frequency and type of sperm chromosomal abnormalities among normal men, *Hum. Genet.,* 77, 108, 1987.
18. **Pellestor, F. and Selle, B.,** Etude cytogenetique du sperme humain, *Med. Sci.,* 5, 244, 1989.
19. **Kupke, K. G. and Muller, U.,** Parental origin of the extra chromosome in trisomy 18, *Am. J. Hum. Genet.,* 38, 724, 1989.
20. **Wramsby, H. and Liedholm, P.,** A gradual fixation method for chromosomal preparations of human oocytes, *Fertil. Steril.,* 41, 736, 1984.
21. **Martin, R. H., Mahadevan, M. M., Taylor, P. J., Hildebrand, K., Long-Simpson, L., Peterson, D., Yamamoto, J., and Fleetham, J.,** Chromosomal analysis of unfertilized human oocytes, *J. Reprod. Fertil.,* 78, 673, 1986.
22. **Wramsby, H., Fredga, K., and Liedholm, P.,** Chromosome analysis of human oocytes recovered from preovulatory follicles in stimulated cycles, *N. Engl. J. Med.,* 316, 121, 1987.

23. **Tarin, J. J., Gomez, E., Sampaio, M., Ruiz, M., Remohi, J., and Pellicer, A.,** Cytogenetic analysis of human oocytes from fertile women, *Hum. Reprod.*, 6, 110, 1991.
24. **Michelmann, H. W. and Mettler, L.,** Cytogenetic investigations on human oocytes and early human embryonic stages, *Fertil. Steril.*, 43, 320, 1985.
25. **Wramsby, H. and Fredga, K.,** Chromosome analysis of human oocytes failing to cleave after insemination *in vitro*, *Hum. Reprod.*, 2, 137, 1987.
26. **Veiga, A., Calderon, G., Santalo, J., Barri, P. N., and Egozcue, J.,** Chromosome studies in oocytes and zygotes from an IVF programme, *Hum. Reprod.*, 2, 425, 1987.
27. **Bongso, A., Ng, S. C., Ratnam, S., Sathananthan, H., and Wong, P.C.,** Chromosome anomalies in human oocytes failing to fertilize after insemination *in vitro*, *Hum. Reprod.*, 3, 645, 1988.
28. **Van Blerkom, J. and Henry, G. I.,** Cytogenetic analysis of living human oocytes: cellular basis and developmental consequences of perturbations in chromosomal organisation and complement, *Hum. Reprod.*, 3, 777, 1988.
29. **Djalali, M., Rosenbusch, B., Wolf, M., and Sterzik, K.,** Cytogenetics of unfertilized human oocytes, *J. Reprod. Fertil.*, 84, 647, 1988.
30. **Papadopoulos, G., Randall, J., and Templeton, A. A.,** The frequency of chromosome anomalies in human unfertilized oocytes and uncleaved zygotes after insemination *in vitro*, *Hum. Reprod.*, 4, 568, 1989.
31. **Ma, S., Kalousek, D. K., Zouves, C., Yuen, B. H., Gomel, V., and Moon, S.,** Chromosome analysis of human oocytes failing to fertilize *in vitro*, *Fertil. Steril.*, 51, 992, 1989.
32. **Pieters, M. H. E. C., Geraedts, J. P. M., Dumoulin, J. C. M., Evers, J. L. H., Bras, M., Kornips, F. H. A. C., and Menheeve, P. P. C. A.,** Cytogenetic analysis of *in vitro* fertilization failures, *Hum. Genet.*, 81, 367, 1989.
33. **Epstein, C. J.,** Mouse monosomies and trisomies as experimental systems for studying mammalian aneuploidy, *Trends Genet.*, 1, 129, 1985.
34. **Schatten, H., Schatten, G., Mazia, D., Balczon, R., and Simerly, C.,** Behaviour of centrosomes during fertilization and cell division in mouse oocytes and in sea urchin eggs, *Proc. Natl. Acad. Sci. U.S.A.*, 83, 105, 1986.
35. **Kola, I. and Trounson, A. O.,** Dispermic human fertilization. Violation of expected cellular behaviour, in *The Cell Biology of Fertilization*, Schatten, G. and Schatten, H., Eds., Academic Press, New York, 277, 1989.
36. **Sathananthan, H., Kola, I., Osborn, J., Trounson, A., Ng, S. C., Bongso, A., and Ratnam, S. S.,** Centrioles in the beginning of human development, *Proc. Natl. Acad. Sci. U.S.A.*, 88, 4806, 1991.
37. **Sathananthan, A. H. and Chen, C.,** Sperm-oocyte membrane fusion in the human during monospermic fertilization, *Gamete Res.*, 15, 177, 1986.
38. **Trounson, A. O., Rogers, P., Kola, I., and Sathananthan, H.,** Fertilization, development and implantation, in *Textbook of Obstetrics*, Turnbull, A. and Chamberlain, G., Eds., Churchill Livingstone, London, 1989, 49.
39. **Sathananthan, A. H., Ng, S. C., Trounson, A. O., Laws-King, A., and Ratnam, S. S.,** Human microfertilization by injection of single or multiple sperm: ultrastructure, *Hum. Reprod.*, 4, 574, 1989.
40. **Shaw, J. M., Kola, I., MacFarlane, D., and Trounson, A. O.,** The chromosomal integrity of rapidly frozen 2-cell mouse embryos is influenced by the dimethylsulphoxide concentration and straw-handling, *J. Reprod. Fertil.*, 91, 9, 1991.
41. **Kola, I.,** Embryo and fetal abnormalities in IVF, *Birth*, 15, 145, 1988.
42. **Wiswedel, K., Bosschieter, J. R., Ronen, J., Nelson, M., Kola, I., and DeJong, P.,** Chromosomal analysis of unfertilized oocytes and cleavage-arrested human embryos in *in vitro* fertilization, *S. Afr. J. Sci.*, 85, 186, 1989.
43. **Mailhes, J. B.,** Incidence of aneuploidy in rodents, in *Aneuploidy Part A: Incidence and Aetiology*, Vig, B.K. and Sandberg, A.A., Eds., Alan R. Liss, New York, 1987, 128.
44. **Mikamo, K. and Kamiguchi, Y.,** Primary incidences of spontaneous chromosomal anomalies and their origins and causal mechanisms in the Chinese hamster, *Mutat. Res.*, 108, 265, 1983.
45. **Latt, S. A.,** Sister chromatid exchange formation, *Annu. Rev. Genet.*, 15, 11, 1981.

Chapter 10

ASSESSMENT OF EMBRYO METABOLISM AND VIABILITY

David K. Gardner and Henry J. Leese

TABLE OF CONTENTS

I. Introduction 196

II. Methods of Assessing Embryo Viability 196
    A. Assessment of Morphology 196
    B. Development in Culture 197
    C. Dye Exclusion 197
    D. Fluorescence of Degenerate Cells 197
    E. Production of Fluorescent Metabolites 198
    F. Production of Platelet Activating Factor 198
    G. Nutrient Uptake Measurements 199

III. Fluorometric Assays 199
    A. Principles of Fluorometric Assays 199
    B. Enzymatic Cycling 201
    C. Bioluminescence Assays 201
    D. Microspectrofluorometric Methods 202

IV. Procedure for Measuring the Uptake of Nutrients by Single Human Embryos 202
    A. Embryo Incubation 202
    B. Metabolite Assays 203
        1. Pyruvate 203
        2. Glucose 205
        3. Lactate 205
    C. Nutrient Uptake and Metabolite Release by Single Human Embryos 205
    D. Embryo Metabolism and Viability 206

References 208

I. INTRODUCTION

Since the birth of Louise Brown in 1978, hundreds of IVF clinics have been established worldwide, resulting in the births of over 20,000 babies. However, although most clinics have high rates of oocyte recovery, fertilization, and embryo development in culture, the proportion of embryos which implant after transfer is low. It has been calculated that 30% of human oocytes fertilized *in vivo* go to term.[1] By contrast, when a single embryo is replaced after fertilization *in vitro*, the average success rate is only 10%.[2] It appears that embryonic loss is accentuated by fertilization and culture *in vitro*. This situation is partially alleviated by the replacement of two or more embryos, in which case the incidence of a successful pregnancy rises to around 20%, although the success rate per embryo transferred is decreased.

With the routine use of exogenous gonadotrophins to stimulate the production of multiple oocytes, clinics are faced with the decision of which of the resulting embryos to replace in the mother and which to cryopreserve. There is an obvious clinical need to be able to select those embryos most likely to implant after replacement in the uterus.[3,4]

It is the aim of this chapter to review methods of assessing embryo viability, and then describe in detail the noninvasive assessment of metabolism and its possible role in the selection of embryos for transfer. "Viability" is defined as the ability of an embryo to give rise to a live offspring after transfer.

II. METHODS OF ASSESSING EMBRYO VIABILITY

Several procedures for determining the viability of preimplantation mammalian embryos have been used:

1. Assessment of morphology
2. Development in culture
3. Dye exclusion
4. Fluorescence of degenerate cells
5. Production of fluorescent metabolites
6. Production of platelet activating factor
7. Nutrient uptake measurements

A. ASSESSMENT OF MORPHOLOGY

The general appearance of embryos has long been used to assess their viability and has been the basis of scoring systems to quantify the extent of development.[5,6] In practice, however, the scoring of embryos, particularly postcompaction, is notoriously difficult. One dilemma faced by the embryologist is that embryos which appear normal under the microscope may be multinucleate or have intracellular abnormalities. By the same token, the appearance of cytoplasmic fragments or blebs are not inconsistent with viability.

B. DEVELOPMENT IN CULTURE

Morphological appearance combined with an assessment of the extent and rate of development in culture is more indicative of embryo viability than morphology alone, since the culture of preimplantation embryos for even a short period can eliminate those incapable of further development. In an extensive study, Cummins et al.[6] used both rate of development and morphological appearance to score human embryos prior to transfer. Analysis of 1539 embryo replacements showed that developmental rate and morphology of the embryos were significantly associated with each other. Although both criteria were useful in predicting the success of embryo transfer, morphological assessment of embryos was found to be a better index of viability than cleavage rate. In a similar study, Mohr et al.[7] observed that at all stages of development, embryos which resulted in a pregnancy were the most rapidly dividing ones. However, Lopata et al.[8] re-examined the data from several clinics and found that even those embryos which were the slowest to divide could also be viable. They concluded that "Although circumstantial evidence suggests that populations of rapidly growing human embryos contain a higher percentage of viable embryos than slowly developing populations, it is clear that speed of cleavage is not, in itself, an intrinsic indication of embryo viability."

The difficulties of using rate of development to score embryos are compounded by the observations of Shire and Whitten,[9,10] who demonstrated that the cleavage rate of mouse embryos *in vitro* was strain dependent. Whether this is the case for human embryos may be difficult to resolve due to the heterogeneity of the population, so this becomes a further problem of using rate of cleavage to score human embryos.

C. DYE EXCLUSION

In 1914, Evans and Schulman[11] found that the survival of cultured tumor cells was related to their ability to exclude the dye trypan blue. Since then, dye exclusion methods have been used to test viability in a wide variety of cells. The exclusion of such dyes by living cells has been regarded as a test of membrane integrity.[12-14] Bellve[15] used eosin Y to examine the viability of mouse embryos derived from donor mice exposed to heat stress. Accumulation of the dye by a given blastomere was followed by visible necrosis of the cell about 12 h later. In the hamster it has been shown that there is a high correlation between the ability of embryos to exclude trypan blue and their uptake of (^{3}H) Uridine.[16]

D. FLUORESCENCE OF DEGENERATE CELLS

Certain dyes have a high affinity for DNA. One example is 4′,6′-diamindino-2-phenylindole (DAPI), which stains nuclei and other DNA-containing structures. Schilling et al.,[17] using rabbit and bovine embryos, showed that DAPI stained only the nuclei of degenerate blastomeres. Nearly 90% of the embryos which did not fluoresce continued to develop, while those which contained fluorescing nuclei in most of their blastomeres did not. It was later shown that

DAPI-negative rabbit embryos were more likely to develop *in utero* after transfer than control embryos.[18] For bovine embryos, however, the use of DAPI was less reliable than morphological observation in predicting the success of embryo transfer.[19]

E. PRODUCTION OF FLUORESCENT METABOLITES

Rotman and Papermaster[20] showed that the fluorescent products produced by the enzymatic hydrolysis of fluorogenic substrates, such as fluorescein derivatives, were only retained by cells with intact plasma membranes. In a study on the use of fluorescein diacetate (FDA) to assess the viability of preimplantation mouse embryos, Mohr and Trounson[21] found that embryos grown under inadequate culture conditions lost the ability to accumulate intracellular fluorescein. FDA has been used to score human embryos produced by *in vitro* fertilization.[7] Embryos grown in suboptimal media showed low fluorescence, while embryos grown in more optimal conditions fluoresced strongly. It is important to realize that the results of using such dyes only reflect basic cell functions rather than developmental potential. Basic cell functions may be retained by embryos which are grossly abnormal, for example those with anucleate or multinucleate blastomeres. This complicates the use of dyes as predictors of pregnancy outcome. When Kola and Folb[22] used FDA to assess the viability of mouse blastocysts which had been exposed to chlorpromazine *in vivo*, no changes in viability were apparent, even at concentrations of chlorpromazine that inhibited subsequent development *in vitro* and *in vivo*.

A further drawback of this approach is the necessity of incubating embryos with a nonphysiological compound and of exposing them to UV light to excite the accumulated dye. Even though studies using FDA have shown that such exposures do not prevent cleavage *in vitro* or subsequent implantation and development *in utero*,[21,23-25] the use of fluorescent dyes is likely to be restricted to those human embryos not destined for replacement. Data from such experiments could, however, be useful in improving culture methods.

F. PRODUCTION OF PLATELET ACTIVATING FACTOR

O'Neill and Saunders[26] showed that, after the culture of human embryos, media contained a factor that reduced the platelet count of spleenectomized mice and was strongly correlated with embryo viability. Embryo derived platelet activating factor (PAF), an ether phospholipid, was assayed in the culture media in which 97 fertilized and 16 unfertilized oocytes had been incubated. Media derived from unfertilized oocytes did not alter the platelet count, whereas that from the zygotes which subsequently resulted in pregnancy caused a 35% reduction. Supplementation of embryo culture medium with exogenous PAF increased mouse blastocyst cell number and subsequent embryo viability after transfer,[27] while the addition of PAF antagonists to the culture medium significantly reduced blastocyst development *in vitro* and *in vivo*.[28,29] However, recent work has indicated that there are problems with assay reproducibility and that a more consistent assay may be required.[30-32]

G. NUTRIENT UPTAKE MEASUREMENTS

Mouse zygotes in culture (and probably those of many other mammals) have a requirement for pyruvate to satisfy their energy requirements.[33] Lactate acts synergistically with pyruvate from the 2-cell stage.[34] Glucose as the sole energy substrate in the medium is unable to support development until the 4-cell stage.[35] The use of nutritional measurements as possible indicators of embryo viability was first examined, using bovine blastocysts, by Renard et al.[36] It was found that day-10 blastocysts which had a glucose uptake greater than 5 µg/h developed better both *in vitro* and *in utero* than embryos with an uptake below this value. Unfortunately, it was not possible to measure the uptake of glucose by earlier stages (day-7 or day-8) due to the insensitivity of the spectrophotometric method used. Rieger,[37] using 1-^{14}C-glucose, showed that morphologically normal day-7 bovine embryos took up significantly more glucose than degenerating ones.

The development of microchemical techniques (to be described in detail below) has enabled the nutrition and metabolism of single oocytes and preimplantation embryos to be studied noninvasively. The work has been carried out on mouse[38-42] and human embryos,[43-46] and confirms the findings of culture experiments, in that pyruvate is consumed preferentially by the early preimplantation stages before glucose becomes the predominant substrate for the blastocyst. Using a microfluorometric technique, Gardner and Leese[40] measured the uptake of glucose by single mouse blastocysts (day-4 of development) prior to transfer to recipient females. It was found that those embryos which went to term after transfer had a significantly higher glucose uptake *in vitro* than those embryos which failed to develop.

This approach need not necessarily be confined to pyruvate and glucose. Figure 1 provides a summary of other potential substrates, metabolites and enzymes whose measurement might be diagnostic of embryo health. A microchemical assay has recently been developed to study amino acid uptake by single mouse embryos.[47] Several amino acids can be measured fluorometrically, e.g., ala, glu, gln, asp, asn, ser, thr, and aminobutyric acid.

III. FLUOROMETRIC ASSAYS

An account of a variety of procedures which may be used for the assessment of embryo metabolism is given below, followed by a detailed description of the procedure used routinely in our laboratories to monitor nutrient uptake by single human embryos. The use of other more invasive techniques has been described previously.[48]

A. PRINCIPLES OF FLUOROMETRIC ASSAYS

The assays are based on the generation or consumption of the reduced pyridine nucleotides, NADH and NADPH in coupled enzymatic reactions. These nucleotides fluoresce when excited with light at 340 nm, whereas the oxidized forms, NAD$^+$ and NADP$^+$ do not. Thus the reaction:

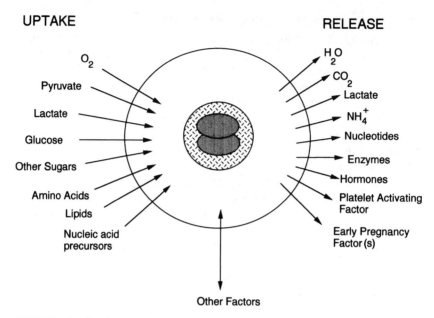

FIGURE 1. Possible factors which might form the basis of a noninvasive test of embryo viability.

$$\text{Pyruvate} + \text{NADH} + \text{H}^+ \xrightarrow{\text{Lactate dehydrogenase}} \text{Lactate} + \text{NAD}^+ \quad (1)$$

may be followed by monitoring the drop in fluorescence, or optical density at 340 nm, as NADH is converted to NAD^+.

Depending on the assay conditions, the decrease in fluorescence is proportional to the amount of pyruvate in the reaction mixture, while the rate at which the fluorescence falls is proportional to the activity of lactate dehydrogenase. Although there is a linear relationship between NAD(P)H and fluorescence over a wide range of concentrations, there is not a strict proportionality via an extinction coefficient (i.e., the Lambert-Beer law does not apply), and it is usual to run a series of standards with each assay performed.

Glucose may be measured by monitoring the increase in fluorescence due to the generation of NADPH in the following reactions:

$$\text{Glucose} + \text{ATP} \xrightarrow{\text{Hexokinase}} \text{Glucose 6-phosphate} + \text{ADP} \quad (2)$$

$$\text{Glucose 6-phosphate} + \text{NADP}^+ \xrightarrow{\text{Glucose 6-phosphate dehydrogenase}} \text{6-phosphogluconate} + \text{NADPH} + \text{H}^+ \quad (3)$$

The number of metabolites and enzymes which may be measured using enzymatic reactions coupled to the generation or consumption of NAD(P)H is very great. Full details of such assays may be found in Bergmeyer and Gawehn[49] and in Lowry and Passonneau.[50]

Reactions are conventionally carried out in cuvettes and the fluorescence or absorbance measured in a fluorimeter or spectrophotometer. While such methods are sufficiently sensitive for metabolic measurements on large numbers of embryos, assays on single or small numbers of embryos require different approaches. Some of these are described below.

B. ENZYMATIC CYCLING

Enzymatic cycling may be used to amplify very small quantities of NAD^+, $NADP^+$, NADH, and NADPH so that they may be measured by conventional fluorimetry. As an example, the NAD^+ generated in the reduction of pyruvate in reaction (1) may be amplified using the following two reactions in a so-called "NAD" cycle:

$$NAD^+ + lactate \xrightarrow{\text{Lactate dehydrogenase}} NADH + pyruvate + H^+ \quad (4)$$

$$NADH + H^+ + ketoglutarate + NH_3 \xrightarrow{\text{Glutamate dehydrogenase}} NAD^+ + glutamate \quad (5)$$

As a result, pyruvate and glutamate are formed in yields up to 6,000- to 8,000-fold per h. The reactions are stopped and either of the products, pyruvate or glutamate is measured by reversing reaction (4) and measuring the NAD^+ fluorimetrically in strong alkali. Related systems have been described for the amplification of the other pyridine nucleotides, such that metabolite concentrations in the range 10^{-13} to 10^{-15} mole may be measured. Full details of these ingenious methods have been provided by Lowry and Passonneau.[50] They have been applied to the measurement of enzymes and metabolites in single mouse embryos[51-53] and in human oocytes.[54]

C. BIOLUMINESCENCE ASSAYS

The bioluminescence firefly luciferin luciferase reaction has been used for many years in the measurement of picomole quantities of ATP:

$$NAD(P)H + FMN + H^+ \xrightarrow{\text{Oxidoreductase}} FMNH_2 + NAD(P)^+$$

$$FMNH_2 + O_2 + RCHO \xrightarrow{\text{Bacterial Luciferase}} FMN + RCOOH + H_2O + Light$$

Using appropriate coupling enzymes, assays based on this principle have been developed for: D-glucose, L(+) and D(−) lactate, 6-phosphogluconate, L-malate, L-alanine, L-glutamate, and glucose 6-phosphate.[55-58] To the best of our knowledge, these assays have yet to be used to measure the consumption of nutrients or the formation of products by single or small groups of embryos.

D. MICROSPECTROFLUOROMETRIC METHODS

In these methods, NAD(P)H and other fluorochromes are measured directly in small droplets of medium, or in single cells, using a quantitative fluorescence microscope.[59,60] The procedure is a one-step determination and is far simpler and less time-consuming than enzymatic cycling. The sample whose fluorescence is to be quantified is visualized under a conventional light source and then activated momentarily with UV light from a mercury source.

Most systems use "epi-illumination," in which the exciting incident light passes onto the specimen or sample through the microscope objective, which acts as a condenser. The fluorescence (which is always of longer wavelength) passes back through the objective and is transmitted via a dichroic mirror, also known as an interference mirror, to a photomultiplier, and the output is displayed on a photometer. Dichroic mirrors reflect a high percentage of the exciting light onto the specimen while allowing the fluorescence emission to pass through. In this way, the exciting and emitted light are kept separate.

Incident light fluorescence results in a better alignment of illumination, more efficient excitation, and less fading of fluorochromes than transmitted light fluorescence. The system in use in our laboratories uses a Diavert or Fluovert inverted microscope with MPV Compact Photometer/Photomultiplier (Leica (Instruments) Ltd.). Such systems are capable of quantifying the fluorescence of samples a few picoliters in volume.

A variety of incubation chambers capable of being mounted on a microscope stage have been described. Rotman[59] sprayed drops of medium 0.1 to 40 μm in diameter onto siliconized microscope slides under mineral oil. Mroz and Lechene[61] carried out reactions in droplets of medium contained in capillary tubes. Hemocytometer slides have also been used.[62,63] For work on single mouse embryos, we have performed reactions in defined volumes of medium in the nanoliter range, dispensed from calibrated glass micropipettes, constructed on a microforge.[64] The droplets are held on siliconized microscope slides under mineral oil. However, for human embryos, volumes in the range 1 to 10 μl can be employed together with extended incubation periods, enabling the use of commercially available micropipettes. Assay reactions are carried out in microliter drops of reaction mixture under mineral oil on siliconized microscope slides. Slides are siliconized by immersing them for 30 sec in 2% v/v dimethyldichlorosilane solution (BDH Chemicals, Poole, Dorset, U.K.).

IV. PROCEDURE FOR MEASURING THE UPTAKE OF NUTRIENTS BY SINGLE HUMAN EMBRYOS

A. EMBRYO INCUBATION

The principal nutrients consumed by early human embryos to satisfy their energy requirements are pyruvate and glucose. Their consumption may conveniently be measured by incubating single embryos in a few microliters of medium for up to 24 h. The incubation time can be reduced by decreasing the incubation volume accordingly.

Any adherent cumulus cells are removed from the embryos by taking them up gently into a finely drawn Pasteur pipette with an internal diameter just larger than the zona pellucida. The embryos are washed through several changes of modified medium containing reduced levels of metabolites and supplemented with 4 mg/ml BSA. Conventional embryo culture media are characterized by serum levels of glucose (around 5 mM) and a relatively high lactate concentration (around 25 mM) (see Chapter 5). However, to measure glucose consumption from an initial concentration of 5 mM would be very difficult, if not impossible, since over a 24 h period, the concentration in a 4 µl droplet would only fall from 5 mM to about 4.90 mM (or by 2%). Using an initial concentration of 1 mM or lower results in a final concentration of about 0.90 mM, amounting to a medium depletion of 10% or more. This difference may be measured reliably. Similarly, it would be difficult to detect the production of lactate by an embryo in the presence of 25 mM lactate. Therefore, in studies concerned with the production of lactate by human embryos, lactate is omitted from the medium.

After washing, embryos are incubated individually in 4 µl droplets of defined medium under liquid paraffin in a gas phase of 5% CO_2. At daily intervals, the embryos are removed from the droplets in the minimum of medium into the tip of an oil-filled drawn Pasteur pipette, washed through three changes of fresh medium, and transferred to a new 4 µl droplets for the next incubation period. The medium remaining in the original droplet and 4 µl control medium from an adjacent embryo-free droplet, incubated in exactly the same manner, are taken up into 10 µl capillary tubes. Samples of medium are then coded to disguise their identity. If the samples are not to be analyzed immediately, they are stored at –70°C (Figure 2). There is negligible breakdown of metabolites during storage for several days under these conditions, or during 24 h incubation at 37°C.

B. METABOLITE ASSAYS
1. Pyruvate
Pyruvate assay: reaction (1)

The reaction mixture has the following composition: 0.095 mM NADH and 28 U/ml LDH in EPPS buffer, pH 8.0.

If micropipettes are to be used, assays can be housed in nanoliter droplets on a siliconized slide overlaid with mineral oil (heavy white grade, Sigma Diagnostics, St. Louis, U.S.A.). Although this approach requires the use of a micromanipulator to maneuver the pipettes, it has the advantage that many samples at a time can be analyzed. To prepare the micropipettes, capillary tubing (o.d. 1.0 mm, i.d. 0.8 mm) is heated in a low flame and pulled by hand. The tubing is then snapped apart and a hook made from the broken ends by gentle heating. The tubing is then positioned in a microforge and a constriction made above the hook using the heated filament of the forge. A small paperclip

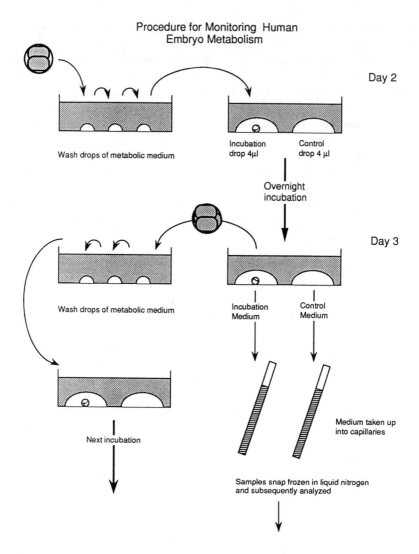

FIGURE 2. Collection of culture medium for metabolite analysis. Human embryos are cultured overnight in defined medium and then transferred to fresh drops. The incubation medium is then taken up and stored in capillary tubes at −70°C prior to analysis.

is attached to the hook, and the heated filament advanced to a position just below the constriction. The weight on the hook pulls the heated glass tubing to a point, which is easily snapped square with a pair of watchmaker's forceps. The pipette can then be mounted in 16-gauge stainless steel tubing and fixed in position with sealing wax. Uptake and release of fluid from the micropipette is achieved by connection to an air-filled syringe, in turn attached by plastic tubing to the stainless steel mount. Such micropipettes should then be cleaned thoroughly with acetone and siliconized. The volume between the tip of the pipette and the constriction can then be calibrated using tritiated water. Such pipettes can be used indefinitely.

Ten nanoliter droplets of reagent are positioned on a siliconized microscope slide, under mineral oil, which is then placed on the stage of the fluorescence microscope. The mineral oil is pre-equilibrated for 12 h with 0.9% NaCl. The microdrops are then brought into focus under a ×20 objective. The fluorescence of each droplet is then measured in turn using an automatic shutter, which closes off the visual light source and exposes the pyridine nucleotides to the UV source. Drops are routinely exposed for 0.25 sec, since there is no detectable photo-oxidation of NADH or NADPH during this time. The photometer scale is linear and extends from 0 to 900 arbitrary units. One nanoliter samples of standard pyruvate solutions or unknown samples are then added to each droplet. The reaction is rapid since the equilibrium favors lactate formation and goes to completion in less than 5 min. The final readings are recorded. A linear relationship is obtained between fluorescence and pyruvate concentration in the range 0 to 1.0 mM (Figure 3).

Alternatively, the reactions can be housed in microliter drops in glass wells on siliconized microscope slides filled with mineral oil. The wells are prepared from perspex tubing 15 mm in diameter and 4 mm deep, attached to a glass slide prior to siliconization. Four 9 μl droplets of reaction mixture are added to the wells using appropriate micropipettes or microsyringes (SMI, Hamilton, SGE). The droplets adopt the shape of flattened spheres. The slide is then placed on the microscope stage, and the edge of a given droplet brought into sharp focus. If the other three droplets have been pipetted accurately, they will also be in sharp focus. We routinely use a ×10 objective and ×6.3 eyepiece. The microscope stage is then moved so that the field of view from which the fluorescence is to be measured is in the center of the droplet. After the initial fluorescence is measured, a 1 μl sample is added.

2. Glucose

Glucose assay: reaction (2)

The procedure is similar to that used for the pyruvate assay, except that NADPH formation as opposed to NADH oxidation is measured (Figure 3). The reaction mixture has the following composition: 1.25 mM NADP$^+$; 0.5 mM ATP, 12 U/ml hexokinase, 6 U/ml G6PDH in EPPS buffer pH 8.0.

3. Lactate

Lactate assay: reaction (1)

The reaction mixture has the following composition: 4.76 mM NAD$^+$, 100 U/ml lactate dehydrogenase, 2.6 mM EDTA in glycine-hydrazine buffer, pH 9.4.

C. NUTRIENT UPTAKE AND METABOLITE RELEASE BY SINGLE HUMAN EMBRYOS

Using these methods, data on the uptake of pyruvate and glucose and on the production of lactate by human embryos has been obtained.[45,46] Qualitatively,

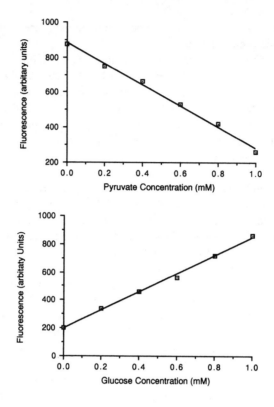

FIGURE 3. Typical standard curves for pyruvate and glucose. As the pyridine nucleotides are oxidized and reduced, there is a corresponding decrease and increase in fluorescence.

the uptake pattern is similar to that in the mouse, though the human embryo takes up considerably more glucose and pyruvate at each stage of development, even allowing for the difference in embryo volume between the two species. The pyruvate uptake of arrested embryos is lower than those which develop normally, and only normal embryos exhibit the characteristic increase in glucose uptake at the blastocyst stage (Figure 4).

D. EMBRYO METABOLISM AND VIABILITY

The question remains as to whether these noninvasive methods have the potential to select for those human embryos more likely to implant in the uterus. The appropriate studies have yet to be carried out on human embryos; however, studies on the bovine[36] and mouse[40] have indicated that an embryo's metabolic activity is positively correlated with its ability to develop after replacement in the uterus.

Initial studies on the uptake of pyruvate by individual human embryos on successive days of culture prior to transfer on day-3 have revealed that the metabolic activity of an embryo on day-2 of development is correlated ($p < 0.01$) (Figure 5) to its metabolic activity the following day.[65] Such data indicate that

Assessment of Embryo Metabolism and Viability 207

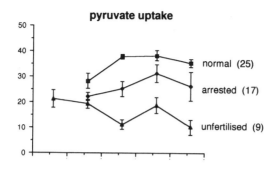
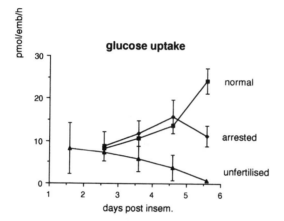

FIGURE 4. The uptake of pyruvate and glucose by single human embryos obtained by IVF and cultured *in vitro*. (From Hardy, K., Hooper, M. A. K., Handyside, A. H., Rutherford, A. J., and Leese, H. J., *Hum. Reprod.*, 4, 188, 1989. With permission.)

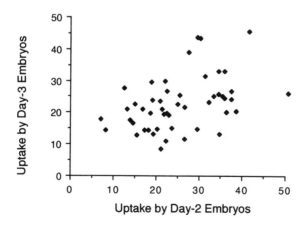

FIGURE 5. The uptake of pyruvate by individual human embryos on successive days of culture. Correlation, r = 0.43, $p < 0.01$.

it may be possible to select human embryos for transfer on the basis of their metabolic activity as early as the 2- to 4-cell stage.

Studying the metabolism of human embryos should not only provide a quantitative test of embryo viability, but will increase our understanding of embryo physiology, thus facilitating the development of more suitable culture conditions.

REFERENCES

1. **Biggers, J. D.,** *In vitro* fertilization and embryo transfer in human beings, *New Engl. J. Med.*, 304, 336, 1981.
2. **Steptoe, P. C., Edwards, R. G., and Walters, D. E.,** Observations on 767 clinical pregnancies and 500 births after human *in vitro* fertilization, *Hum. Reprod.*, 1, 89, 1986.
3. **Plachot, M.,** Choosing the right embryo: the challenge of the nineties, *JIVET*, 6, 193, 1989.
4. **Tesarik, J.,** Viability assessment of preimplantation concepti: a challenge for human embryo research, *Fertil. Steril.*, 52, 364, 1989.
5. **Shea, B. F.,** Evaluating the bovine embryo, *Theriogenology*, 15, 31, 1981.
6. **Cummins, J. M., Breen, T. M., Harrison, K. L., Shaw, J. M., Wilson, L. M., and Hennessey, J. F.,** A formula for scoring human embryo growth rates in *in vitro* fertilization: its value in predicting pregnancy and in comparison with visual estimates of embryo quality, *JIVET*, 3, 284, 1986.
7. **Mohr, L. R., Trounson, A. O., Leeton, J. F., and Wood, C.,** Evaluation of the human egg *in vitro*, in *Fertilization of the Human Egg in vitro*, Beier, H. M. and Linder, H. R., Eds., Springer-Verlag, Berlin, 1983, 211.
8. **Lopata, A., Nayudu, P., Jones, G., and Abramczuk, J.,** The quality of human embryos obtained by in *vitro* fertilization, in *Human In Vitro Fertilization*, Testart, J. and Fryman, R., Eds., INSERM Symposium 24, Elsevier, Holland, 1985.
9. **Shire, J. G. M. and Whitten, W. K.,** Genetic variation in the timing of the first cleavage: Effect of parental genotype, *Biol. Reprod.*, 23, 363, 1980.
10. **Shire, J. G. M. and Whitten, W. K.,** Genetic variation in the timing of cleavage in mice: effect of maternal genotype, *Biol. Reprod.*, 23, 369, 1980.
11. **Evans, H. M. and Schulman, W.,** The action of vital stains belonging to the benzydene group, *Science*, 39, 443, 1914.
12. **Schrek, R.,** A method for counting the viable cells in normal and malignant cell suspensions, *Am. J. Cancer*, 28, 389, 1936.
13. **Holmberg, B.,** On the permeability to lissamine green and other dyes in the course of cell injury and cell death, *Exp. Cell Res.*, 22, 406, 1961.
14. **Malinin, T. I. and Perry, V. P.,** A review of tissue and organ viability assays, *Cryobiology*, 4, 101, 1967.
15. **Bellve, A. R.,** Development of mouse embryos with abnormalities induced by parental heat stress, *J. Reprod. Fertil.*, 35, 393, 1973.
16. **Hutz, R. J., DeMayo, F. J., and Dukelow, W. R.,** The use of vital dyes to assess embryonic viability in the hamster, Mesocricetus Auratus, *Stain Technol.*, 60, 163, 1985.
17. **Schilling, E., Niemann, H., Cheng, S. P., and Doepke, H.-H.,** DAPI — a further fluorescence test for diagnosing the viability of early cow and rabbit embryos, *Zuchthyg.*, 14, 170, 1979.

18. Schilling, E., Niemann, H., and Smidt, D., Evaluation of fresh and frozen cattle embryos by fluorescence microscopy, in *In vitro Fertilization and Embryo Transfer,* Hafez, E.S.E. and Semm, K., Eds., Alan R. Liss, New York, 1982, 349.
19. Renard, J.-P., Menezo, Y., and Heyman, Y., Alternative tests to assess viability of bovine embryos, *Theriogenology,* 17, 106, 1982.
20. Rotman, B. and Papermaster, B. W., Membrane properties of living mammalian cells as studied by enzymatic hydrolysis of fluorogenic esters, *Proc. Natl. Acad. Sci. U.S.A.,* 55, 134, 1966.
21. Mohr, L. R. and Trounson, A. O., The use of fluorescein diacetate to assess embryo viability in the mouse, *J. Reprod. Fertil.,* 58, 189, 1980.
22. Kola, I. and Folb, P. I., Chlorpromazine inhibits the mitotic index, cell number, and formation of mouse blastocysts, and delays implantation of CBA mouse embryos, *J. Reprod. Fertil.,* 76, 527, 1986.
23. Whittingham, D. G., Viability assays, in *Frozen Storage of Laboratory Animals,* Zeilmaker, G.H., Ed., Gustav Fischer, Stuttgart, 1981, 95.
24. Hoppe, R. W. and Bavister, B. D., Evaluation of the fluorescein diacetate (FDA) vital dye viability test with hamster and bovine embryos, *Anim. Reprod. Sci.,* 6, 323, 1984.
25. Pruitt, J. A., Wilson, J. M., Kraemer, D. C., Forrest, D. W., and Evans, J. W., Viability of equine embryos following fluorescein diacetate staining, *Theriogenology,* 29, 291, 1988.
26. O'Neill, C. and Saunders, D. M., Assessment of embryo quality, *Lancet,* ii, 1035, 1984.
27. Ryan, J. P., Spinks, N. R., O'Neill, C., and Wales, R. G., Implantation potential and foetal viability of mouse embryos cultured in media supplemented with platelet-activating factor, *J. Reprod. Fertil.,* 89, 309, 1990.
28. Spinks, N. R. and O'Neill, C., Embryo-derived platelet-activating factor is essential for establishment of pregnancy in the mouse, *Lancet,* i, 106, 1987.
29. Spinks, N. R., Ryan, J. P., and O'Neill, C., Antagonists of embryo-derived platelet-activating factor act by inhibiting the ability of the mouse embryo to implant, *J. Reprod. Fert.,* 88, 241, 1990.
30. Milligan, S. R. and Finn, C. A., Failure to demonstrate platelet activating factor involvement in implantation in mice, *J. Reprod. Fertil.,* 88, 105, 1990.
31. Amiel, M. L., Duquenne, C., Benveniste, J., and Testart, J., Platelet aggregating activity in human embryo culture media free of PAF-acether, *Hum. Reprod.,* 4, 327, 1990.
32. Smal, M. A., Dziadek, M., Cooney, S. J., Attard, M., and Balbo, B. A., Examination for platelet-activating factor production by preimplantation mouse embryos using a specific radioimmunoassay, *J. Reprod. Fertil.,* 90, 419, 1990.
33. Biggers, J. D., Whittingham, G. D., and Donahue, R. P., The pattern of energy metabolism in the mouse oocyte and zygote, *Proc. Natl. Acad. Sci. U.S.A.,* 58, 560, 1967.
34. Brinster, R. L., Studies on the development of mouse embryos *in vitro:* IV Interaction of energy sources, *J. Reprod. Fertil.,* 10, 227, 1965.
35. Brinster, R. L. and Thomson, J. L., Development of eight-cell mouse embryos *in vitro, Exp. Cell Res.,* 42, 308, 1966.
36. Renard, J.-P., Philippon, A., and Menezo, Y., *In vitro* uptake of glucose by bovine blastocysts, *J. Reprod. Fertil.,* 58, 161, 1980.
37. Rieger, D., The measurement of metabolic activity as an approach to evaluating viability and diagnosing sex in early embryos, *Theriogenology,* 21, 138, 1984.
38. Leese, H. J. and Barton, A. M., Pyruvate and glucose uptake by mouse ova and preimplantation mouse embryos, *J. Reprod. Fertil.,* 72, 9, 1984.
39. Gardner, D. K. and Leese, H. J., Non-invasive measurement of nutrient uptake by single cultured preimplantation mouse embryos, *Hum. Reprod.,* 1, 25, 1986.
40. Gardner, D. K. and Leese, H. J., Assessment of embryo viability prior to transfer by the non-invasive measurement of glucose uptake, *J. Exp. Zool.,* 242, 103, 1987.

41. **Gardner, D. K. and Leese, H. J.,** The role of glucose and pyruvate transport in regulating nutrient utilization by preimplantation mouse embryos, *Development,* 104, 423, 1988.
42. **Gardner, D. K. and Leese, H. J.,** Concentrations of nutrients in mouse oviduct fluid and their effects on embryo development and metabolism *in vitro, J. Reprod. Fertil.,* 88, 361, 1990.
43. **Leese, H. J., Hooper, M. A. K., Edwards, R. G., and Ashwood-Smith, M. J.,** Uptake of pyruvate by early human embryos determined by a non-invasive technique, *Hum. Reprod.* 1, 181, 1986.
44. **Hardy, K., Hooper, M. A. K., Handyside, A. H., Rutherford, A. J., and Leese, H. J.,** Non-invasive measurement of glucose and pyruvate uptake by individual human oocytes and early embryos, *Hum. Reprod.,* 4, 188, 1989.
45. **Gott, A. L., Hardy, K., Winston, R. M. L., and Leese, H. J.,** Non-invasive measurement of pyruvate and glucose uptake and lactate production by single human preimplantation embryos, *Hum. Reprod.,* 5, 104, 1990.
46. **Leese, H. J., Gardner, D. K., Gott, A. L., Handyside, A. H., Hardy, K., Hooper, M. A. K., Rutherford, A. J., and Winston, R. M. L.,** Non-invasive biochemical methods for assessing human embryo quality, in *Advances in Assisted Reproductive Technologies,* Mashiah, S., Ed., Plenum Press, New York, 1990, 737.
47. **Gardner, D. K., Clarke, R. N., Lechene, C. P., and Biggers, J. D.,** Development of a noninvasive ultramicrofluorometric method for measuring net uptake of glutamine by single preimplantation mouse embryos, *Gamete Res.,* 24, 427, 1989.
48. **Biggers, J. D., Gardner, D. K., and Leese, H. J.,** Control of carbohydrate metabolism in preimplantation mammalian embryos, in *Growth Factors in Mammalian Development,* Rosenblum, I.Y. and Heyner, S., Eds., CRC Press, Boca Raton, FL, 1989, 19.
49. **Bergmeyer, H. U. and Gawehn, K.,** *Methods of Enzymatic Analysis,* 2nd ed., Academic Press, New York, 1974.
50. **Lowry, O. H. and Passonneau, J. V.,** A flexible system of enzymatic analysis, Academic Press, New York, 1972.
51. **Barbehenn, E. K., Wales, R. G., and Lowry, O. H.,** The explanation for the blockage of glycolysis in early mouse embryos, *Proc. Natl. Acad. Sci. U.S.A.,* 71, 1056, 1974.
52. **Barbehenn, E. K., Wales, R. G., and Lowry, O. H.,** Measurement of metabolites in single preimplantation embryos; a new means to study metabolic control in early embryos, *J. Embryol. Exp. Morphol.,* 43, 29, 1978.
53. **Hsieh, B., Chi, M. M., Knor, J., and Lowry, O. H.,** Enzymes of glycogen metabolism and related metabolites in preimplantation mouse embryos, *Dev. Biol.,* 72, 342, 1979.
54. **Chi, M. M., Manchester, J. K., Yang, V. C., Curato, A. D., Strickler, R. C., and Lowry, O. H.,** Contrast in levels of metabolic enzymes in human and mouse ova, *Biol. Reprod.,* 39, 295, 1988.
55. **Palmisano, J. and Schwartz, J. H.,** Microassays for glucose 6-phosphate and 6-phosphogluconate based on bioluminescent techniques, *Anal. Biochem.,* 126, 409, 1982.
56. **Wienhausen, G. and DeLuca, M.,** Bioluminescent assays of picomole levels of various metabolites using immobilized enzymes, *Anal. Biochem.,* 127, 380, 1982.
57. **Robrish, S. A., Curtis, M. A., Sharer, S. A., and Bowen, W. H.,** The analysis of picomole amounts of L(+) and D(−) lactic acid in samples of dental plaque using bacterial luciferase, *Anal. Biochem.,* 136, 503, 1984.
58. **Idahl, L. A., Sandstrom, P. E., and Sehlin, J.,** Measurement of serum glucose using the luciferin/luciferase system and a liquid scintillation spectrometer, *Anal. Biochem.,* 155, 177, 1986.
59. **Rotman, B.,** Measurement of activity of single molecules of B-D-galactosidase, *Proc. Natl. Acad. Sci. U.S.A.,* 47, 1981, 1961.
60. **Jonkind, J. F., Ploem, J. S., Reuser, A. J. J., and Galjaard, H.,** Enzyme assays at the single cell level using a new type of microfluorimeter, *Histochemistry,* 40, 221, 1974.

61. **Mroz, E. A. and Lechene, C.,** Fluorescence analysis of picolitre samples, *Anal. Biochem.*, 102, 90, 1980.
62. **Rutili G., Arfors, K. E., and Ulfendahl, H. R.,** Fluorescence measurements in nanolitre samples, *Anal. Biochem.*, 72, 539, 1976.
63. **Leese, H. J.,** Non-invasive methods for assessing embryos, *Hum. Reprod.*, 2, 435, 1987.
64. **Leese, H. J., Biggers, J. D., Mroz, E. A., and Lechene, C.,** Nucleotides in a single mammalian ovum or preimplantation embryo, *Anal. Biochem.*, 140, 443, 1984.
65. **Gardner, D. K., Spitzer, A., and Osborn, J. C.,** Development of a complex serum-free medium and its effects on the development and metabolism of the preimplantation human embryo, *Proc. Am. Fertil. Soc.*, 164, 1991.

Chapter 11

CRYOPRESERVATION OF OOCYTES AND EMBRYOS

Jillian M. Shaw, Apichart Oranratnachai, and Alan Trounson

TABLE OF CONTENTS

I. Introduction 214
   A. Background 214
   B. Cryobiological Principles of Slow Cooling 215
      1. Seeding 215
      2. Cryoprotectants 217
   C. Cryobiological Principles of Rapid Cooling 218

II. Materials and Methods 220
   A. General Equipment 220
      1. Containers for Liquid Nitrogen 221
      2. Freezing Straws and Tubes 221
      3. Cryoprotectants and Cryoprotectant Additives 222
      4. Water Baths 222
      5. Other Equipment 222
      6. Solutions 222
      7. Other Considerations 223
   B. Freezing Protocols 223
      1. General Guidelines 223
      2. Propanediol Slow Cooling for Human Embryos 224
      3. Vitrification of Mouse Embryos 226
      4. Rapid 4.5 M DMSO Freezing of Mouse Embryos 226
      5 DMSO Slow Cooling for Mouse Oocytes 230
      6. Vitrification of Mouse Oocytes 231
      7. Rapid 4.5 M DMSO Freezing of Mouse Oocytes 232

III. Discussion 233

Acknowledgments 234

References 234

I. INTRODUCTION

The cryopreservation of gametes and embryos involves an initial exposure to cryoprotectants, cooling to subzero temperatures, storage, thawing, and finally, dilution and removal of the cryoprotectants, with return to a physiologic environment which allows further development. The cells must maintain their structural integrity throughout the cryopreservation procedure. Possibly the single most important principle of cryopreservation is to reduce damage caused by intracellular ice formation. This is usually achieved by dehydrating the cells before or during the cooling procedure. If dehydration is inadequate, large, intracellular crystals of ice may form, which damage the cells. Major factors known to affect survival of cryopreserved cells include the species, developmental stage, cryoprotectants, and method of cryopreservation.

Oocytes and embryos of humans and some, but not all, other mammalian species can be cryopreserved. In human *in vitro* fertilization programs, it is usually human embryos, not unfertilized oocytes, which are cryopreserved. Although it is desirable as it has fewer attendant social, moral and legal problems than embryo freezing, the freezing of unfertilized human oocytes is rarely performed, as the results are inferior to those of embryo freezing. Most currently available cryopreservation procedures for oocytes and embryos cause some reduction in viability as compared to unfrozen controls. The best rapid freezing procedures for the mouse do not cause any significant reduction in viability, and it is clear that future research must aim at improving freezing procedures for the human. This chapter presents the most commonly used protocol for human embryos (propanediol slow cooling), and details several procedures for mouse oocytes and embryos. Those for the mouse illustrate the three major freezing protocols available today (slow cooling, "ultra rapid freezing," and vitrification), and indicate a potential path along which freezing protocols for the human can develop.

A. BACKGROUND

Methods allowing biological tissues to be cryopreserved have been available for decades, but early attempts to freeze mammalian ovarian tissue, oocytes, or embryos met with limited success.[1,2] It was not until 1972 that preimplantation mammalian embryos were successfully cryopreserved. The first successful freezing methods for mammalian embryos were very time consuming, as they depended on slow cooling (1°C/min or less) to low subzero temperatures (around −80°C) before the embryos could be placed in liquid nitrogen.[3,4] Furthermore, embryos needed to be thawed slowly and the cryoprotectant added and removed in many small steps. Slow cooling methods also require freezing equipment which is capable of providing accurate cooling and warming rates. The slow cooling procedure is, however, very versatile and can give good survival rates for embryos over a range of developmental stages for many species. The first IVF pregnancies from cryopreserved human embryos resulted from the slow cooling procedure.[5]

Cryopreservation procedures used for mammalian eggs and embryos have advanced rapidly since 1972. Slow cooling protocols have been simplified, and made less time consuming.[6-9] A number of rapid cooling protocols have also been developed. The rapid freezing protocols allow embryos to be plunged directly into liquid nitrogen or liquid nitrogen vapor from temperatures of 0°C or above.[10-25] Rapid cooling methods usually require the presence of higher concentrations of cryoprotectants than the slow cooling procedures and have been used successfully to preserve oocytes and embryos ranging from the pronuclear to blastocyst stages of development. For the mouse it is now possible to obtain very high survival rates of oocytes with a freezing procedure involving less than 10 sec exposure to the cryoprotectant solution before plunging into liquid nitrogen.[26] Mouse preimplantation embryos can be frozen, with little loss of viability, using a 20 to 40 min (at 0°C) exposure to the cryoprotectant solution before direct transfer to liquid nitrogen.[24,25]

B. CRYOBIOLOGICAL PRINCIPLES OF SLOW COOLING

For many years, the large size of the mammalian oocyte and embryo made them impossible to freeze successfully, as most cooling procedures failed to prevent the lethal formation of intracellular ice crystals. It was not until 1972 that it became possible to freeze oocytes and embryos by slow cooling because of the increased understanding of (a) the reasons why slow (<1°/min) and fast cooling and warming rates differ; (b) the effects of seeding at high sub-zero temperatures (above 7°C); (c) the role of the cryoprotectants; and (d) ways of introducing and removing the cryoprotectant. The importance of each of these points is outlined below.

For every type of cell, there is an optimum rate of cooling. The maximal cooling rate for different cells may vary by several orders of magnitude.[8,27,28] The cooling velocity yielding optimum survival of mouse ova, for example, is about 2000 times less than for human red blood cells. Mathematical models based on observations of cells have been developed to explain and to some extent predict optimum cooling rates.[29-32] Such models have been particularly successful with mouse embryos.

The principal rate-limiting factor which governs the slow cooling procedure is the rate of passage of water through the cell membrane. This depends on (a) the composition and permeability characteristics of the cell membrane; (b) the surface-to-volume ratio of cells; (c) the temperature; and (d) the difference in osmotic pressure between the two sides of the membranes. These factors must be taken into account in dehydrating and rehydrating cells.[30,31] Cells which are cooled too slowly do not survive cryopreservation well because of so-called "solution effects." This is thought to be caused by the prolonged exposure of cells to high concentrations of salts and other solutes.[27,28]

1. Seeding

For some cell types, it is not necessary to manually induce ice formation in the external solution, but for large cells it is very important for consistent rates of success because it prevents supercooling and starts the dehydration process. The highest temperature at which physiological saline solutions and most cryoprotectant solutions used for slow cooling can be made to freeze lies around $-3°C$. If ice formation is not initiated by seeding, the solution will remain unfrozen until a much lower subzero temperature is reached. It is possible for solutions to be supercooled by as much as $15°C$ below the "true" freezing point. This property is important for embryo freezing because ice formation is associated with a rise in temperature as the latent heat of fusion is released, and because ice formation removes water from both the solution and the embryo. When ice formation is initiated at a high subzero temperature, ice spreads slowly through the solution, and there is a slow release of latent heat. This does not harm the embryo. When ice formation occurs in a deeply supercooled solution, however, the ice propagates very rapidly through the solution. This is detrimental to embryos because they remain fully hydrated when ice formation starts, increasing the likelihood of intracellular ice formation. Furthermore, there may be a significant temperature rise within the solution which, unless it is compensated for, will alter the cooling rate.

For most slow cooling protocols for embryos, ice formation is initiated manually, "seeded," at slightly supercooled temperatures (e.g., -5 to $-7°C$). The usual procedure is to make a small portion of the solution very cold, for example, by touching the wall of the container with an object cooled at $-196°C$. After seeding at one point, ice spreads throughout the entire solution.

When solutions are seeded at -5 to $-7°C$, ice crystals do not spread into the cells of the embryo because of the marginally higher osmolarity (lower freezing point) of their intracellular environment. Following seeding, the concentration of the solutes in the nonfrozen fraction gradually increases as water is incorporated into the extracellular ice crystals. The increasing concentration of extracellular solutes generates an osmotic gradient across the cell membrane, which draws water out of the cell causing the cell to dehydrate. By cooling sufficiently slowly, nearly all of the available water can be removed from the cell, with the result that the cell is not damaged when plunged into liquid nitrogen. Although this prevents intracellular ice crystal formation, severe dehydration can be detrimental, especially if cells are thawed rapidly. Thus, in practice, the dehydration process is stopped before this point, and intracellular freezing is induced by placing the container directly into liquid nitrogen. Under these conditions, either small, harmless intracellular ice crystals or glasses (a homogeneous rather than a crystalline solid) form. The plunging temperature is usually between -30 and $-80°C$, and depends on a number of factors, especially the anticipated thawing rate.

The warming rate is critical for the success of slow cooling procedures, because it determines the extent to which ice crystals grow during warming. Most protocols used today terminate the cooling step at temperatures between -30 and $-40°C$, and straws are warmed in air or in a water bath. When straws are plunged after slow cooling to $-80°C$, a slower warming rate ($8°C$ per min) is better.

Optimal warming rates depend on the cell type frozen and, very importantly, on the amount of water in cells when intracellular freezing occurs.[27,28] If a small amount of intracellular water is present when the cell is plunged, small ice crystals can form. Under these circumstances, rapid thawing rates are essential because slow warming rates allow the small ice crystals time to grow into larger, damaging ice crystals. This process is known as recrystallization.

If cells are cooled slowly so that they are nearly completely dehydrated when they are plunged into liquid nitrogen, recrystallization does not occur or is very limited even with slow warming. These cells may, however, be damaged by rapid warming because of extreme, rapid changes in osmolarity in the dehydrated cells. Slow warming, as it gives more time for the cells to rehydrate, is best for severely dehydrated cells. Thus, optimal warming rates depend critically on the cooling procedure.

2. Cryoprotectants

The role of the cryoprotectants is to protect biological materials from damage by ice crystals and high concentrations of solutes.[27,28] All freezing methods developed to date rely on the presence of one or more cryoprotectants. Cryoprotectants and cryoprotectant additives may be divided into two groups, intracellular (penetrating) and extracellular (nonpenetrating) agents. Examples of penetrating cryoprotectants include glycerol, dimethyl sulphoxide (DMSO), ethylene glycol, and 1,2-propanediol (PROH); these have molecular weights of less than 100. The compounds which, as a result of their size or polarity, remain in the extracellular solution include large sugar molecules such as sucrose, ficoll, and raffinose, as well as proteins and lipoproteins. Frequently, egg yolk, milk, and blood serum are used in combination with other cryoprotectants because they contain such molecules.[33]

The mode of action of cryoprotectants is complex. Their protective properties may be attributable to a number of properties. Adding a cryoprotectant causes a slight lowering of the freezing point of the solution, but at the concentrations used for slow cooling procedures, they only lower the freezing point by between 2 and 3°C. Their protective effects stem more from their ability to bond to water and their apparent ability to reduce the toxic effects of high concentrations of other compounds (their so-called colligative properties).[34] Most of the permeating cryoprotectants are very water soluble and have appreciable heats of solution, indicating that they alter water structure by breaking hydrogen bonds. They are also capable of forming hydrogen bonds with water molecules. With glycerol and 1,2-propanediol, the hydrogen bonding is between the hydrogen of the OH groups and the water oxygen. The oxygen on the DMSO molecules bonds with water protons with the release of heat.

Two additional properties of cryoprotectants help protect cells during slow cooling, when the cells are very dehydrated and are surrounded by concentrated salts. The cryoprotectants appear to reduce damage caused by high levels of salt, a property known as salt buffering. At high concentrations, cryoprotectants also help minimize damage by ice formation, as they cause the water to form a glass rather than ice crystals; this is called vitrification.

For slow cooling procedures, cryoprotectant concentrations are usually around 1.5 M, many times higher than any other component in the medium. Thus the cryoprotectants enter the cells by osmosis. While the cryoprotectants readily cross the cell membranes, water usually crosses even more readily, which can lead to problems. Cells placed in a cryoprotectant solution shrink as the water rapidly leaves the cells to dilute the high concentration of extracellular solutes. However, as the cryoprotectant enters the cell, an equilibrium is re-established and the cell will return to (or near) its original size. A more serious problem is created when permeating cryoprotectants need to be removed. When a cell which contains cryoprotectant is placed in medium containing a lower concentration of cryoprotectant, water enters the cells to dilute the cryoprotectant more rapidly than the cryoprotectant can leave the cells. This causes cells to swell, or even burst. This problem can be reduced by removing the cryoprotectant in a series of 3 to 10 steps, of progressively lower concentrations of cryoprotectant (e.g., 1.5, 1.0, 0.5, 0.25 M). This does not prevent the cells from swelling, but it reduces the magnitude of swelling. When cells have returned to their normal size (equilibrated) with a solution they can be moved to the next solution (usually 3 to 10 min/step).

An alternative and a more rapid method for removing cryoprotectants from cells is to use a high concentration of a nonpenetrating molecule such as sucrose (MW 342.3). The high extracellular concentration of the nonpenetrating molecule counterbalances the high concentration of cryoprotectant in the cell, as it reduces the difference in osmolarity between the inside and the outside of the cell. Cells containing cryoprotectant may even shrink when placed in a concentrated sucrose solution (e.g., 1.0 M), indicating that both the cryoprotectant and the water are leaving the cell. The use of high concentrations of sucrose usually allows the cryoprotectant to be removed in one step; thus it is both simpler and faster than those procedures which remove the cryoprotectant by dilution alone.

There are a large number of studies investigating the usefulness of slow cooling procedures for mammalian oocytes.[8,35-37] Several live births have been reported both for the human[38,39] and for other species,[40] but it is becoming increasingly evident that unfertilized eggs can be damaged by temperatures below 37°C or by the cryoprotectant alone.[41-43] As a result, there is now considerable interest in developing rapid cooling procedures, in particular for the mammalian oocyte.

C. CRYOBIOLOGICAL PRINCIPLES OF RAPID COOLING

Slow cooling is carried out at low cryoprotectant concentrations using slow cooling rates. Embryos and oocytes can also be frozen using rapid cooling procedures. Rapid cooling methods can be classified depending on (a) the cryoprotectant concentration and (b) the cooling procedure. "Vitrification" procedures use very high concentrations of cryoprotectant to make the solution and its contents vitrify (form a glass-like solid rather than ice crystals on cooling) and allow this glassy state to be retained during warming.[34,44] Lower cryoprotectant concentrations (intermediate between those used for slow cooling and those used for vitrification) allow ice crystal formation to occur at some stage of the cooling and warming procedure. Procedures which use these lower cryoprotectant concentrations are generally known as rapid freezing or ultrarapid freezing procedures. The methods may use direct or stepwise cooling procedures. In many procedures straws are plunged directly from room temperature or 0°C into liquid nitrogen. Cooling in the vapor phase is also commonly used. Holding steps at other temperatures may also be used.

Vitrification may be defined as a physical process by which a highly concentrated solution of cryoprotectants solidifies during cooling without the formation of ice crystals. The solid, called a glass, retains the normal molecular and ionic distribution of the liquid state and can be considered to be an extremely viscous supercooled liquid.[9,14,34,44,45] Vitrification has certain advantages over freezing because it avoids the damage caused by intracellular ice formation and the osmotic effects caused by extracellular ice formation. The theories behind vitrification as a method for cryopreservation have been described by several workers.[9,14,34] A vitrification solution needs to consist of one or more cryoprotectants in excess of 40% (v/v). The original vitrification solution which consisted of 20.5% DMSO, 15.5% acetamide, 10% propanediol, and 6% ethylene glycol allowed a successful cryopreservation of mouse 8-cell embryos.[44] This solution is, however, toxic to cells at 20°C, so embryos are usually only exposed to the final concentrated solution at low temperatures (0 to 4°C). Revision of the initial composition of vitrification solutions, i.e., combinations of glycerol (6.5 M) and polyethylene glycol (6%) or glycerol (25%) with propanediol (25%), or 40% ethylene glycol, 30% ficoll, and 0.5 M sucrose, have reduced their toxicity and have made the method a little easier to use.[46] Vitrification and other rapid freezing protocols have been used for mammalian oocytes, but the results are very variable, and there is considerable evidence for cryoprotectant toxicity.[8,47,48] The introduction of very short exposure times for oocyte freezing may, however, overcome the problems of cryoprotectant toxicity, as excellent fertilization rates and developmental rates *in vivo* have been achieved by using only a 5 to 10 sec equilibration period.[26]

In addition to vitrification procedures, there are now a number of rapid freezing procedures for embryos. The "rapid" or "ultrarapid" freezing procedures generally use lower solute concentrations in conjunction with short exposure times to reduce the problems of cryoprotectant toxicity.[23,49] Although rapid freezing procedures can be used with cryoprotectant concentrations as low as those used for slow cooling procedures (1 to 1.5 M), some studies have indicated that they give better results when used with cryoprotectant concentrations of around 4 to 4.5 M.[16,25] The lower concentrations were associated with chromosomal aberrations, possibly as a result of ice forming in the solution during cooling. Solutions which contain relatively high (35%) concentrations of solutes will vitrify on cooling but form ice during the warming step.

At lower concentrations, ice forms during the cooling phase. The extent to which crystallization occurs increases as the solute concentration is reduced.

It is possible that most cell types can be cryopreserved by rapid cooling techniques if nontoxic conditions can be identified for exposure of the cells to concentrations of cryoprotectants high enough to vitrify or to produce innocuous ice during cooling or warming.

Rapid cooling methods do not follow the equilibrium curve for cooling and cell water content.[9] They rely on the presence of high concentrations of cryoprotectants and cryoprotectant additives, such as acetamide, polyethylene glycol, or sucrose. The additives perform various functions; large non-permeating molecules such as sucrose, Ficoll, and PEG reduce the water content of the cell, and the acetamide is added as it is thought to reduce the toxicity of cryoprotective agents such as DMSO. High concentrations of cryoprotectant will on their own cause cells to dehydrate because water diffuses out of the cell faster than the cryoprotectant can enter the cell. The high intracellular concentrations of cryoprotectant in the fully equilibrated cell have the potential to be toxic to cells, in particular at higher temperatures. Lowering the temperature of exposure of cells to cryoprotectant to around 0°C reduces toxicity and slows the rate of diffusion of cryoprotectant across the cell membrane. By carefully selecting the duration of exposure to the cryoprotectant solution, selecting the composition of the cryoprotectant solution, or adjusting the temperature of exposure it is possible to identify windows with lower toxicity, which will improve the survival of cryopreserved cells. When the total solute concentration exceeds 40%, the solutions will tend to vitrify (form a glass) instead of crystallizing when rapidly cooled. Vitrification avoids the occurrence of lethal intracellular ice and osmotic effects caused by freezing of the extracellular solution.

II. MATERIALS AND METHODS

A. GENERAL EQUIPMENT

Freezing procedures require liquid nitrogen. The volume of liquid nitrogen needed will depend on the freezing procedure chosen, the type of biological freezer, the size and specifications of the storage tanks, and the frequency of use of the equipment. It is usual to use 20 to 100 liters each week. Liquid nitrogen is potentially dangerous, and must be handled with care. Pure nitrogen gas can asphyxiate living organisms. Tanks must therefore be kept in a well-ventilated area to remove the nitrogen gas which evaporates from the tanks. Eye and hand protection should be worn to prevent frostbite. Liquid nitrogen spills are difficult to avoid, and it is important to consider that most types of laboratory floor coverings will crack when liquid nitrogen is spilled on them. Spills of liquid nitrogen which saturate a person's clothing require immediate action, i.e., that he remove the affected clothing and shoes immediately.

1. Containers for Liquid Nitrogen

Liquid nitrogen will evaporate from storage tanks at a rate determined by the efficiency of the storage tank. When purchasing a tank for liquid nitrogen, the required storage capacity should be considered as well as its weight (when full), the neck width, insulation properties, and whether the materials are going to be stored in goblets or on canes. Wide-necked tanks are more convenient as storage containers but tend to allow faster evaporation of the liquid nitrogen. The insulation properties of a storage tank can decline very markedly with age. Old or second hand tanks may, as a result, be uneconomical. A spare tank can be useful when searching for lost straws or goblets. The spare tank enables the canisters with frozen materials to be placed in the backup tank while the storage tank is thoroughly searched (or emptied). In addition to the storage tanks, a small container is required to hold and carry liquid nitrogen. A wide-necked stainless steel container of approximately 1 l capacity is ideal, but polystyrene containers or other well-insulated containers provide a much cheaper and acceptable alternative. We do not recommend evacuated glass vacuum flasks, because they are potentially very dangerous because they may explode, causing injury from glass fragments and liquid nitrogen burns.

2. Freezing Straws and Tubes

Oocytes and embryos are usually frozen in plastic straws, plastic tubes, or glass ampoules. Plastic 0.25 ml bovine insemination straws IMV AA 201, or similar straws, e.g., IMV ZA 029 or IMV ZA 142 (IMV, L'Aigle, France) are normally available from suppliers of veterinary products or of products for artificial breeding of domestic animals. Straws are available in a range of colors and can be used as supplied by the manufacturer. We do not sterilize or wash plastic straws before use because we have found that sterilization of these insemination straws by irradiation can have detrimental effects on the freezing properties of the straws.[50] Straws may, if required, be sterilized using ethylene oxide. Nunc cryotubes (1 ml 375353) with caps are available from scientific suppliers. Sample tubes with pop tops, such as those used for standard biochemical procedures, can be used, but they become very brittle in liquid nitrogen. If they are used, we recommend that the tops not be used, or that the tops be perforated before use to prevent explosions. Glass vials have the advantage that embryos can be seen through the side, but they are more fragile than cryotubes and can explode if not properly sealed.

Straws can be sealed by heat, polyvinyl alcohol (cold water soluble, e.g., Sigma P-8136), or Polyvinylpyrrolidone powder (Sigma PVP). Heat sealers, such as those used to seal plastic bags or autoclave bags, can usually be used to seal plastic insemination straws; the temperature of the sealer should be approximately 95°C. Glass vials can be either flame sealed or sealed by pushing a plastic tube over the neck of the vial. The plastic tubes should be heated in boiling water to soften them before being pushed onto the vial.

Materials from the same patient or experiment are usually stored together in storage goblets or on canes. To prevent the goblets or the straws or vials inside them from floating away, it is advisable to place a heavy object (e.g., a coin or a pellet of lead) in the goblet and to wedge tissue paper into the opening.

3. Cryoprotectants and Cryoprotectant Additives

The cryoprotectants and cryoprotectant additives used in this chapter are dimethyl sulfoxide (DMSO) $CH_3.SO.CH_3$ M.W. 78.13 (Sigma D 8779, or D 2650), propane-1,2-diol (1,2-propanediol or propylene glycol) $CH_3.CH(OH).CH_2OH$ M.W. 76.10 (Sigma P 1009), acetamide $CH_3.CO.NH_2$ M.W. 59.07 (Sigma A 0500), polyethylene glycol (PEG) M.W. 8000 (Sigma P 2139), sucrose M.W. 342.3 (Sigma S 9378), and Ficoll M.W. 70 000 (Sigma F 2878). These chemicals should be stored and handled as indicated. It is advisable to read the specification sheets for each chemical; these sheets can be obtained from the supplier or local distributor.

4. Water Bath

Stirred water baths with accurate temperature control can be obtained from scientific suppliers.

5. Other Equipment

Other equipment used for most freezing protocols includes (1) marker pens with fine tips, used to label dishes, straws and tubes. These must be resistant to water; (2) accurate timers which, ideally, have a countdown alarm; (3) sharp scissors, needed to give a clean cut when removing the ends of straws; (4) syringes (0.5 to 1 ml) with flexible tubing, with a diameter the same as that of the straw, needed to aspirate and eject solutions from straws; (5) glass pipettes, used to handle embryos. Glass Pasteur pipettes can be finely drawn over a flame to give an opening only slightly larger than the embryos. These should be attached to mouth pipettes or to a rubber bulb; (6) to search for straws or goblets lost in the liquid nitrogen, a torch and tongs with very long handles or blades; (7) large artery forceps or the equivalent, useful to manipulate straws and tubes within liquid nitrogen.

Slow cooling procedures require a biological freezer. This can be home-made, or purchased ready made, from major scientific, medical, or agricultural suppliers. There are many varieties available, in a wide range of price brackets. The price is determined by the machine's complexity, whether it is manual or automatic, whether it is self-seeding or not, and if it can be programmed. The price is not necessarily a guarantee of reliability.

6. Solutions

Hepes buffered Medium M2[51] pH 7.2 to 7.4, is usually used for the handling of oocytes and embryos and for the cryopreservation solutions. Other buffers, such as Dulbecco's phosphate buffered saline, may also be used. Buffers may be made or purchased.

7. Other Considerations

Before beginning a human embryo cryopreservation program, consideration needs to be given to the establishment and running costs, recordkeeping, patient consent forms, storage levies, and storage times.

1. Costs may include the purchase of a biological freezer, storage tanks, protective mask and gloves, and an appropriate floor covering resistant to liquid nitrogen spills. Running costs include liquid nitrogen and liquid nitrogen delivery fees;
2. It is important to ensure that an appropriate recordkeeping system is in place before any embryos are frozen. It is also essential that all straws, ampoules, or tubes are clearly labelled (with non-water soluble markers) and their position in the storage tank is recorded;
3. For human oocyte or embryo freezing, patient consent forms approved by the governing institution are generally required;
4. Decisions also need to be made concerning (a) how many and what quality of embryos should be transferred in the collection vs. subsequent cycles, (b) whether frozen embryos should be returned in natural cycles or cycles with some stimulation, (c) what degree of monitoring there should be in the replacement cycles, and (d) the timing of the replacement relative to the age of the embryos;
5. It is helpful to devise incentive schemes to encourage couples to return promptly to have their frozen embryos replaced (e.g., storage levies). To prevent the accumulation of "unwanted" embryos, there should be a policy governing the maximum length of time that the embryos should be kept in storage, and how the "unwanted" embryos should be disposed of.

B. FREEZING PROTOCOLS
1. General Guidelines

All procedures outlined below require the following equipment: finely drawn glass pipettes, a marker pen, timers, liquid nitrogen in a container, a water bath, 35 mm petri dishes, cryoprotectant solution, buffer, and equilibrated culture medium into which the oocytes or embryos are placed after the thawing procedure is complete. The procedures which use straws also require a heat sealer (or sealing compound), a pair of sharp scissors, and a small syringe with flexible tubing, which can be used to expel the contents of the straw.

The following are some general rules for freezing and thawing:

1. Always clearly label tubes, straws, and goblets or canes, with a fine tipped indelible marker pen; labelling should be completed before freezing is started;
2. All embryos should be collected and moved in a way which minimizes the volume of fluid accompanying the embryo. This is usually done using a drawn Pasteur pipette with an opening just wider than the embryo, and by having air bubbles or oil in front of and behind the embryo;

3. Fresh pipettes should be used for each new solution;
4. Good records must be kept;
5. The liquid nitrogen level in the storage tanks must be maintained;
6. Always take care when removing straws and tubes from storage, as they may be filled with liquid nitrogen. Liquid nitrogen inside straws or vials rapidly expands when they are removed from the storage tank. The rapidly expanding gas can cause straws and ampoules to explode, so appropriate safety precautions are absolutely essential. The danger can be reduced by holding the straw or tube in the vapor phase just above the liquid nitrogen until all liquid nitrogen has evaporated.

2. Propanediol Slow Cooling for Human Embryos

This procedure is used quite successfully for human embryos at early stages of development. Embryos are equilibrated with propanediol, and slow cooled in straws. They are thawed rapidly, and are rehydrated in several steps. For the cooling procedure, allow 2 to 4 h, for the thawing procedure allow 45 to 60 min.

The following provides the detailed procedure:

1. Start by checking your embryos. Most IVF groups have found that poor embryos do not survive freezing well, and therefore only freeze healthy looking embryos;
2. Check the freezer and, if necessary, start it to get the chamber temperature to +20°C;
3. Using buffer containing 20% serum makeup and filter, sterilize a 1.5 M propanediol solution (e.g., 1.1 ml propanediol to 8.9 ml buffer), and a 1.5 M propanediol +0.1 M sucrose solution (add 1.1 ml propanediol and 8.9 ml buffer to 0.342 g sucrose). Add 1 to 2 ml of the 1.5 M propanediol solution to one labeled 35 mm petri dish and 1 to 2 ml 1.5 M propanediol +0.1 M sucrose to another 35 mm petri dish;
4. Take a labeled straw with the appropriate dimensions for your freezing apparatus, pre-rinsed in 1.5 M propanediol with 0.1 M sucrose;
5. Place the embryo(s) in the dish with 1.5 M propanediol, for 10 to 15 min at room temperature. Then move the embryo(s) to the dish with 1.5 M propanediol +0.1 M sucrose. The embryos should then be loaded into the straws immediately by either using the syringe and tubing to aspirate the solution containing the embryo into the straw, or by collecting the embryo in the pipette and loading it into a cryoprotectant bead in the straw;
6. The straw should be sealed and then placed in the freezing chamber (20°C);
7. As soon as the last straw has been loaded, start the cooling procedure. It is essential that all loading be complete within 15 min.
    a. Cool at 2°C/min to −8°C;
    b. Hold for 10 min at −8°C; seed (at a point well away from the embryos) the straws a few minutes into this hold period. Check that the ice

spreads over to the section with embryos and that this ice does not melt. Ice must be visible in all straws before proceeding;
c. Cool at –0.3°C/min to –30°C;
d. Cool at –50°C/min to –150°C;
e. Hold for 2 h at –150°C, then transfer to your small liquid nitrogen canister.

Insert the straws into marked goblets (precooled to –196°C). Before putting the goblet in the tank, it may be necessary to wedge the straws inside it by stuffing tissue paper in the top; this prevents straws from floating out of the goblet. Do not let the straws warm up during any of these transfer procedures;
8. Make sure all paperwork is completed.

Certain equipment and steps should be used in the thawing procedure.
Have ready marked dishes (petri dishes or a multiwell dish), a waterbath at 30°C, scissors, a syringe with tubing, tissues, and a timer. For this post-thaw rehydration procedure, it is more convenient to use labelled nunc 4-well dishes than 35 mm petri dishes. The dishes/wells should contain at least 0.6 ml of the following solutions:

1. 1.0 M propanediol + 0.2 M sucrose in buffer
2. 0.5 M propanediol + 0.2 M sucrose in buffer
3. 0.2 M sucrose in buffer
4. Buffer alone

The following are the steps of the procedure:

1. Start timer, remove straw from LN, wipe dry with a tissue, and hold (by end not containing embryos) in air for a total of 30 sec, then plunge into a 30°C waterbath for 40 to 50 sec;
2. Remove from water, wipe dry, cut seals off both ends of the straw, and gently (to ensure that all liquid stays in the straw) attach 1 ml syringe with tubing;
3. Gently expel into 1.0 M propanediol + 0.2 M sucrose. If the embryo is not found, suck the solution back into the straw and let it rest for 5 min, then try expelling the contents again. Look for the embryo and isolated zonae; if the embryo is still unaccounted for, then vigorously suck the solution up and down the straw until it is found or deemed lost;
4. After 10 min in solution 1, the embryos should be moved to solution 2 for 5 min, then solution 3 for 10 min and solution 4 for 10 min at room temperature; then move the whole nunc dish to 37°C for 10 min;
5. The embryo is now ready to be placed in culture medium with 20% serum, for continued culture or transfer;
6. If the embryo(s) survived, arrange for embryo transfer.

3. Vitrification of Mouse Embryos

This rapid freezing procedure is a modification of the vitrification procedure developed by Kasai et al.[46] for morula stage mouse embryos. Embryos are equilibrated with a 40% ethylene glycol, 30% Ficoll 70,000, 0.5 M sucrose solution at 20°C for 2 to 5 min and then plunged into liquid nitrogen. They are thawed rapidly, washed in a 0.5 M sucrose solution followed by buffer, then cultured. For the cooling procedure, allow 2 to 5 min; for the warming procedure, allow 5 to 10 min.

In addition to general equipment listed above (see Section II.B.1), this procedure requires cryoprotectant solution containing ethylene glycol, Ficoll, and sucrose, and a wash solution containing 0.5 M sucrose. All embryo handling procedures are carried out at room temperature (20°C).

The following are details of the freezing procedure:

1. Prepare the cryoprotectant solution. The final solution contains 40% by volume ethylene glycol, 18% w/v Ficoll (70,000), and 0.3 M sucrose;
2. Label the insemination straws and fill them with 20 to 30 μl cryoprotectant solution;
3. The container that the straws are going to be plunged into must contain at least 5 cm of liquid nitrogen;
4. Embryos are collected in a minimal volume of buffer in a finely drawn glass pipette and then inserted into the cryoprotectant in the straw;
5. Seal the straw and, after a total equilibration period of 2 to 5 min, plunge the straw into liquid nitrogen.

The following are details of the thawing procedure:

1. Move straws from the storage tank to a canister containing at least 5 cm liquid nitrogen;
2. Ensure that no liquid nitrogen is trapped in the straw; if necessary hold the straw in the vapor phase;
3. Rapidly immerse the straw fully in water at 20°C;
4. As soon as the solution has liquefied, expel the contents gently into a dish containing 0.5 M sucrose;
5. After 5 min, transfer the embryos to a dish containing buffer.

4. Rapid 4.5 M DMSO Freezing of Mouse Embryos

This procedure is suitable for preimplantation mouse embryos (pronuclear to blastocyst stage) but is best for mouse embryos before compaction.[24,25] Embryos are equilibrated with a 4.5 M DMSO, 0.25 M sucrose solution at 20 or 0°C, and then plunged into liquid nitrogen. They are thawed rapidly, washed in a 0.25 M sucrose solution followed by buffer, then cultured. For the cooling procedure, allow 3 to 40 min; for the warming procedure, allow 10 to 20 min.

In addition to general equipment listed above (see Section II.B.1), this procedure requires cryoprotectant solution containing 4.5 M DMSO and 0.25

M sucrose, and wash solution containing 0.25 M sucrose. If the prefreeze equilibration procedure is carried out at 0°C the following additional equipment is needed: an ice bath at 0°C, a thermometer, and to prevent temperature fluctuations inside the straw while the embryos are being inserted, insulating material or a precooled metal block which fits around the straw. The metal blocks produced by Cryogenetic Technology are ideal (cryoprism, Cryogenetic Technology, Soquel, CA).

The following are details of the freezing procedure:

1. Make up cryoprotectant solution by weighing out 0.86 g sucrose into a 10 ml graduated container, e.g., a Falcon 2001 tube. Add 5 ml buffer containing 8 mg crystalline bovine serum albumin/ml (BSA). When the sucrose has dissolved, add 3.3 ml dimethyl sulphoxide (DMSO). If the DMSO is all added at once, the solution may become cloudy; this can be avoided by adding several smaller aliquots (e.g., 1.1 ml DMSO) and mixing the solution thoroughly after each addition. The final volume should then be made up to 10 ml with buffer;
2. The freezing properties of the cryoprotectant solution used for this procedure must be checked before it is used on embryos. This is done by aspirating 25 µl cryoprotectant into a 250 µl insemination straw, sealing it, and then plunging the straw into liquid nitrogen. The plunged cryoprotectant solution should be transparent (i.e., vitrified), it must not be cloudy or have opaque areas (ice), as this indicates a too low cryoprotectant concentration. If ice forms, the solution must be remade. The cryoprotectant solution can retain its freezing properties for at least one month if stored at −18 to −20°C, but the solution must be discarded if it ceases to vitrify when plunged into liquid nitrogen;
3. Decide which equilibration temperature to use. The optimum equilibration temperature for mouse embryos differs depending on the stage of development. Two and eight-cell embryos can be frozen after equilibration at either 20 or 0°C, but blastocyst stage mouse embryos must be equilibrated at 0°C. Equilibration at 0°C gives marginally better results,[24] but it is a more difficult procedure.

The following steps comprise the procedure for equilibration at 20°C:

4. Collect embryos into a dish with buffer;
5. Transfer the embryos with a minimal amount of buffer into the cryoprotectant solution (30 µl) in the insemination straw, using a finely drawn glass pipette (usually 10 to 20 embryos per straw);
6. Heat seal the straw at one end as close to the cryoprotectant bead as possible (preferably 2 mm). If straws are frozen with a large air space between the seal and the CP bead, the bead is sucked towards the seal when the straw is plunged (as the cold causes the air to shrink); this gives very nonuniform survival;

7. As soon as the straw is sealed, it should be laid horizontally on the bench, to ensure that all embryos have time to sink onto the inner surface of the straw;
8. After 2 to 3 min, plunge the straw into liquid nitrogen.

For equilibration at 0°C, the procedure is largely as described above, except that for work at 0°C, the straws containing cryoprotectant should be precooled and should be heat sealed at both ends to prevent water from entering. Cool the loaded, sealed straws in a water/ice bath at 0 or 1°C. Try to reduce temperature changes in the cryoprotectant bead while the straws are removed from the bath to insert the embryos. This can be achieved by wrapping the straw in foam or clamping the straw into a molded metal block at 0°C (e.g., the "cryoprism" see above). After inserting the embryos, the straw is resealed and returned to the 0°C waterbath. At the end of the equilibration period (6 to 10 min for pronuclear embryos; 20 to 40 min for all other stages), straws are removed from the waterbath, rapidly wiped dry, and immediately plunged into liquid nitrogen. For the best results, it is essential that the cryoprotectant bead in the straw (at 0°C) does not warm up while the embryos are inserted or when the straws are plunged at the end of the equilibration period. If possible, place a thermocouple in dummy straws and perform the whole procedure to check for temperature changes.

The following are details of the thawing procedure:

1. Before placing straw in the waterbath, hold the straw in the vapor phase until there is no liquid nitrogen left inside the straw;
2. Thaw the straw by rapidly moving it from the liquid nitrogen (or LN2 vapor) into a water bath at 35 to 37°C;
3. As soon as the cryoprotectant solution melts (3 sec), remove the straw from the water, rapidly wipe it dry, and cut off the sealed end;
4. Expel the thawed solution gently but rapidly into the bottom of a dish with 2.5 to 3 ml of medium M2 containing 0.25 M sucrose (0.86 g/10 ml) at room temperature (as an approximate guide, there should be 1 ml sucrose solution for each 10 µl cryoprotectant solution expelled from the straw. To reduce accidental embryo losses, it is best to stop the straw from flicking as the seal is removed by holding the straw firmly near the seal while it is being cut and the syringe with tubing attached.);
5. The contents of the dish should not be agitated for the first 3 min, as this causes rapid changes in osmolarity and reduces embryo viability;
6. After 5 to 10 min, the embryos can be transferred to a dish with buffer to remove the sucrose;
7. After 10 min in the buffer, the embryos can be transferred to droplets of culture medium.

Certain other notes should be made for the 4.5 M DMSO procedure. The concentration of DMSO must not be reduced below 33%, as this allows ice to

TABLE 1
Troubleshooting for the 4.5 M DMSO Rapid Freezing Procedure

Problem	Solution
Straw develops cracks on freezing	Try smaller beads of solution
Cryoprotectant cracks on freezing	Sucrose concentration may be too high
Straw explodes on thawing	Hold straw in vapor until all LN2 has evaporated
Water enters straw	Improve seal, use new straws as old straws seal poorly
CP turns milky on adding DMSO	Add DMSO stepwise, mix well each time
CP turns milky on freezing	Not enough cryoprotectant, CP solution old
CP bead moves on freezing	Air space too big, seal closer to bead Seal insufficient
Bubbles in straw and embryos on thawing	Straw batch, straw irradiation
Embryos stick in straw	Add more BSA, or change BSA batch
CP flicks out of straw	Hold close to end being cut
Writing comes off	Use permanent ink
Embryo swells in post-thaw solution(s)	Solution agitated too much Incorrect composition of solutions Do not have less than 1 ml 0.25 M sucrose per 10 µl expelled cryoprotectant
Zona lysis	Indicates poor freezing conditions Straw or BSA batch, straw irradiation
Poor embryo recovery rates	Embryo insertion technique needs to be improved, straws flicked when the seal is removed. Batch of BSA not optimal, try another supplier.

form when the straw is plunged into liquid nitrogen. Ice formation during cooling has been linked to chromosomal damage in mouse embryos. If this freezing procedure is performed correctly, the majority of embryos should be found after freezing, the blastomeres and zonae should be intact, and the embryos should resume development within 24 h in culture. Some potential problems, and their remedies are listed in Table 1. It is important to remember that frozen embryos cannot "perform" better than nonfrozen embryos; thus embryos of a mouse strain which develop poorly if collected at or before the 2-cell stage should be collected after the 2-cell stage. Furthermore, the success of embryo transfers generally declines as time in culture is increased. Embryos frozen at the pronuclear or 2-cell stage should therefore be transferred to the oviducts of day 1 recipients, rather than being cultured and transferred to the uterus. This 4.5 M DMSO freezing procedure is not well suited for mouse oocytes.

The following section discusses oocyte freezing protocols. Mice ovulate approximately 12 to 14 h after the administration of hCG. The oocytes should be collected within 2 h of ovulation to minimize their susceptibility to parthenogenetic activation.[43] Oocytes can be collected from the oviduct and frozen, either as intact cumulus masses or following removal of the cumulus using hyaluronidase solution. The results of cumulus intact and cumulus denuded oocytes may differ. Optimal results with unfertilized oocytes require both good freezing and good *in vitro* fertilization procedures. The success rates for mouse *in vitro* fertilization can fluctuate widely; thus it is advisable to practice on nonfrozen mouse oocytes until consistent IVF results can be obtained. One mouse IVF protocol is outlined below.

The day before the IVF procedure, prepare the following solutions and let them equilibrate overnight at 37°C 5% CO_2: (a) a dish with modified T6 + BSA (lactate and pyruvate free) (250 µl per pair of cauda) under oil, (b) modified T6 + BSA (20 µl) under oil, (c) culture drops (20 µl), and, if needed, (d) hyaluronidase solution (250 µl). It is very important not to let the sperm cool down at any stage. The cauda from each male should be placed immediately into the warm 250 µl drop of mT6. The cauda should be cut rapidly into pieces and the dish then returned to the incubator to allow the sperm to swim out of the ducts. Groups of eggs are placed in the 20 µl drops in the incubator for 10 min before insemination. Using a prewarmed pipette tip, aspirate 1 µl of the sperm solution and add it to the egg drop. The sperm quality starts to deteriorate after 3 to 4 h. The oocytes should be moved to a culture drop 1 to 3 h after insemination. The addition of fetal calf serum (FCS) to the collection, sucrose, wash, and insemination solutions may help reduce problems with zona hardening.

5. DMSO Slow Cooling for Mouse Oocytes

Cumulus enclosed or cumulus denuded oocytes are slow cooled to a low subzero temperature before being placed in liquid nitrogen. For the cooling step, allow approximately 190 min; for the thawing step, allow at least 30 min.

This procedure requires the following equipment: a 0°C icebath, a biological freezer, glass vials and plastic caps, a container with boiling water, a wide bore pipette to remove solutions from the vial, cryoprotectant solution with 3 *M* DMSO, and buffer.

The following are details of the procedure:

1. Prepare a 0°C icebath and precool a sterile 3.0 *M* DMSO solution and labelled glass vials containing 0.3 ml buffer;
2. Check the biological freezer and precool it to 0°C;
3. Place oocytes or cumulus masses in the precooled buffer at 0°C for 10 min;
4. Slowly add 0.3 ml of the 3.0 *M* DMSO solution to the oocytes, cap the vials, and equilibrate for 15 min;
5. Place the vials in the biological freezer and start the cooling program.

Cool from 0°C to –7°C at 0.5°C per min. At –7°C, wait 5 min to ensure that the core temperature of the straw is at 7°C.

Seed the sample (away from the oocytes) by touching the sucrose fraction with a metal object precooled in liquid nitrogen. Confirm that ice formation has occurred and has spread through the solution. Maintain the temperature at −7°C for about 10 min after the solution containing the embryos has frozen.

Cool at 0.5°C per min to −80°C.
Cool rapidly to −196°C.
The following are details of the thawing procedure.

1. Precool the biological freezer to −80°C;
2. Make sure there is no liquid nitrogen trapped inside the ampoule. If there is, hold the ampoule in the liquid nitrogen vapor phase until it has all evaporated. This reduces the risk of the ampoule exploding;
3. Cut the end of the cap off and then place the vial in the biological freezer for the thawing procedure;
4. Warm the vials at 8°C per min to +4°C;
5. Slowly add 2.4 ml buffer at 4°C;
6. Allow the diluted contents to return to room temperature and let it equilibrate for 20 min;
7. Remove the eggs or cumulus masses from the vial and wash them in two changes of buffer before placing the eggs in culture.

6. Vitrification of Mouse Oocytes

This procedure, described by Nakagata,[26] is appropriate for cumulus denuded but not cumulus enclosed mouse oocytes. Oocytes are equilibrated with a vitrification solution for less than 10 sec and then plunged into liquid nitrogen. They are thawed rapidly while simultaneously adding the diluent (0.3 M sucrose). For the cooling procedure, allow 10 sec; for the warming procedure, allow 10 min.

This procedure requires a micropipettor to measure out volumes of 20 to 30 μl, labelled 0.5 ml freezing tubes, a waterbath at 37°C, syringe and needle, equilibrated HTF containing 20% fetal calf serum, cryoprotectant in PBS, 0.3 M sucrose solution + 20% FCS and PBS + 20% FCS. The freezing and thawing procedures are carried out at room temperature.

The following are details of the procedure:

1. Make up cryoprotectant solution, in a tube (e.g., Falcon 2001). Weigh out 1.97 g DMSO (2.53 M), 1.39 g acetamide (2.36 M), 0.9 g propanediol (1.19 M), and 0.54 g polyethylene glycol (5.4%). Make up to 10 ml with PBS containing 16 g/ml BSA. The acetamide gives this solution a low pH, but this need not be adjusted. Solutions should be made up on the day of use;
2. Collect the cumulus masses from the oviducts, and place them in a hyaluronidase solution which does not activate oocytes. Once the cumulus has dissolved, wash the oocytes in several changes of equilibrated HTF containing 20% fetal calf serum (at 37°C, covered by liquid paraffin).

Culture the washed oocytes in HTF + 20% FCS for 20 min. The oocytes are now ready to be frozen;
3. Insert 20 to 30 µl cryoprotectant solution into labeled 0.5 ml cryo tubes;
4. Insert small numbers of oocytes (<10) into the cryoprotectant. It is essential that no excess fluid accompany the oocytes; therefore, use a pipette only marginally wider than the oocytes, and use beads of oil or air, rather than medium, above and below the bead with the oocytes;
5. Cap the tube, tap the tube against the bench several times to ensure that all fluid is in the bottom of the tube, and then insert it into the liquid nitrogen.

Below are details of the thawing procedure:

1. Have ready a 37°C waterbath, and a 1 ml syringe containing 0.3 to 0.4 ml of a 0.3 M sucrose solution;
2. Lift the cryo tube into the LN2 vapor to let the liquid nitrogen escape, and then remove the cap;
3. Place the lower part of the tube in the waterbath, and after a few seconds, when the solution just starts to change its appearance, inject the sucrose solution. This should be done so that all the cryoprotectant is mixed up as it thaws;
4. Use a clean Pasteur pipette to move the contents of the tube into a petri dish;
5. Collect all oocytes as soon as possible, wash them in an excess of fresh 0.3 M sucrose, followed by a rinse in buffer, and then place them into culture drops;
6. After 5 to 15 min in medium (HTF + 20% FCS), the oocytes can be placed in the insemination drops.

This procedure can also be carried out using plastic 0.25 ml insemination straws. The procedures are then the same as outlined below for rapid DMSO oocyte freezing. Excellent results can also be obtained using VS1, which has a slightly higher cryoprotectant concentration (DMSO 2.62 M, acetamide 2.62 M, propylene glycol 1.3 M, polyethylene glycol 6% wt/vol).

7. Rapid 4.5 M DMSO Freezing of Mouse Oocytes

This procedure only differs from the rapid freezing method for mouse embryos, in that it uses shorter equilibration times, a higher sucrose concentration in the cryoprotectant, and straws frozen in the vapor phase rather than being plunged into liquid nitrogen. It is suitable for cumulus denuded and cumulus enclosed mouse oocytes.

For most steps, the freezing procedure is identical to that outlined for embryo freezing.

1. 10 ml of the oocyte cryoprotectant solution contains 1.72 g sucrose and 3.3 ml DMSO;

2. Oocytes with or without cumulus are transferred with a minimal amount of buffer into the cryoprotectant solution (30 µl) in the insemination straw, using a finely drawn glass pipette (usually 10 oocytes per straw);
3. Heat seal the straw at one end as close to the cryoprotectant bead as possible (preferably 2 mm);
4. The total equilibration time for oocytes with cumulus is 20 to 30 sec, and for oocytes without cumulus 8 to 20 sec. To increase the mixing of the oocytes with the cryoprotectant within this very short equilibration time, it is possible to flick the straw gently after it has been sealed, allowing the air bubbles that this creates to move through the cryoprotectant;
5. At the end of the equilibration period, the straws are cooled in the vapor phase of the liquid nitrogen. This reduces damage caused by the cryoprotectant cracking on cooling and warming. Vapor cooling can be achieved by floating a polystyrene raft (0.5 to 1 cm thick) on the surface of the liquid nitrogen.

The following thawing procedure can be used:

1. Before placing straw in the waterbath, hold the straw in the vapor phase until there is no liquid nitrogen left inside the straw;
2. Thaw the straw by moving it rapidly from the liquid nitrogen (or LN2 vapor) into a water bath at 35 to 37°C;
3. As soon as the cryoprotectant solution melts (3 sec), remove the straw from the water, rapidly wipe it dry, and cut off the sealed end;
4. Expel the thawed solution gently but rapidly into the bottom of a dish with 2.5 to 3 ml of medium M2 containing 0.25 M sucrose (0.86 g/10 ml) at room temperature;
5. The contents of the dish should not be agitated for the first 3 min, as this causes rapid changes in osmolarity and reduces oocyte viability;
6. After 5 to 10 min, the oocytes can be transferred to a dish with buffer; remove the sucrose;
7. After 10 min in the buffer, the oocytes can be transferred to droplets of insemination medium.

III. DISCUSSION

The freezing protocols in this chapter represent a small selection of the range of options which are available. The protocol for human embryos is very widely used and achieves relatively consistent results. A number of other freezing protocols have been used for human embryos, including rapid cooling procedures, but the success rates have been low, and few ongoing pregnancies or live births have been achieved. For the species on which most research has been performed, the mouse, freezing procedures have been optimized to the extent that the development of frozen thawed embryos, *in vitro* and *in vivo*, is not statistically reduced as compared to their nonfrozen controls.[24] It has yet to be established whether freezing protocols can be optimized to this extent for mouse oocytes and eggs and embryos of other species. Freezing procedures suited to a particular species are not necessarily suitable for other cell stages or other species. The reason for these differences probably reflects differences in cell volume, membrane permeability, and composition, tolerance to cryoprotectant toxicity, lipid content, and other as yet unrecognized factors.

It is likely that oocytes and embryos of some species will prove to be much more difficult to cryopreserve than those of the mouse, but advances in our understanding of cryobiology may ultimately result in freezing protocols to suit oocytes and embryos of most species, including man.

ACKNOWLEDGMENTS

We would like to thank Dr. M. Wood and Dr. G. Jones for information on the mouse and human slow cooling protocols.

REFERENCES

1. **Green, S. H., Smith, A. U., and Zuckerman, S.**, The numbers of oocytes in ovarian autografts after freezing and thawing, *J. Endocrinol.*, 13, 330, 1956.
2. **Parrott, D. M. V.**, The fertility of mice with orthotopic ovarian grafts derived from frozen tissue, *J. Reprod. Fertil.* 1, 230, 1960.
3. **Whittingham, D. G., Leibo, S. P., and Mazur, P.**, Survival of mouse embryos frozen to −196°C and −269°C, *Science,* 178, 411, 1972.
4. **Wilmut, I.**, The effect of cooling rate, warming rate, cryoprotective agent, and stage of development on survival of mouse embryos during freezing and thawing, *Life Sci.,* 11, 1071, 1972.
5. **Trounson, A. and Mohr, L.**, Human pregnancy following cryopreservation, thawing and transfer of an eight-cell embryo, *Nature,* 305, 707, 1983.
6. **Willadsen, S. M.**, Factors affecting the survival of sheep embryos during freezing and thawing, in *CIBA Foundation Symposium 52, "The Freezing of Mammalian Embryos"*, Elliot, K. and Whelan, J., Eds., Elsevier/North Holland, Amsterdam, 1977.
7. **Whittingham, D. G., Wood, M., Farrant, J., Lee, H., and Halsey, J. A.**, Survival of frozen mouse embryos after rapid thawing from −196°C, *J. Reprod. Fertil.,* 56, 11, 1979.
8. **Friedler, S., Giudice, L. C., and Lamb, E. J.**, Cryopreservation of embryos and ova, *Fertil. Steril.,* 49, 743, 1988.
9. **Mazur, P.**, Equilibrium, quasi-equilibrium, and nonequilibrium freezing of mammalian embryos, *Cell Biophysiol.,* 17, 53, 1990.
10. **Biery, K. A., Seidel, G. E., Jr., and Elsden, R. P.**, Cryopreservation of mouse embryos by direct plunging into liquid nitrogen, *Theriogenology,* 25, 140, 1986.
11. **Miyamoto, H. and Ishibashi, T.**, Liquid nitrogen vapor freezing of mouse embryos, *J. Reprod. Fertil.,* 78, 471, 1986.
12. **Szell, A. and Shelton, J. N.**, Sucrose dilution of glycerol from mouse embryos frozen rapidly in liquid nitrogen vapour, *J. Reprod. Fertil.,* 76, 401, 1986.

13. **Szell, A. and Shelton, J. N.**, Osmotic and cryoprotective effects of glycerol-sucrose solutions on day-3 mouse embryos, *J. Reprod. Fertil.*, 80, 309, 1987.
14. **Rall, W.F.**, Factors affecting the survival of mouse embryos cryopreserved by vitrification, *Cryobiology,* 24, 387, 1987.
15. **Rall, W. F., Wood, M. J., Kirby, C., and Whittingham, D. G.**, Development of mouse embryos cryopreserved by vitrification, *J. Reprod. Fertil.*, 80, 499, 1987.
16. **Trounson, A., Peura, A., and Kirby, C.**, Ultra-rapid freezing: a new low cost and effective method of embryo cryopreservation, *Fertil. Steril.*, 48, 843, 1987.
17. **Trounson, A., Peura, A., Freemann, L., and Kirby, C.**, Ultrarapid freezing of early cleavage stage human embryos and eight-cell mouse embryos, *Fertil. Steril.*, 49, 822, 1988.
18. **Bongso, A., Ng, S. C., Sathananthan, H., Lee, M.-L., Mok, H., Wong, P. C., and Ratnam, S.**, Chromosome analysis of two-cell mouse embryos frozen by slow and ultrarapid methods using two different cryoprotectants, *Fertil. Steril.*, 49, 908, 1988.
19. **Reinthaller, A., Kainz, Ch., Deutinger, J., and Bieglmayer, Ch.**, Development of mouse embryos following conventional and ultra rapid cryopreservation, *Arch. Gynecol. Obstet.*, 244, 33, 1988.
20. **Wilson, L. and Quinn, P.**, Development of mouse embryos cryopreserved by an ultra-rapid method of freezing, *Hum. Reprod.*, 4, 86, 1989.
21. **Takahashi, Y. and Kanagawa, H.**, Effect of equilibration period on the viability of frozen-thawed mouse morulae after rapid freezing, *Mol. Reprod. Develop.*, 26, 105, 1990.
22. **Van der Auwera, I., Cornillie, F., Ongkowidjojo, R., Pijnenborg, R., and Koninckx, P. R.**, Cryopreservation of pronucleate mouse ova: slow versus ultrarapid freezing, *Hum. Reprod.*, 5, 619, 1990.
23. **Trounson, A.**, Cryopreservation, *Brit. Med Bull.*, 46, 695, 1990.
24. **Shaw, J. M., Diotallevi, L., and Trounson, A. O.**, A simple rapid dimethyl sulphoxide freezing technique for the cryopreservation of one-cell to blastocyst stage preimplantation mouse embryos, *Reprod. Fertil. Dev.*, 3, 621, 1991.
25. **Shaw, J. M., Kola, I., MacFarlane, D.R., and Trounson, A.**, An association between chromosomal abnormalities in rapidly frozen 2-cell mouse embryos and the ice-forming properties of the cryoprotective solution, *J. Reprod. Fert.*, 91, 9, 1991.
26. **Nakagata, N.**, High survival rate of unfertilized mouse oocytes after vitrification, *J. Reprod. Fertil.*, 87, 479, 1989.
27. **Elliot, K. and Whelan, J.**, Eds., *CIBA Foundation Symposium 52, The Freezing of Mammalian Embryos,* Elsevier/North Holland, Amsterdam, 1977.
28. **Ashwood-Smith, M. J. and Farrant, J.**, Eds., *Low Temperature Preservation in Medicine and Biology,* Pitman Press, Bath, 1980.
29. **Leibo, S. P., McGrath, J. J., and Cravalho, E. G.**, Microscopic observation of intracellular ice formation in unfertilized mouse ova as a function of cooling rate, *Cryobiology,* 15, 257, 1978.
30. **Leibo, S.**, Water permeability and its activation energy of fertilized and unfertilized mouse ova, *J. Membr. Biol.*, 53, 179, 1980.
31. **Jackowski, S., Leibo, S. P., and Mazur, P.**, Glycerol permeabilities of fertilized and unfertilized mouse ova, *J. Exp. Zool.*, 212, 329, 1980.
32. **Mazur, P., Rall, W. F., and Leibo, S. P.**, Kinetics of water loss and the likelihood of intracellular freezing in mouse ova, *Cell Biophysiol.*, 6, 197, 1984.
33. **Kasai, M., Niwa, K., and Iritani, A.**, Effects of various cryoprotective agents on the survival of unfrozen and frozen mouse embryos, *J. Reprod. Fertil.*, 63, 175, 1981.
34. **Fahy, G. M.**, Vitrification, in *Low Temperature Biotechnology: Emerging Applications and Engineering Contributions,* McGrath, J. J. and Diller, K. R., Eds., BED-Vol. 10/HTD Vol. 98, 1989.
35. **Glenister, P. H., Wood, M. J., Kirby, C., and Whittingham, D. G.**, The incidence of chromosome anomalies in first-cleavage mouse embryos obtained from frozen-thawed oocytes fertilized in vitro, *Gamete Res.*, 16, 205, 1987.

36. **Trounson, A. and Kirby, C.,** Problems in the cryopreservation of unfertilized eggs by slow cooling in dimethyl sulfoxide, *Fertil. Steril.,* 52, 778, 1989.
37. **Carroll, J., Depypere, H., and Matthews, C. D.,** Freeze-thaw-induced changes of the zona pellucida explains decreased rates of fertilization in frozen-thawed mouse oocytes, *J. Reprod. Fertil.,* 90, 547, 1990.
38. **Chen, C..** Pregnancy after human oocyte cryopreservation, *Lancet,* 1, 884, 1986.
39. **Van Uem, J. F., Siebzehnrubl, E. R., Schuh, B., Koch, R., Trotnow, S., and Lang, N.,** Birth after cryopreservation of unfertilized oocytes, *Lancet* 1, 752, 1987.
40. **Schroeder, A. C., Champlin, A. K., Mobraaten, L. E., and Eppig, J. J.,** Developmental capacity of mouse oocytes cryopreserved before and after maturation in vitro, *J. Reprod. Fertil.,* 89, 43, 1990.
41. **Johnson, M. H.,** The effect on fertilization of exposure of mouse oocytes to dimethyl sulfoxide: an optimal protocol, *J. In Vitro Fertil. Embryo Transfer,* 6, 168, 1989.
42. **Pensis, M., Loumaye, E., and Psalti, I.,** Screening of conditions for rapid freezing of human oocytes: preliminary study toward their cryopreservation, *Fertil. Steril.,* 52, 787, 1989.
43. **Shaw, J. M. and Trounson, A. O.,** Parthenogenetic activation of unfertilized mouse oocytes by exposure to 1,2-propanediol is influenced by temperature, oocyte age and cumulus removal, *Gamete Res.,* 24, 269 1989.
44. **Rall, W. F. and Fahy, G. M.,** Ice-free cryopreservation of mouse embryos at −196°C by vitrification, *Nature,* 313, 573, 1985.
45. **Fahy, G. M., MacFarlane, D. R., Angell, C. A., and Meryman, H. T.,** Vitrification as an approach to cryopreservation, *Cryobiology,* 21, 407, 1984.
46. **Kasai, M., Komi, J. H., Takakamo, A., Tsudera, H., Sakurai, T., and Machida, T.,** A simple method for mouse embryo cryopreservation in a low toxicity vitrification solution, without appreciable loss of viability, *J. Reprod. Fertil.,* 89, 91, 1990.
47. **Kono, T. and Tsunoda, Y.,** Ovicidal effects of vitrification solution and the vitrification-warming cycle and establishment of the proportion of toxic effects on nuclei and cytoplasm of mouse oocytes, *Cryobiology,* 25, 197, 1988.
48. **Kola, I., Kirby, C., Shaw, J., Davey, A., and Trounson, A.,** Vitrification of mouse oocytes results in aneuploid zygotes and malformed fetuses, *Teratology,* 38, 467, 1988.
49. **Fahy, G. M.,** The relevance of cryoprotectant "toxicity" to cryobiology, *Cryobiology,* 23, 1, 1986.
50. **Shaw, J. M., Diotallevi, L., and Trounson, A. O.,** Ultrarapid embryo freezing: effect of dissolved gas and pH of the freezing solution and straw irradiation, *Hum. Reprod.,* 3, 905, 1988.
51. **Quinn, P., Barros, C., and Whittingham, D. G.,** Preservation of hamster oocytes to assay the fertilizing capacity of human spermatozoa *J. Reprod. Fertil.,* 66, 161, 1982.

Chapter 12

ULTRASTRUCTURE IN FERTILIZATION AND EMBRYO DEVELOPMENT

A. Henry Sathananthan

TABLE OF CONTENTS

I. Introduction 238

II. TEM Techniques 238
    A. Sperm Preparation 238
    B. Oocytes and Embryos 239
    C. Rapid Processing and Embedding Procedure 239

III. Sperm Structure and Function 240
    A. Effects of Centrifugation, Washing, and Layering 240
    B. Acrosome Reaction 240
    C. Sperm Morphology 241
    D. Frozen Sperm 241
    E. Immotile Sperm 243

IV. Oocyte Maturation 243

V. Organization of Gametes 247

VI. Fertilization *In Vitro* 248

VII. Inheritance of Paternal Centrioles 251

VIII. Early Embryonic Development 252

IX. Co-Culture of Embryos 254

References 258

I. INTRODUCTION

Assisted reproductive technology (ART) has advanced considerably since the first baby was born in England by *in vitro* fertilization (IVF) in 1978. Transmission electron microscopy (TEM) is being used in some research centers in ART for the assessment of gametes, fertilization, embryos, and the reproductive tract in the treatment of human infertility. Though it is time consuming, expensive, and invasive, it has played a significant role in our research programs in the development of techniques associated with ART and in understanding human gamete structure and function, fertilization, and early development, including aberrant features of these processes in the event of reproductive failure (see reviews in references 1–8). TEM is both precise and objective when compared to routine assessment by light microscopy (LM) and has been a very valuable research tool in our hands. The events that occur in the first week of human development (from conception to implantation), hitherto little known *in vivo*, have now been documented and the fine structure of gametes and embryos defined. This became possible with the advent of IVF and associated technologies.

Our research with TEM commenced in 1977 at the Queen Victoria Medical Centre, Melbourne, when we published some of the earliest pictures of human conception.[1,9,10] Thereafter, TEM was used routinely at the Monash Medical Centre, Melbourne and at affiliated research centers in Singapore. This has led to some important discoveries, particularly in gamete membrane fusion and interaction, microfertilization, and the inheritance of paternal centrioles in the human embryo. This paper reviews the contributions made by TEM in the development and understanding of various aspects of ART over the past decade in relation to the treatment of infertility. Since the procedures employed in routine TEM are universally known, our methods of handling sperm, oocytes, and embryos are presented.

II. TEM TECHNIQUES

A. SPERM PREPARATION

Sperm structure and function are assessed in pellets or at the egg surface after various procedures in ART. The pellets are centrifuged at 160 to 350 × *g* after each experimental procedure (see below) and fixed in standard fixative: 3% glutaraldehyde in 0.1 *M* cacodylate buffer (pH 7.2 to 7.3). This fixative is routinely used for gametes and embryos in order to compare their structure with those of somatic cells. The fixative is stable for 3 to 6 months and only needs to be stored at 4°C. Fixation is usually carried out at room temperature. Gelatin, agar, or agarose are not used to support the pellet. Once fixed, the material is stored in a cold room at 4°C until further processing. Usually processing is carried out rapidly soon after fixation.

B. OOCYTES AND EMBRYOS

Oocytes are fixed with the cumulus intact or after its removal with 0.1% bovine hyaluronidase using standard fixative, usually at room temperature. Removal of the cumulus facilitates quick serial sectioning of the oocyte. When preservation of the spindle is required, the fixative is warmed to 37°C in an oven before fixation. Similarly, for cooling experiments, the fixative is chilled to 0°C, before fixation. Embryos are fixed with remaining cumulus cells after ART. All fixed material is stored at 4°C or transported in fixative in small vials.

C. RAPID PROCESSING AND EMBEDDING PROCEDURE

1. Post-fixation: Glutaraldehyde is washed out in distilled water (10 min), and the specimens are post-fixed in 1% aqueous osmium tetroxide (20 to 30 min).
2. Dehydration:
   - 70% Ethyl Alcohol   10 min
   - 90% Ethyl Alcohol   5 to 10 min
   - 100% Ethyl Alcohol   5 to 10 min (two changes)
   - Acetone   5 to 10 min (two changes)
3. Embedding:
   - Acetone: Araldite mixture* (1:1)   10 to 15 min
   - Araldite mixture   3 h to overnight
   - Flat embed and orientate in Araldite in plastic or rubber molds
   - Polymerize in 60°C oven 24 to 48 h

*Araldite mixture is prepared fresh as follows:
Fluka AG Durcupan–ACM (Switzerland) is used for most specimens.

| AM | 5 ml | C | 0.3 ml |
| B | 5 ml | D | 0.3 ml |

Mix thoroughly before use and store if required at −20°C.
(NB. Epon resin or Epon/Araldite mixtures may be used as alternatives.)

4. Serial Sectioning:
   - Blocks are cut with a fine saw and mounted on wooden or resin stubs.
   - Alternative series of thick sections (1 µm) and thin sections (~70 nm) are cut using glass and diamond (Diatome) knives, respectively. LKB and Reichert ultramicrotomes are used for sectioning.
5. Staining and Microscopy:
   - Thick sections are stained with toluidine blue or methylene blue (in borax) at 70°C for LM.
   - Thin sections are stained (10 min) with alcoholic uranyl acetate (saturated solution in 70% alcohol) followed by Reynolds' lead citrate (10 min). Stains are washed out in distilled water.
   - In our studies, Philips (301 and 400T) and Jeol 1200 EX electron microscopes are used.

III. SPERM STRUCTURE AND FUNCTION

Assessment of sperm quality for ART has been an integral component of TEM work, in addition to laboratory assessment by LM and computerized sperm analysis by Cellsoft. The effects of centrifugation, washing, and layering of sperm by "swim-up" in various culture media used in ART are being evaluated.[11] Sperm were studied in pellets and also during penetration of egg-vestments to assess the physiological acrosome reaction (AR) and their capacity to penetrate the zona pellucida (ZP).[12]

A. EFFECTS OF CENTRIFUGATION, WASHING, AND LAYERING

TEM examination of sperm after processing for ART reveals some changes in sperm membrane structure. Sperm are usually washed and pelleted with medium at $350 \times g$ for 10 min during routine IVF. Centrifugation of semen without medium in order to pellet the sperm at $160 \times g$ or $350 \times g$ causes some swelling and rupture of the plasma membrane (PM) in about 80% of acrosome-intact sperm examined. Semen fixed without centrifugation also show such changes but to a lesser extent. This may be due to osmotic changes during the fixation process,[8,11] since the sperm PM is known to be difficult to fix for TEM. Sperm washed, centrifuged, and layered in IVF culture media (Earle's, Whittingham's T6, and Ham's F10) for 10 to 15 min also show similar changes, with further swelling and disruption of the PM. Such changes are also evident after Ficoll[13] or Percoll[14] separation with centrifugation. Sperm from male factor patients washed and pelleted in IVF media for sperm microinjection at higher speeds 3352 or $11,400 \times g$ may show considerable wrinkling of the acrosome or complete loss of PM. There is about a 5% decrease in motility after high-speed centrifugation, although the tails are still intact.[11]

B. ACROSOME REACTION

The early stages of the sperm acrosome can only be visualized by TEM. Our routine TEM studies have been on motile sperm harvested after washing, centrifugation, and "swim-up" in various culture media or after Ficoll or Percoll separation.[13,14] Both normospermic and severe oligo-asthenospermic sperm pellets were evaluated for morphology as well as for the sperm AR. Sperm pellets were examined 1 to 6 h after incubation at 37°C. The AR in culture media has been documented,[16,17] where partial decondensation of acrosome matrix followed by formation of vesicles within the acrosome during the early stages of the AR was observed, which is a deviation from the usual mammalian pattern.[18] The vesicles originate from the outer acrosomal membrane (OAM) alone or from both the PM and OAM, while the classical AR (see below) was observed consistently at the anterior end of the equatorial segment.[16] This sequence of events was observed in our pelleted sperm, capacitated in culture media.[11]

Chen and Sathananthan[12] reported the physiological AR at the surface of the oocyte, 1 to 3 h after insemination (Figures 1 and 2). In this study, the sister oocytes fertilized normally and produced viable IVF pregnancies. The classical AR, as observed in other mammals,[18] often occurs at the surface of the ZP, where vesiculation results by the intermittent fusion of the PM and OAM during the AR. Vesiculation may occur in two stages — the acrosome cap reacting first, followed by the equatorial segment of the acrosome.[19] Sperm initially bind to the surface of the ZP by their PM (Figure 1), and both acrosome-intact and acrosome-reacting sperm have been seen entering the ZP and penetrating between the cumulus cells. However, only acrosome-reacted sperm can penetrate the thickness of the ZP and enter the PVS,[19,20] to fuse with the oocyte (Figure 3). Recent studies have also shown that the ZP, oocyte-cumulus complexes, and follicular fluid induce the human AR.[21-24] The classical AR has also been reported in human sperm initiated by human follicular fluid.[23,24] The incidence of the AR varies with the method of induction employed. Capacitation, a physiological process, is a prerequisite for increasing the rate of the AR, which is usually assessed by staining for LM and by immunofluorescence.[25-27] The most reliable and objective method of assessment is by TEM. In the first 1 to 6 h, 10% sperm show evidence of the AR in pellets, which increase to about 15% after 24 h.[17] In the presence of cumulus-oocyte complexes, 31% of sperm initiated or completed the AR, 14 to 18 h after incubation.[22] Yudin et al.[23] capacitated sperm for 6 h and initiated the AR with human follicular fluid in 3 min in 40% of sperm. Sperm incubated and left overnight (24 h) at room temperature may show a higher incidence of the AR in T6 medium.[11] The rate of sperm capacitation and the incidence of the AR also seem to vary with the donor, even after overnight incubation. The best method for assessing the AR is to combine fluorescence with TEM[26] (Figure 4).

C. SPERM MORPHOLOGY

Sperm morphology has recently come into focus as a salient factor in IVF,[28,29] while motility appears to be the most important factor influencing the outcome of IVF.[30,31] Subtle sperm abnormalities that cannot be detected by LM can best be visualized by TEM.[32-34] Sperm abnormalities include defects of the acrosome, nucleus, midpiece, and tail components. Abnormal sperm with nuclear defects can penetrate the ZP, the PVS, and even the oocyte.[2,5,35,36] Whether such penetration will result in genetic defects or abnormal development has yet to be established.[15] Acrosomal, midpiece, and tail defects will, no doubt, affect sperm penetration of the egg vestments, since both the sperm AR and motility are involved in this process. Several workers have surveyed sperm tail defects in patients with absent or impaired motility[37-39] and have found a variety of axonemal aberrations deviating from the normal "9 + 2" organization of microtubules.

D. FROZEN SPERM

Some TEM studies on freezing of sperm have been conducted in conjunction with our clinical procedures.[8,11] The effects of routine freezing with

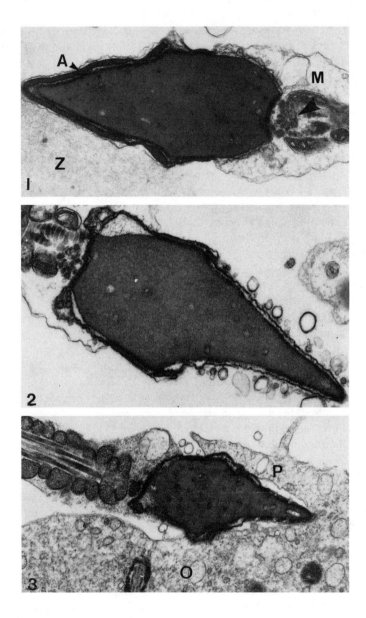

FIGURE 1. Sperm-binding: sperm PM bound to the surface of the ZP (Z). Note intact acrosome (A) and centriole in the neck region (arrow). M = midpiece. (Original magnification × 35,700.) (From Chen, C. and Sathananthan, A. H., *Arch. Androl.*, 16, 183, 1986. With permission.)
FIGURE 2. Sperm-AR: vesiculating sperm entering the ZP. The PM and outer acrosome membranes have fused, and the acrosome contents have been discharged. P = postacrosomal region. (Original magnification × 35,700.) (From Chen, C. and Sathananthan, A. H., *Arch. Androl.*, 16, 183, 1986. With permission.) **FIGURE 3.** Sperm-egg fusion: the postacrosomal region (midsegment) of the spermhead PM has fused with the oolemma. The egg has engulfed the spermhead by means of a process (P). O = ooplasm. (Original magnification × 19,600.) (From Sathananthan, A. H., Ng, S. C., Edirisinghe, R., Ratnam, S. S., and Wong, P. C., *Gamete Res.*, 15, 317, 1986. With permission.)

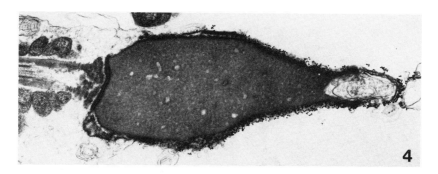

FIGURE 4. AR detected by concanavalin A-gold labeling: acrosome reacted sperm showing gold particles conjugated with Con A predominantly bound to the inner acrosome membrane. Sperm with intact acrosomes are not labeled. (Original magnification × 35,700.)

various cryoprotectants include subtle demembranation which may occur in some sperm.[40-42] Cryotreatment alters the viability, motility, and acrosomal function of sperm.[43] The PM and acrosome are most vulnerable to freeze-thaw. Spermheads with intact acrosomes with or without PM, those with swollen acrosomes and with loss of matrix, those with disrupted acrosomes, where both PM and outer acrosome membranes are absent or disrupted, and nude sperm without any surface membranes are the major types categorized by TEM.[11,41] However, the sperm AR does seem to occur in well-preserved frozen-thawed sperm, which resembles that observed in nonfrozen capacitated sperm in pellets.[11] This is not surprising since frozen sperm are used successfully for artificial insemination both *in vivo* and *in vitro*.[43] Further, cryopreserved sperm could well be used for microinjection and other procedures in ART.

E. IMMOTILE SPERM

The ultrastructure of sperm from five patients with immotile sperm was evaluated.[11] One of these donors had a few wriggling sperm with no forward progression, while another had many dead sperm. Two patients had chronic bronchitis with bronchial asthma, while the others had no associated clinical condition. The percentage of abnormal forms was high in four of the samples, and all possible distortions of the tail axoneme, fibrous sheath, midpiece, neck, and spermhead were evident. Dynein arms were lacking in the axonemes of two donors, while immature sperm, white blood cells, and bacteria were prevalent in two cases. However, there were sperm with normal heads, some undergoing the AR. Ultrastructural and clinical features associated with this syndrome have been reported.[44] Fertilization and embryo development have resulted after micromanipulation of immotile sperm from one patient, but there was no pregnancy after embryo transfer.[45,46]

IV. OOCYTE MATURATION

Preovulatory oocyte maturation is one of the prerequisites for successful IVF. In gonadotrophin stimulated cycles, multiple oocytes are recovered at

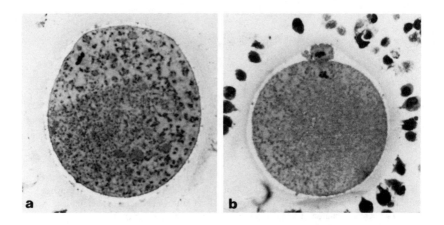

FIGURE 5. Light micrographs of thick sections of oocytes. (a) Metaphase I oocyte: note spindle with chromosomes at periphery; (b) Metaphase II oocyte: the chromosomes are in the ooplasm and in the first polar body. Note a few cumulus cells outside ZP. Both oocytes were cooled before fixation. (Original magnification × 600.) (From Sathananthan, A. H., Trounson, A. O., Freeman, L., and Brady, T., *Hum. Reprod.*, 3, 968, 1988. With permission.)

different stages of maturation, and it is necessary to culture some of these oocytes before insemination to ensure full maturity (see Chapter 3). Oocyte maturation includes both nuclear and cytoplasmic maturation of the germ cell and also involves the interaction of the surrounding follicle cells with the maturing oocyte via the ZP. The morphological events leading to oocyte maturation have been well documented.[2,4,20,47-51]

One of our priorities in IVF was to examine the stages of preovulatory oocyte maturation after gonadotrophin stimulation and to establish the fertilizability of the mature oocyte *in vitro*. Since the intermediate stages of maturation from the germinal vesicle (GV) stage to metaphase II (MII) cannot be visualized easily by phase-contrast or Nomarski optics, these had to be documented by TEM.[2,4,51] Occasionally GV oocytes are recovered during IVF, and GV breakdown occurs *in vitro*,[47] when the oocyte resumes meiosis (Figure 5). Maturation progresses from the GV stage (Figure 6) through metaphase I (Figure 7), the first polar body is abstricted, and meiosis is again arrested at MII (Figures 8 and 9), when the egg is ovulated. The second maturation division is completed at fertilization (Figure 10). Cortical maturation of the oocyte involves proliferation and migration of cortical granules (CG) beneath the oocyte cell membrane (oolemma).[52] This aspect of oocyte maturation is as significant as nuclear maturation and led to the crucial finding that oocytes should be matured *in vitro* for 3 to 6 h before insemination for IVF.[53] CG originate from Golgi membranes and microfilaments (MF) beneath the oolemma composed of actin seem to play a role in the surface migration of CG.[54] Recently, actin has been demonstrated by immunofluorescence in the egg cortex.[55] Cumulus cell structure and cumulus-oocyte interaction also reflect the state of preovulatory maturation. Gap junctions and desmosomes have been demonstrated between cumulus cell processes and the oocyte.[2,4,51] It is

Ultrastructure of Fertilization and Embryo Development 245

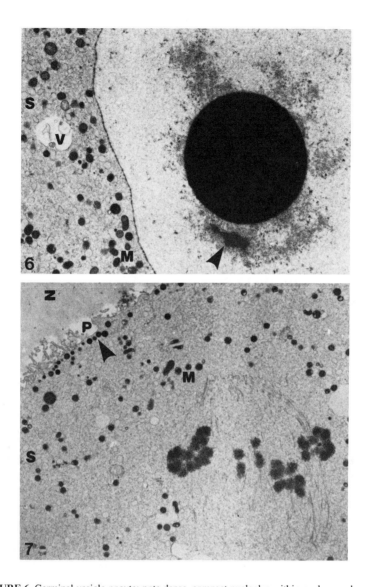

FIGURE 6. Germinal vesicle oocyte: note dense, compact nucleolus within nucleus and nuclear pores on envelope. M = mitochondria, S = vesicular SER, V = vacuole. (Original magnification × 11,900.) **FIGURE 7.** Metaphase I oocyte: the chromosomes are seen in pairs on the spindle and CG are at the surface (arrow). M = mitochondria, P = perivitelline space, S = vesicular SER, Z = ZP. (Original magnification × 7,000.) (From Sathananthan, A. H., *Gamete Res.*, 12, 385, 1985. With permission.)

also believed that the ZP undergoes a maturational process.[56] The architecture of the ZP, the gelatinous glycoprotein shell around the oocyte, is being investigated both by TEM and SEM.[57,58] It consists of fine fibrils and granules embedded in an amorphous matrix[2] and changes in its fine structure have been reported during oocyte maturation from MI to MII.[57] Familiari et al.[58] have

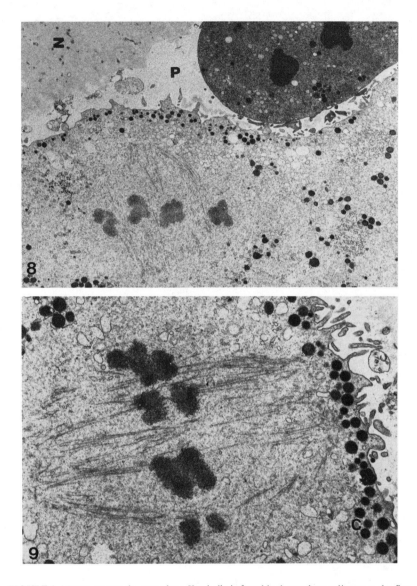

FIGURE 8. Mature oocyte: the metaphase II spindle is found in the ooplasm adjacent to the first polar body. P = perivitelline space; Z = ZP. (Original magnification × 7,000.) **FIGURE 9.** Metaphase II spindle of a mature oocyte: the spindle is barrel-shaped and consists of microtubules. The centrosomes are not well defined at the spindle poles, while chromosomes are located on the spindle equator. C = cortical granules. (Original magnification × 15,400.) (From Sathananthan, A. H., Trounson, A. O., Freeman, L., and Brady, T., *Hum. Reprod.*, 3, 968, 1988. With permission.)

demonstrated the surface architecture of the ZP using SEM. The ZP is antigenic and species specific and allows only human sperm to penetrate through it. Three glycoproteins have been identified in the ZP of mouse oocytes, one of which (ZP3) binds to sperm and induces the AR.[59] The identification of specific glycoproteins that compose the human ZP is a priority in oocyte

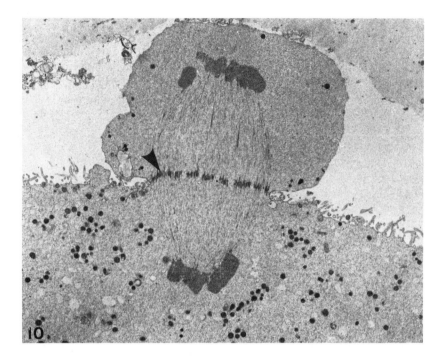

FIGURE 10. Fertilized ovum (3 h postinsemination): abstriction of the second polar body at fertilization. Note chromosomes at both ends of the telophase II spindle and dense interbody at constriction (arrow). (Original magnification × 7,000.) (From Sathananthan, A. H., *Gamete Res.*, 12, 385, 1985. With permission.)

research. The origin of the ZP is controversial in that it is believed to be secreted both by the oocyte and the cumulus during oocyte maturation.[56] Zona material is occasionally found in pockets of the oolemma,[2] which might indicate its origin from the oocyte. Possible endocytosis or exocytosis of this material has also been observed in human oocytes, while this material has been demonstrated between cumulus cells as well.[2]

V. ORGANIZATION OF GAMETES

The general ultrastructural organization of the human oocyte has been well documented,[2] and most of the cellular organelles have been identified and their functions determined. The structure of the MII spindle of the mature oocyte has been also investigated.[4,50,51,61] Meiotic spindles are barrel-shaped, anastral, and composed of numerous microtubules (MT) (Figures 9 and 10). Centrioles are not present, and MT organizing centers are ill-defined at spindle poles.[61] Sperm ultrastructure and spermatogenesis are portrayed in an excellent atlas by Holstein and Roosen-Runge.[62]

Abnormal features of the oocyte have been reviewed.[3,7] The effects of prolonged culture and the subtle changes that occur during postmaturation and aging were defined.[2,63] Most culture media show similar effects on oocyte ultrastructure, and the organelles most vulnerable are the vesicular smooth endoplasmic reticulum (SER) which shows progressive swelling and becomes vacuolar on prolonged culture. Postmature or aging oocytes show loss of surface microvilli, centripetal migration of CG, and large conglomerations of CG. Their spindles are deep seated, have fewer MT, and may show some displacement of chromosomes. Some oocytes show a hypertrophy of aggregates of smaller elements of SER,[64] which are known to be sensitive to gonadotrophins. Studies are now being pursued with natural cycle oocytes to determine the extent of this hypertrophy. Large amounts of gonadotrophins are given to patients to induce superovulation, but only 8 to 10% of embryos transferred after IVF result in viable pregnancies.[65] This may be due in part to the poor quality of oocytes retrieved for ART.

VI. FERTILIZATION *IN VITRO*

Our significant contributions to human embryology have been in gamete fusion and interaction (see reviews in references 2 and 5). The earliest pictures of human conception were documented 3 h after insemination in 1979 at Monash University.[1,9,10] These findings were most welcome by the pioneering IVF teams in England and Australia at the time, when the first IVF babies were being born. Sperm-egg membrane fusion and early events of sperm penetration and incorporation can be precisely visualized by TEM (Figures 3 and 11). During gamete interaction, the oolemma fuses with the post acrosomal region of the spermhead PM, followed by sperm incorporation.[35,66,67] The maternal chromosomes condense to form a female pronucleus (Figure 12) after the second polar body is abstricted (Figure 10). In 1982, we demonstrated the cortical and zona reactions in human oocytes at fertilization (Figures 13 through 16), which establish a primary block to polyspermy at the level of the ZP.[68] The exocytosis of CG and the interaction of their contents with the inner part of the ZP cause a chemical hardening of the ZP, establishing this primary sperm block.[1,2,5,20] Supernumerary sperm freely penetrate the outer ZP[12,52] (Figure 16) but are seen rarely in the deeper regions of the zona. Sperm binding to the ZP and the various stages of the AR and sperm penetration were also documented in these studies (Figures 1 and 2). Only acrosome-vesiculating or acrosome-reacted sperm can fuse with the oocyte (Figure 3).[35]

The first pictures of sperm-oocyte membrane fusion and sperm incorporation (1 to 3 h after insemination) were published in 1986.[35,66] The fusogenic mid-region of the spermhead was defined (Figure 3), and gamete membrane fusion evidently occurs along the anterior half of the postacrosomal segment,[5,35] while the spermhead is engulfed by a tongue-like process of the cortical ooplasm and then phagocytosed. During monospermic fertilization, sperm are incorporated tail first, and we concluded that sperm motility is not essential for gamete fusion.[66,67] This crucial finding had applications later in the treatment by microinjection[46] of patients with immotile cilia syndrome

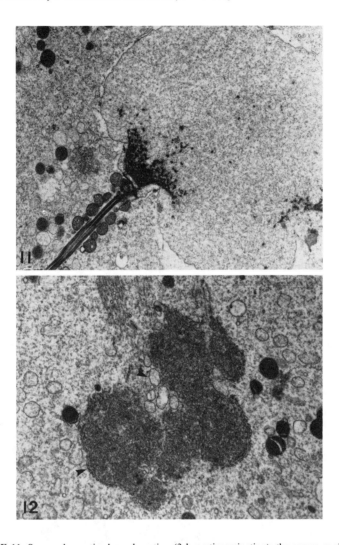

FIGURE 11. Sperm chromatin decondensation (3 h postinsemination): the sperm nucleus has expanded in the ooplasm, while the midpiece is still intact. The nuclear envelope is dismantling. (Original magnification × 15,400.) (From Sathananthan, A. H., Ng, S. C., Edirisinghe, R., Ratnam, S. S., and Wong, P. C., *Gamete Res.,* 15, 37, 1986. With permission.) **FIGURE 12.** Condensation of egg chromatin (3 h postinsemination): the female pronucleus is developing at the inner pole of the telophase II spindle. Elements of SER are forming the pronuclear envelope (arrows). (Original magnification × 27,300.)

(see Chapter 7). Gamete membrane fusion may also occur when sperm show structural head defects, particularly in their nuclei.[69] In most instances, the sperm midpiece and tail are incorporated into the ooplasm, and the midpiece remains attached to the developing male pronucleus (Figure 11). The tail is usually incorporated in zipper-like fashion.[35] Sperm nuclear decondensation and early pronuclear formation have been reported, both during monospermic

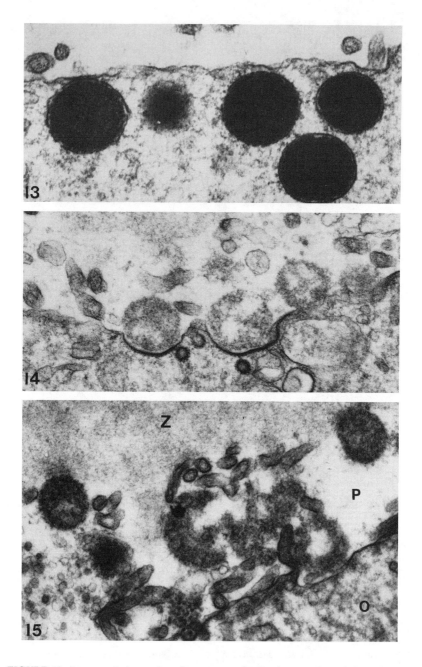

FIGURE 13. Intact cortical granules of a mature unfertilized oocyte beneath its oolemma.
FIGURE 14. Exocytosis of cortical granules at fertilization (3 h postinsemination). **FIGURE 15.** Interaction of cortical granule secretory products with the inner region of the zona. O = ooplasm, P = perivitelline space, Z = ZP. (From Sathananthan, A. H., in *In Vitro Fertilization and Embryo Transfer,* Trounson, A. O. and Wood, C., Eds., Churchill Livingstone, London, 1984, 131. With permission.)

Ultrastructure of Fertilization and Embryo Development 251

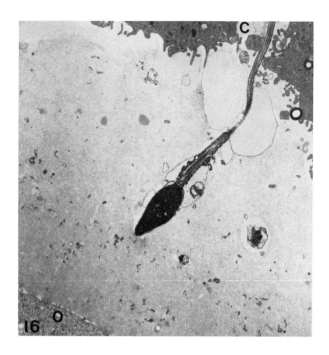

FIGURE 16. Block to polyspermy: sperm penetrating the ZP of a fertilized ovum blocked just outside the inner zona, which is denser and more compact than its outer region. C = cumulus, O = oocyte. (Original magnification × 7,000.) (From Sathananthan, A. H., Trounson, A. O., and Wood, C., *J. Androl.*, 3, 356, 1982. With permission.)

and polyspermic fertilization[9,35] and after microfertilization.[36] A few decondensing spermheads have nuclear defects.[36] The later stages of pronuclear formation and association are usually assessed by LM 12 to 16 h after insemination, a routine procedure in IVF. The fine structural features of bipronuclear and tripronuclear ova (Figures 17 through 19) have been documented.[2,20,36,67,70,71] Fertilization in ART procedures is often positively confirmed by identifying remnants of sperm tails in the ooplasm and CG contents in the PVS, to rule out parthenogenetic activation. We also have shown that tripronuclear ova could be formed by penetration of two sperm simultaneously.[36]

VII. INHERITANCE OF PATERNAL CENTRIOLES

Our most significant contribution to fundamental human embryology is the recent discovery of centrioles in 1-cell human embryos at syngamy.[72] At this stage, maternal and paternal chromosomes come together to establish the embryonic genome at the culmination of fertilization. It was shown that sperm centrioles contributed to the formation of the first mitotic spindle, confirming Boveri's theory of centriolar inheritance in sea urchin development, postulated

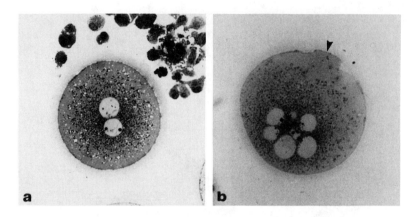

FIGURE 17. Light micrographs of fertilized ova. (a) Normal bipronuclear ovum. (b) Abnormal polyspermic ovum. Note incomplete abstriction of the second polar body (arrow). (Original magnification × 400.)

in 1900.[73] It is widely accepted in mammals that maternal centrosomes organize the mitotic spindle in cleaving embryos. This is largely based on studies on mouse fertilization. Mammalian oocytes, including those of the human, have no centrioles but have osmiophilic centrosomes.[73] The sperm has a single functional centriole associated with osmiophilic material (Figure 1). Sperm centrioles were demonstrated at one of the poles of the first mitotic spindle of monospermic as well as dispermic embryos (Figure 20). This study also demonstrated for the first time tripolar spindles at syngamy, obtained from developing tripronuclear human 1-cell embryos,[72] which would explain how some triploid embryos become diploid during early cleavage.[74] Such fundamental differences in fertilization and other disparities in the early embryology of the mouse and the human question the validity of the mouse research model, which is extensively used to develop various techniques of ART. It is further evident that the ultrastructure of the mouse oocyte and embryo[75] is significantly different from that of the human oocyte and embryo,[2] which must reflect differences in their biochemistry and physiology. An alternative model for research in ART needs to be developed due to the ethical concerns of using human embryos for research (see Chapter 15).

VIII. EARLY EMBRYONIC DEVELOPMENT

The fine structure of early human embryos has not been documented fully since research on preimplantation embryos (2-cell to blastocyst) has always been restricted, even in the early days of IVF. Nevertheless, the normality of early cleavage-stage embryos, cultured *in vitro* for embryo transfer, had to be established.[1,2,76-78] Culture conditions are still suboptimal and have not improved embryo quality significantly over the years. Embryos assessed as being "normal" with the LM (Figure 21) may invariably show ultrastructural defects highlighting the subjective nature of such

Ultrastructure of Fertilization and Embryo Development

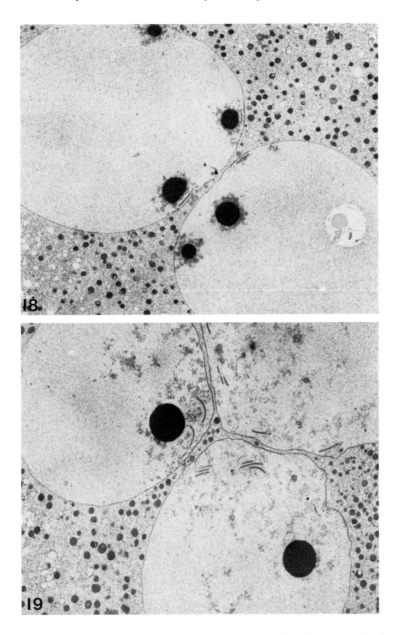

FIGURE 18. Bipronuclear ovum: the two pronuclei are closely associated in the central ooplasm. Note dense nucleoli. **FIGURE 19.** Tripronclear ovum: two of the three pronuclei may have originated from sperm.

assessment.[72,76,77,79] Prolonged culture of embryos beyond the 4-cell stage often induces subtle structural changes similar to those reported for oocytes,[63] when progressive vacuolation, loss of microvillous and pinocytotic activity, and clumping of organelles become evident. Considerable pinocytotic and lysosomal activity is observed in early blastomeres, indicating

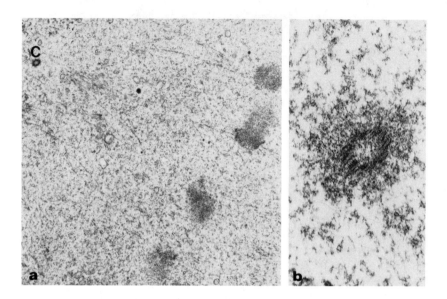

FIGURE 20. Fertilized ovum at syngamy. (a) Half the first mitotic spindle shows a sperm centriole at one pole. Microtubules extend from the pole to the chromosomes. (Original magnification × 13,200.) (From Sathananthan, A. H., Kola, I., Osborne, J., Trounson, A., Ng, S. C., Bongso, A., and Ratnam, S. S., *Proc. Natl. Acad. Sci. U.S.A.*, 88, 4806, 1991. With permission.) (b) Sperm centriole with surrounding centrosomal substance at spindle pole (compare with Figures 1 and 11).

that there is uptake of protein from the culture medium and consequent intracellular digestion. The formation of desmosome-like cell junctions between blastomeres occurs as early as the 2- or 4-cell stage,[2,77,79,80] and compaction is evident at the 8-cell stage.[76,79] Centrioles were detected previously at the 8-cell stage,[79] but 2- to 4-cell embryos must now be examined for centrioles, since their recent discovery at syngamy.[72] Nuclear activation at the time of embryonic genome expression can also be visualized by TEM when the nucleoli become granular and reticulated (Figures 21 through 26), and this occurs between the 4- and 8-cell stages in human embryos.[79,82] Cavitation of the morula and the process of blastocyst hatching have been reported recently.[79]

IX. CO-CULTURE OF EMBRYOS

It is now becoming increasingly apparent that the natural environment of the embryo, such as the fallopian tube or uterus, must be simulated during early embryo development. Physiological media similar to human tubal fluid and those incorporating amniotic fluid have been used to culture embryos[83] (see Chapters 5 and 11). Further, co-culture of early embryos with human tubal, endometrial cells or vero cells have also been attempted.[84-86] Even embryos co-cultured with human ampullary cells as-

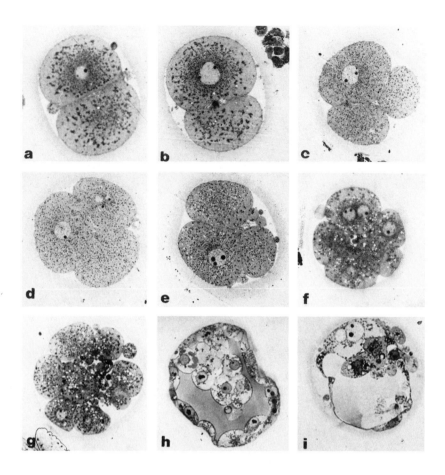

FIGURE 21. Light micrographs of early embryos co-cultured with human ampullary cells; (a) and (b) 2-cell embryo, (c) 4-cell embryo, (d) abnormal 4-cell embryo with micronuclei, (e) 6-cell embryo with fragments, (f) abnormal 8-cell embryo with binucleate blastomere, (g) 10-cell embryo with fragments, (h) early blastocyst with trophoblast and inner cell mass, (i) abnormal blastocyst. (Original magnification × 400.) (From Sathananthan, A. H., Bongso, A., Ng, S. C., Ho, J., Mok, H., and Ratnam, S., *Hum. Reprod.*, 5, 309, 1990. With permission.)

sessed by TEM show some of the pathological features similar to those cultured in IVF media.[79] These defects include multinucleation of blastomeres, formation of micronuclei, and internal fragmentation of blastomeres, which cannot be detected by routine assessment of whole embyros by phase or Nomarski microscopy.

Multinucleation and fragmentation also have been reported in embryos developed *in vivo* flushed from the genital tract.[80] The fate of multinucleated cells has not been determined, but fragments formed during early cleavage are clearly excluded during the process of blastocyst hatching.[79] Several attempts have been made to culture embryos to blastocysts before embryo transfer with some success,[83,85,87,88] as is the practice in farm

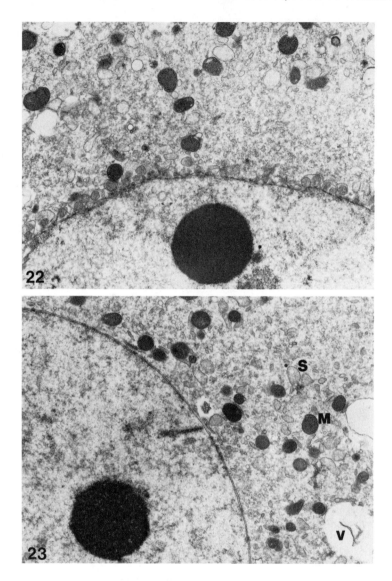

FIGURE 22. Blastomere of 4-cell embryo. Note dense compact nucleolus and blebs on nuclear envelope. (Original magnification × 17,500.) (From Sathananthan, A. H., Bongso, A., Ng, S. C., Ho, J., Mok, H., and Ratnam, S., *Hum. Reprod.*, 5, 309, 1990. With permission.) **FIGURE 23.** Blastomere of 8-cell embryo. Note partially granular nucleolus. M = mitochondria, S = vesicular SER, V = vacuole. (Original magnification × 17,500.)

animals. Some initial studies also have been reported during implantation of the human blastocyst *in vitro*.[89] Reviews on abnormal nuclear configurations and the pathology of IVF embryos assessed by TEM have been published.[2,3,7,71] Some ultrastructural features of early embryos are shown in Figures 22 through 26.

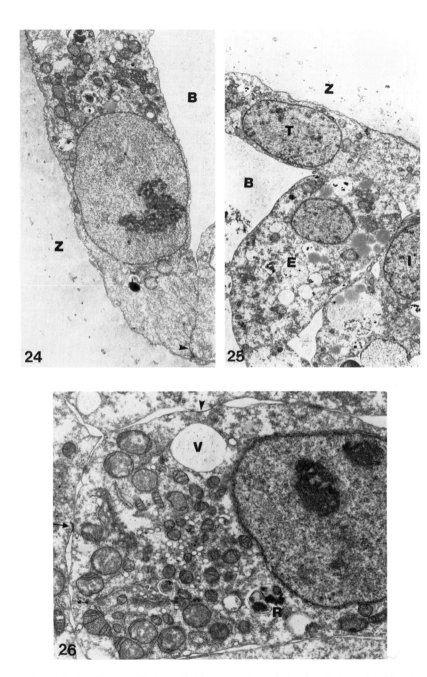

FIGURE 24. Trophoblast cell of an early blastocyst. Note reticulated nucleolus and cell junction (arrow). (Original magnification × 8,050.) **FIGURE 25.** Endodermal cell (E) of a late blastocyst. B = blastocele, I = inner cell mass, T = trophoblast cell, Z = ZP. (Original magnification × 8,050.) **FIGURE 26.** Embryoblast cell from inner cell mass of late blastocyst. Note cell junctions (arrows) with adjacent cells and appearance of rough endoplasmic reticulum (arrow). R = residual body, V = vacuole. (Original magnification × 17,500.)

REFERENCES

1. **Sathananthan, A. H.**, Ultrastructural morphology of fertilization and early cleavage in the human, in *In Vitro Fertilization and Embryo Transfer.*, Trounson, A. O. and Wood, C., Eds., Churchill Livingstone, London, 1984, 131.
2. **Sathananthan, A. H., Trounson, A. O., and Wood, C.**, *Atlas of Fine Structure of Human Sperm Penetration, Eggs and Embryos Cultured In Vitro*, Praeger, Philadelphia, 1986.
3. **Sathananthan, A. H.**, Abnormal nuclear configurations encountered in human IVF and possible genetic implications, *Assisted Reprod. Technol./Androl.*, 1, 115, 1990.
4. **Sathananthan, A. H., Trounson, A. O., and Ng, S. C.**, Maturation of the human oocyte, in *Ultrastructure of the Ovary: Physiology and Pathology*, Familiari, G., Makabe, S., Motta, P. M., Eds., Plenum, New York, 1990, 29.
5. **Sathananthan, A. H., Ng, S. C., Trounson, A. O., Ratnam, S. S., and Bongso, T. A.**, Human sperm-oocyte fusion, in *Mechanism of Fertilization: Plants to Humans*, Dale, B., Ed., Plenum, New York, 1990, 329.
6. **Sathananthan, A. H. and Trounson, A.**, The microinjection technique and the role of the acrosome reaction in microfertilization, in *Advances in Assisted Reproductive Techniques*, Mashiach, S., Ben Rafael, Z., Laufer, N., and Schenker, J.G., Eds., Plenum, New York, 1990, 825.
7. **Sathananthan, A. H.**, The pathology of *in vitro* fertilization, in *Diagnostic Ultrastructure of Neoplastic Diseases*, Papadimitriou, J.M., Henderson, D.W., and Spagnola, D., Eds., Churchill Livingstone, Edinburgh, 1991, 435.
8. **Sathananthan, A. H., Ng, S. C., Trounson, A., and Ratnam, S. S.**, Transmission electron microscopy in the assessment of infertility for assisted reproductive technology, in *Contributions to Obstetrics and Gynaecology*, Vol. 1, Ratnam, S.S., Ng, S.C., Sen, D.K., and Arulkumaran, S., Eds., Churchill Livingstone, London, 1991, 61.
9. **Lopata, A., Sathananthan, A. H., McBain, J. C., Johnston, W. I. H., and Spiers, A. L.**, The ultrastructure of the preovulatory human egg fertilized in vitro, *Fertil. Steril.*, 33, 12, 1980.
10. **Edwards, R. G.**, *Conception in the Human Female*, Academic Press, London, 1980.
11. **Sathananthan, A. H., Ng, S. C., Ho, J., Tok, V., and Ratnam S. S.**, Ultrastructural assessment of human sperm for techniques in assisted reproductive technology, unpublished data, 1991.
12. **Chen, C. and Sathananthan, A. H.**, Early penetration of human sperm through the vestments of human eggs in vitro, *Arch. Androl.*, 16, 183, 1986.
13. **Bongso, A., Ng, S. C., Mok, H., Lim, H. L., Teo, H. L., Wong, P. C., and Ratnam, S. S.**, Improved sperm concentration, motility and fertilization rates following Ficoll treatment of sperm in a human in vitro fertilization program, *Fertil. Steril.*, 51, 850, 1989.
14. **Dravland, J. E. and Mortimer, D.**, A simple discontinuous Percoll gradient procedure for washing human spermatozoa, *IRCS Med. Sci.*, 13, 16, 1985.
15. **Ng, S. C., Bongso, A., Sathananthan, A. H., and Ratnam, S. S.**, Micro-insemination of human oocytes, in *Advances in Assisted Reproductive Technologies*, Mashiach, S., Ben Rafael, Z., Laufer, N., and Schenker, J. G., Eds., Plenum, New York, 1990, 840.
16. **Nagae, T., Yanagimachi, R., and Srivastava, P. N.**, Acrosome reaction in human spermatozoa, *Fertil. Steril.*, 45, 701, 1986.
17. **Stock, C. E. and Fraser, L. R.**, The acrosome reaction in human sperm from men of proven fertility, *Hum. Reprod.*, 2, 109, 1987.
18. **Yanagimachi, R.**, Mammalian fertilization, in *The Physiology of Reproduction*, Knobil, E. and Neill, J., Eds., Academic Press, New York, 1988, 135.
19. **Sathananthan, A. H., Trounson, A. O., and Wood, C.**, Ultrastructural observations on the penetration of sperm into human eggs, *J. Androl.*, 3, 356, 1982.
20. **Soupart, P.**, Fertilization, in *Human Reproduction: Conception and Contraception*, Hafez, E.S.E., Ed., Harper & Row, New York, 1980, 453.
21. **Cross, N. L., Morales, P., and Overstreet, J. W.**, Induction of acrosome reaction by the human zona pellucida, *Biol. Reprod.*, 38, 235, 1988.
22. **Stock, C. E., Bates, R., and Kindsay, K. S.**, Human oocyte–cumulus complexes stimulate the human acrosome reaction, *J. Reprod. Fertil.*, 86, 723, 1989.

23. Yudin, A. I., Gottlieb, W., and Meizel, S., Ultrastructural studies of the early events of the human sperm acrosome reaction as initiated by human follicular fluid, *Gamete Res.*, 20, 11, 1988.
24. Suarez, S. S., Wolf, D. P., and Meizel, S., Induction of the acrosome reaction in human spermatozoa by a fraction of human follicular fluid, *Gamete Res.*, 14, 107, 1986.
25. Talbot, P. and Chacon, R. S., A triple staining technique for evaluation of normal acrosome reactions of human sperm, *J. Exp. Zool.*, 215, 201, 1981.
26. Holden, C. A., Hyne, R. V., Sathananthan, A. H., and Trounson, A. O., Assessment of the human sperm acrosome reaction using concanavalin A lectin, *Mol. Reprod. Dev.*, 25, 247, 1990.
27. Moore, H. D. M., Smith, C. A., Hartman, T. D., and Bye, A. P., Visualization and characterization of the acrosome reaction of human spermatozoa by immunolocalization with monoclonal antibody, *Gamete Res.*, 17, 245, 1987.
28. Kruger, T. F., Acosta, A. A., Simmons, K. F., Swanson R. J., Matta, J. F., and Oehninger, S., Predictive values of abnormal sperm morphology in in vitro fertilization, *Fertil. Steril.*, 49, 112, 1988.
29. Jinno, M., Kabayashi, T., Sugimura, K., Nozawa, S., Katayama, E., and Iida, E., IVF/sperm morphology, *Mol. Androl.*, 2, 161, 1990.
30. Mahadevan, M. M. and Trounson, A. O., The influence of seminal characteristics in the success rate of human in vitro fertilization, *Fertil. Steril.*, 42, 400, 1984.
31. Bongso, T. A., Ng, S. C., Mok, H., Lim, N. N., Teo, H. L., Wong, P. C., and Ratnam, S. S., Effect of sperm motility on human in vitro fertilization, *Arch. Androl.*, 22, 185, 1989.
32. Bartoov, B., Eltes, F., Weissenberg, R., and Lunefeld, B., Morphological characterization of abnormal human spermatozoa using transmission electron microscopy, *Arch. Androl.*, 5, 305, 1980.
33. Zamboni, L., The ultrastructural pathology of the spermatozoon as a cause of infertility: the role of electron microscopy in the evaluation of semen quality, *Fertil. Steril.*, 48, 711, 1987.
34. Dadoune, J. P., Ultrastructural abnormalities of human spermatozoa, *Hum. Reprod.*, 3, 311, 1988.
35. Sathananthan, A. H., Ng, S. C., Edirisinghe, R., Ratnam, S. S., and Wong, P. C., Sperm–oocyte interaction in the human during polyspermic fertilization in vitro, *Gamete Res.*, 15, 317, 1986.
36. Sathananthan, A. H., Ng, S. C., Trounson, A. O., Laws-King, A., Bongso, A., and Ratnam, S. S., Human microfertilization by injection of single or multiple sperm: ultrastructure, *Hum. Reprod.*, 4, 574, 1989.
37. Ryder, T. A., Mobberley, M. A., and Hughes, L., A survey of the ultrastructural defects associated with absent or impaired human sperm motility, *Fertil. Steril.*, 53, 556, 1990.
38. Williamson, R. A., Koehler, J. K., Smith, W. D., and Stenchever, M. A., Ultrastructural sperm tail defects associated with sperm immotility, *Fertil. Steril.*, 41, 103, 1984.
39. Hancock, A. S. and de Kretser, D. M., The axonemal ultrastructure of spermatozoa from men with asthenospermia, in press.
40. Mahadevan, M. M. and Trounson, A. O., Relationship of the fine structure of the sperm head to fertility of frozen human semen, *Fertil. Steril.*, 41, 287, 1984.
41. Barthelemy, C., Royere, D., Hammahah, S., Lebos, C., Tharanne, M. J., and Lansac, J., Ultrastructural changes in membranes and acrosome of human sperm during cryopreservation, *Arch. Androl.*, 25, 29, 1990.
42. Mack, S. R. and Zaneveld, L. J. D., Acrosomal enzymes and ultrastructure of unfrozen and cryotreated human spermatozoa, *Gamete Res.*, 18, 375, 1987.
43. Wolf, D., Sperm cryopreservation: state of the art, *J. In Vitro. Fertil. Embryo Transfer*, 6, 325, 1989.
44. Palmblad, J., Mossberg, B., and Afzelius, B. A., Ultrastructural cellular and clinical features of the immotile cilia syndrome, *Annu. Rev. Med.*, 35, 481, 1984.
45. Ng, S. C., Sathananthan, A. H., Edirisinghe, W. R., Ho, K. C., Wong, P. C., Ratnam, S. S., and Ganatra, S., Fertilization of a human egg with sperm from a patient with immotile cilia syndrome: case report, in *Advances in Fertility and Sterility*, Ratnam, S.S., Teoh, E.S., and Anandakumar, C., Eds., Parthenon, Lancaster, 4, 71, 1987.

46. **Bongso, T. A., Sathananthan, A. H., Wong, P.C., Ratnam, S. S., Ng, S. C., Anandakumar, C., and Ganatra, S.,** Human fertilization by microinjection of immotile sperm, *Hum. Reprod.,* 4, 175, 1989.
47. **Zamboni, L., Thompson, R. S., and Moore-Smith, D.,** Fine morphology of human oocyte maturation in vitro, *Biol. Reprod.,* 7, 425, 1972.
48. **Suzuki, S., Kitai, H., Tojo, R., Seki, K., Oba, M., Fujiwara, T., and Iizuka, R.,** Ultrastructure and some biologic properties of human oocytes and granulosa cells cultured in vitro, *Fertil. Steril.,* 35, 142, 1981.
49. **Sundstrom, P., Nilsson, B. D., Liedholm, P., and Larsson, E.,** Ultrastructural characteristics of human oocytes fixed at follicular puncture or after culture, *J. In Vitro Fertil. Embryo Transfer,* 2, 195, 1985.
50. **Szollosi, D., Mandelbaum, J., Plachot, M., Salat-Baroux, J., and Cohen, J.,** Ultrastructure of the human preovulatory oocyte, *J. In Vitro Fertil. Embryo Transfer,* 3, 232, 1986.
51. **Sathananthan, A. H.,** Maturation of the human oocyte in vitro: nuclear events during meiosis (an ultrastructural study), *Gamete Res.,* 12, 385, 1985.
52. **Sathananthan, A. H. and Trounson. A. O.,** Ultrastructural observations on cortical granules in human follicular oocytes cultured in vitro, *Gamete Res.,* 5, 191, 1982.
53. **Trounson, A. O., Mohr, L. R., Wood, C., and Leeton, J. F.,** Effect of delayed insemination in vitro fertilization, culture and transfer of human embryos, *J. Reprod. Fertil.,* 64, 285, 1982.
54. **Sathananthan, A. H., Ng, S. C., Chia, C. M., Law, H. Y., and Edirisinghe, R. W.,** The origin and distribution of cortical granules in human follicular oocytes, *Ann. N.Y. Acad. Sci.,* 442, 251, 1985.
55. **Pickering, S. J., Johnson, M. H., Braude, P. R., and Houliston, E.,** Cytoskeletal organization in fresh, aged and spontaneously activated human oocytes, *Hum. Reprod.,* 3, 978, 1988.
56. **Dietl, J.,** Ultrstructural aspects of the developing mammalian zona pellucida, in *The Mammalian Egg Coat,* Dietl, J., Ed., Springer-Verlag, Berlin, 1989, 49.
57. **Tesarik, J., Pilka, L., and Travnik, P.,** Zona pellucida resistance to sperm penetration before completion of human oocyte maturation, *J. Reprod. Fertil.,* 83, 487, 1988.
58. **Familiari, G., Nottola, S. A., Micara, G., Aragona, C., and Motta, P. M.,** Is the sperm-binding capability of the zona pellucida linked to its surface structure? A scanning electron microscopic study of human in vitro fertilization, *J. In Vitro Fertil. Embryo Transfer,* 5, 134, 1988.
59. **Wassarman, P.,** Cellular and molecular elements of mammalian fertilization. in *Mechanism of Fertilization: Plants to Humans,* Dale, B., Ed., Nato ASI Series H: Cell Biology, Vol. 45, 1990, 305.
60. **Phillips, D. M.,** Structure and function of the zona pellucida, in *Ultrastructure of the Ovary,* Familiari G., Makabe, S., and Motta, P. M., Eds., Kluwer, Boston, 1991, 63.
61. **Sathananthan, A. H., Trounson, A. O., Freeman, L., and Brady, T.,** The effects of cooling human oocytes, *Hum. Reprod.,* 3, 968, 1988.
62. **Holstein, A. F. and Roosen-Runge, E. C.,** *Atlas of Human Spermatogenesis.* Grosse Verlag, Berlin, 1980.
63. **Sathananthan, A. H. and Trounson, A. O.,** Effects of culture and cryopreservation on human oocyte and embryo ultrastructure and function, in *Ultrastructure of Human Gametogenesis and Early Embryogenesis,* Van Blerkom, J. and Motta, P.M., Eds., Kluwer Academic, Philadelphia, 1988, 181.
64. **Sathananthan, A. H., Ng, S. C., Ratnam, S. S., Edirisinghe, W. R., and Law, H. Y.,** Are we overstimulating in IVF?, *Singapore J. Obstet. Gynecol.,* 19, 83, 1988.
65. **Voluntary Licensing Authority,** *The Second Report of the Voluntary Licensing Authority for Human In Vitro Fertilization and Embryology,* VLA, London, 1987.
66. **Sathananthan, A. H. and Chen, C.,** Sperm-oocyte membrane fusion in the human during monospermic fertilization, *Gamete Res.,* 15, 177, 1986.
67. **Sathananthan, A. H., Trounson, A., and Freemann, L.,** Morphology and fertilizability of frozen oocytes, *Gamete Res.,* 16, 343, 1987.
68. **Sathananthan, A. H. and Trounson, A. O.,** Cortical granule release and zona interaction in monospermic and polyspermic human ova fertilized in vitro, *Gamete Res.,* 6, 225, 1982.

69. **Sathananthan, A. H., Ng, S. C., Trounson, A., Bongso, A., Ho, J., and Ratnam, S. S.,** Role of electron microscopy in assisted reproductive technology (review), *J. Med. Lab. Sci.,* 4, 91, 1990.
70. **Sathananthan, A. H. and Trounson, A. O.,** Human pronuclear ovum: fine structure of monospermic and polyspermic fertilization in vitro, *Gamete Res.,* 12, 385, 1985.
71. **Van Blerkom, J.,** Developmental failure in human reproduction associated with preovulatory oogenesis and preimplantation embryogenesis, in *Ultrastructure of Human Gametogenesis and Early Embryogenesis,* Van Blerkom, J. and Motta, P.M., Eds., Kluwer Academic, Philadelphia, 1989, 125.
72. **Sathananthan, A. H., Kola, I., Osborne, J., Trounson, A., Ng, S. C., Bongso, A., and Ratnam, S. S.,** Centrioles in the beginning of human development, *Proc. Natl. Acad. Sci. U.S.A.,* 88, 4806, 1991.
73. **Mazia, D.,** The chromosome cycle and the centrosome cycle in the mitotic cycle, *Int. Rev. Cyto.,* 100, 49, 1987.
74. **Kola, I., Trounson, A. O., Dawson, G., and Rogers, P.,** Pronuclear human oocytes: altered cleavage patterns and subsequent karyotypic analysis of embryos, *Biol. Reprod.,* 37, 395, 1987.
75. **Dvorak, M., Cech, S., Stastna, J., Tesarik, J., and Travnik, P.,** *The Differentiation of Preimplantation Mouse Embryos,* Purkyne Univ. Press, Brno, 1985.
76. **Sathananthan, A. H., Wood, C., and Leeton, J.,** Ultrastructural evaluation of 8–16 cell human embryos cultured in vitro, *Micron,* 13, 193, 1982.
77. **Trounson, A.O. and Sathananthan, A.H.,** The application of electron microscopy in the evaluation of 2–4 cell human embryos cultured in vitro for embryo transfer, *J. In Vitro Fertil. Embryo Transfer,* 1, 153, 1984.
78. **Sundstrom, P., Nilsson, D., and Liedholm, P.,** Cleavage rate and morphology of early human embryos obtained after artificial fertilization and culture, *Acta Obstet. Gynecol. Scand.,* 60, 109, 1981.
79. **Sathananthan, A. H., Bongso, A., Ng, S. C., Ho, J., Mok, H., and Ratnam, S.,** Ultrastructure of preimplantation human embryos co-cultured with human ampullary cells, *Hum. Reprod.,* 5, 309, 1990.
80. **Pereda, J.,** Ultrastructural observation of early human eggs. Analysis of four concepti, in *Developments in Ultrastructure of Reproduction,* Motta, P.M., Ed., Alan Liss, New York, 367, 1989.
81. **Tesarik, J., Kopecny, V., Plachot, M., and Mandelbaum, J.,** Early morphological signs of embryonic gene expression in human preimplantation development as revealed by quantitative electron microscopy, *Dev. Biol.,* 128, 15, 1988.
82. **Lopata, A., Kohlman, D., and Johnston, I.,** The fine structure of normal and abnormal human embryos developed in culture, in *Fertilization of the Human Egg in Vitro,* Beier, H. M. and Lindner, H. R., Eds., Springer-Verlag, Berlin, 1983, 189.
83. **Trounson, A.,** Fertilization and embryo culture, in *Clinical In Vitro Fertilization.,* Wood, C. and Trounson, A., Eds., Springer-Verlag, Berlin, 1989, 127.
84. **Bongso, A., Ng, S. C., Sathananthan, A. H., Pohlian, N., Rauff, M., and Ratnam, S. S.,** Improved quality of human embryos when co-cultured with human ampullary cells, *Hum. Reprod.,* 4, 706, 1989.
85. **Bongso, A., Ng, S. C., and Ratnam, S. S.,** Co-cultures: their relevance to assisted reproduction, *Hum. Reprod.,* in press, 1991.
86. **Menezo, Y. and Ouhibi, N.,** Embryo co-culture, *Asst. Reprod.Technol./Androl.,* 1, 297, 1990.
87. **Fehilly, C. B., Cohen, J., Simons, R. F., Fishel, S. B., and Edwards, R. G.,** Cryopreservation of cleaving embryos and expanded blastocysts in the human: a comparative study, *Fertil. Steril.,* 44, 638, 1985.
88. **Mohr, L. R. and Trounson, A. O.,** Comparative ultrastructure of the hatched human, mouse and bovine blastocysts, *J. Reprod. Fertil.,* 66, 499, 1984.
89. **Lindenberg, S. and Hyttel, P.,** In vitro studies of the peri-implantation phase of human embryos, in *Ultrastructure of Human Gametogenesis and Early Embryogenesis,* Van Blerkom, J. and Motta, P.M., Eds., Kluwer Academic, Philadelphia, 1988, 201.

Chapter 13

UTERINE RECEPTIVITY

Peter Rogers

TABLE OF CONTENTS

I. Introduction 264

II. Knowledge from Animal Studies on Uterine Receptivity 264

III. Theoretical Calculations of Human Uterine Receptivity 266
    A. The Natural Cycle 266
    B. Uterine Receptivity and Embryo Viability during Stimulated IVF Cycles 266
    C. The Relative Importance of Uterine Receptivity and Oocyte Quality: Data from Oocyte Donation 267

IV. Endocrine Requirements for Human Uterine Receptivity 268
    A. Follicular Phase Estradiol Levels 269
    B. The Need for Luteal Support 270

V. Morphological Studies: The Search for a Receptive Endometrium 271
    A. Endometrial Morphology and the Luteal Phase Defect 272
    B. The Effects of Ovarian Stimulation on Endometrial Morphology 273
    C. Ultrasound Studies of the Endometrium 274
    D. Human Uterine Epithelial Tight Junctions 274

VI. The Contribution of Studies with Agonadal Women Receiving Hormone Replacement Therapy for IVF to Our Understanding of Uterine Receptivity in the Human 275
    A. Fixed and Variable Length Hormone Replacement Cycles 275
    B. The Human Implantation Window 276

VII. Strategies for Improving Uterine Receptivity 278

References 280

I. INTRODUCTION

The aim of this chapter is to bring the reader up to date with current thinking about the role of uterine receptivity in present day *in vitro* fertilization (IVF) and to identify the limited number of strategies that are being used to influence it.

Despite recent advances in reproductive medicine, the role played by uterine receptivity in contributing to human infertility remains unclear. The primary reason for this lies in our fundamental lack of knowledge of the basic mechanisms by which uterine receptivity is controlled. Understanding of the local processes involved in mammalian implantation remains an elusive goal for present day reproductive research, not the least because of the wide degree of variability seen from one species to the next. Add to this the major practical and ethical constraints that govern research among humans in a field like implantation, and it is perhaps less surprising that comparatively little is known about this crucial area.

The emergence of IVF as a routine clinical treatment for infertility has provided an important avenue for focusing basic and clinical research on the human reproductive processes from gametogenesis through to fertilization and implantation. In particular, attention is now being paid to the role of the nonreceptive uterus in preventing embryo implantation following ovarian hyperstimulation, since it is now apparent that implantation failure is the major impediment to higher IVF pregnancy rates.

II. KNOWLEDGE FROM ANIMAL STUDIES ON UTERINE RECEPTIVITY

Understanding of the basic mechanisms controlling implantation is complicated by the wide variability that exists from species to species in the manner by which the embryo comes into contact with the endometrium.[1] Despite this variability, current thinking, while not ignoring the role of the blastocyst, favors the view that it is the uterus, appropriately conditioned by ovarian hormones, that predominantly determines the success of implantation.[2] Among well-studied species such as laboratory rodents, it has been shown that the uterus becomes receptive to the implanting blastocyst for a short period of time a few days after the commencement of continuous progesterone (P_4) administration.[3,4] Priming estrogen prior to this P_4 is not essential, although a small amount of estrogen must be given at some time after the commencement of P_4 for an implantation receptive uterus to be established. These and other studies have led to the concept of an "implantation window," defined as the period of time when the uterus is receptive to the implanting blastocyst. In addition to the receptive state, it has also been postulated that the uterus goes through "implantation neutral" and "implantation hostile" states.[5] During the neutral phase, the embryo can survive in the uterus but will not implant, while during the hostile phase, the embryo is actively destroyed. How the uterus effects these receptive, neutral, and hostile states remains largely unclear, although embryo-toxic compounds have been demonstrated in uterine flushings from rats and mice taken at times other than when implantation normally occurs,[5,6] and there is a suggestion that similar embryo-toxic compounds occur in the human.[7] Other studies have implicated a major role for the uterine epithelium in preventing implantation, unless the correct hormonal priming has occurred.[8] In this work, the embryo was only able to implant in the unprimed mouse uterus once the epithelium had been removed.

Further support for the hypothesis that the uterus is the major controlling partner in the implantation process comes from numerous studies demonstrating that mammalian embryos can initiate implantation-type vascular reactions in nonuterine tissues with a high degree of success, regardless of the sex or hormonal status of the host. Ectopic sites that have been studied in this way include the anterior chamber of the eye,[9,10] the kidney,[11] the testis,[12] and the spleen.[13] Although tissues from ectopic sites respond differently to the implanting embryo from those in uterine sites, and despite the fact that subsequent embryo development is often disorganized, the study of ectopic implantation can provide valuable insights into normal intrauterine implantation.[10,14] Indeed, normal development to term has been reported in the human following ectopic implantation.[15]

A number of mammalian species (including some of the marsupials) utilize embryonic diapause or delayed implantation to maximize reproductive efficiency.[16] During diapause, blastocyst development is arrested by the uterus until conditions are suitable for pregnancy to continue. That control over diapause is entirely a uterine phenomenon can easily be shown by removing the blastocyst from the uterine environment, at which time normal development will recommence.[17] Conversely, recent studies in cattle have shown that under certain conditions, the uterus can induce the preimplantation embryo to accelerate its development in order to "catch up" to the uterus and be ready to implant at the optimal time in terms of uterine receptivity.[18]

In summary, these and other animal studies have led to a number of important concepts concerning embryo implantation. It is believed that, assuming a normal embryo, the uterus is the primary force in controlling the success of implantation, and that the period of time during which the uterus is receptive for implantation is the "implantation window." Finally, the term "synchrony" is used to describe the situation where the early embryo and the uterus are both developing at a rate so that they will be ready to commence implantation at the same time. In other words, the length of the implantation window is defined as the amount of embryo-uterine developmental asynchrony that can be tolerated while still allowing successful implantation.

III. THEORETICAL CALCULATIONS OF HUMAN UTERINE RECEPTIVITY

A. THE NATURAL CYCLE

Estimates of maximum human fecundability (defined as a percentage of women who will produce a full-term infant per menstrual cycle during which frequent intercourse occurs) range from 14.4 to 31.8% for various populations and age groups of women.[19] Under normal circumstances, a number of factors may contribute to this low success rate, including anovulation, intercourse at the wrong time, reduced semen quality, failure of egg or sperm transport, fertilization failure, embryonic mortality, and lack of uterine receptivity.[20] Of these potential factors, it is probable that embryonic mortality contributes significantly,[21] as a result of both chromosomal[22] and other developmental abnormalities within the embryo. Evidence to support this has recently been gathered in a study looking at the incidence of dizygotic twins resulting from twin ovulations in natural cycles.[23] This work suggests that in the natural conception cycle, uterine factors may not play the major role in implantation failure.

B. UTERINE RECEPTIVITY AND EMBRYO VIABILITY DURING STIMULATED IVF CYCLES

The large amount of human implantation data produced following superovulation and multiple embryo transfer by various IVF groups has provided an avenue for exploring the relative contributions of embryonic and uterine factors to implantation failure in stimulated cycles.[24,25] These studies were based on a hypothetical two parameter model for implantation proposed by Speirs et al.[26] This model assumed that each embryo had a probability (E) of survival, and that, in any given patient, there was a probability (U) that the uterus would be receptive. Thus, when a single embryo was transferred, the probability of pregnancy was represented by the product $U \times E$. This simplistic model made a number of assumptions: that U and E were independent, that U and E were the only factors influencing implantation, that one embryo successfully implanting did not influence the chance of other embryos implanting, and that the probabilities U and E did not alter significantly within each IVF group with time.

Five large sets of IVF data were analyzed using this mathematical model for implantation, and values for U and E calculated using maximum-likelihood methods (Table 1). When these values for U and E were used to construct tables of predicted singleton and multiple implantation rates following embryo transfer for each IVF group, only two of the five predicted sets of data deviated significantly from the actual observed results (Queen Elizabeth and Norfolk). These results suggested that the U-E model may in fact be a good approximation of the biological events that control implantation. If this is the case, then it is quite evident that low uterine receptivity is playing a significant role in implantation failure in human IVF. It is also of interest to note that

TABLE 1
Estimates for Uterine Receptivity (U) and Embryo Viability (E) Based on Implantation Data from Five IVF Groups

IVF Group	Uterine receptivity (U)	Embryo viability (E)
Monash, Melbourne	0.31 ± 0.07	0.32 ± 0.06
Royal Women's, Melbourne	0.42 ± 0.11	0.23 ± 0.05
Queen Elizabeth, Adelaide	0.42 ± 0.17	0.28 ± 0.10
Norfolk, Virginia	0.64 ± 0.22	0.21 ± 0.08
Bourne Hall, Cambridge[a]	0.36	0.43

Note: ± simultaneous 95% confidence limits.

[a] From Walters, D. E., Edwards, D. G., and Meistrich, M. L., *J. Reprod. Fertil.*, 74, 557, 1985.

From Rogers, P. A. W., Milne, B. J., and Trounson, A. O., *J. In Vitro Fertil. Embryo Transfer*, 3, 93, 1986.

Norfolk, the only IVF clinic at that time not using the anti-estrogen, clomiphene citrate (CC) as a superovulation drug, had a theoretical uterine receptivity of 0.64. By contrast, the four IVF groups that used CC had significantly lower theoretical uterine receptivity values, ranging from 0.31 to 0.42. It would be of interest to repeat the same statistical analyses on more recent sets of IVF pregnancy data generated from programs using gonadotrophin releasing hormone analogue (GnRH-a) superovulation protocols that avoid CC.

If these theoretical values for uterine receptivity following superovulation for IVF are correct, then two major conclusions may be drawn. First, as has been shown in a number of other species, the human uterus has selective mechanisms by which the implanting embryo can be accepted or rejected. Second, if IVF pregnancy rates are going to be improved significantly, then it will be necessary to address the problem of low uterine receptivity. This is particularly important since problems with low embryo viability can be overcome to some extent by replacing more embryos, whereas uterine receptivity is always fixed for each patient and will rapidly become the dominant negative factor controlling the overall pregnancy rate once three or more good embryos are transferred to the uterus.

C. THE RELATIVE IMPORTANCE OF UTERINE RECEPTIVITY AND OOCYTE QUALITY: DATA FROM OOCYTE DONATION

Oocyte and embryo donation provide an important new avenue for investigating the relative contributions of uterine and embryonic factors to human infertility. In a recent study involving oocyte donation to 35 infertile women over the age of 40, 15 ongoing pregnancies were achieved by using oocytes donated from younger women[27] (the average age of donors was 33.4 years). The conclusions from this study were that (1) the primary determinant of age-related decline in female fertility is poor oocyte quality, with endometrial receptivity having a secondary though important role, and (2) that the aging uterus can adequately sustain pregnancy even when reproductive potential is artificially prolonged into the late 40s. While this first conclusion is clearly valid for the outcome of the study, it is important to note that the 35 older women who were oocyte recipients were specifically selected on the basis of their infertility, and do not represent the normal age-matched population. The authors point out in their discussion that a better study design would have included reciprocal donation by older individuals to younger recipients. Thus, a more valid conclusion from this study might be that, "In chronically infertile women that have failed to achieve pregnancy by other means (including ovulation induction and IVF), oocyte donation can provide an effective means of doing so." In other words, there is almost certainly a subset of women in whom infertility is due entirely to defective oocytes. Thus, conclusions regarding the role that aging plays in the reduction of both oocyte viability and uterine receptivity in the normal population cannot be drawn validly from this study.

In another study that reported 100 cycles of oocyte donation, an analysis has been made of factors affecting the outcome.[28] This work involved 68 donors, 82 recipients and resulted in 27 clinical pregnancies. The major conclusions were as follows:

1. The age of the recipient significantly affects pregnancy rate, falling from 50% in the 25 to 29 year age group to 9.7% in the 45 to 49 age group;
2. The pregnancy rate in patients with primary ovarian failure (50%, 8/16) was significantly higher than in patients with secondary ovarian failure (18%, 9/50);
3. The pregnancy rate was significantly greater when parous donors were used (33%, 23/69) compared to non-parous donors (13%, 4/31);
4. The number of gametes/embryos transferred significantly affected the pregnancy rate regardless of the treatment used, rising from 11% with one or two transferred to 33% with three or four;
5. The age of the donors did not affect the pregnancy rate.

Although the number of subjects is relatively small, the observation that oocytes from parous women give higher pregnancy rates supports the concept outlined in the previous paragraph that oocyte quality may vary significantly from individual to individual, and may thus be the dominant factor causing infertility in some women. In addition, this study provides evidence that, independent of donor age, recipient age has a significant effect on pregnancy outcome, presumably through reduced uterine receptivity.

IV. ENDOCRINE REQUIREMENTS FOR HUMAN UTERINE RECEPTIVITY

Prior to IVF and embryo transfer becoming routine clinical treatments for human infertility, very little data were available concerning the sequence and amounts of estrogen and progesterone necessary to prepare the human endometrium for implantation. Studies of circulating estradiol (E_2) and P_4 and progesterone levels during the normal menstrual cycle show wide variability from woman to woman.[29] However, there is little understanding of how these varying levels of E_2 and P_4 within the wide normal range may influence receptivity. Although it is known that excessive E_2 administered post-ovulation can prevent implantation,[30] very little is known about the pre- and peri-implantation levels of E_2 and P_4 required for successful implantation. In one study looking at 527 cycles in 67 subfertile patients, it was found that significantly more viable pregnancies occurred among patients with an E_2 to P_4 ratio in the range of 7.63 to 12.22 (calculated as E_2 in pmol/l divided by P_4 in nmol/l).[31] Steroid levels were measured in circulating blood taken at the presumed time of implantation.

IVF has generated large amounts of accurate endocrine data on the circulating levels of E_2 and P_4 during stimulated cycles.[32] In addition, receptive cycles are clearly identified by pregnancy following embryo transfer. Unfortunately, this major increase in previously difficult to obtain data has tended to confuse rather than clarify the situation. As with the variability seen in the natural cycle, pregnancies have been achieved by numerous IVF groups using a wide range of stimulation-protocols that have resulted in an even wider range of circulating E_2 and P_4 levels.

A. FOLLICULAR PHASE ESTRADIOL LEVELS

While it may never be possible to define absolute limits for follicular E_2 levels that will give optimum uterine receptivity, attempts have been made to identify both the normal follicular E_2 range and the E_2 profiles that are thought to indicate a higher prospect of pregnancy.[33,34] The first of these studies analyzed the follicular E_2 pattern in 102 consecutive IVF conception cycles in patients receiving a standardized clomiphene citrate/human menopausal gonadotrophin (CC/HMG) superovulation regimen. From this work, a median E_2 response with 5th and 95th percentiles was derived for each day of the follicular phase. This allowed the authors to prospectively identify patients within the 5 to 95th percentiles; a range of plasma E_2 values they then defined as a valid marker of satisfactory folliculogenesis. However, this study did not comment on the E_2 profiles of nonpregnant patients receiving the same ovarian stimulation. Presumably, if the values for the 5 to 95th percentiles are roughly similar in conception and nonconception cycles, then little can be concluded from this work about the effects of follicular E_2 on the final prospects of achieving pregnancy or the effects it may have on uterine receptivity. Indeed, the same group has reported that in 45 out of 662 IVF patients from whom more than seven oocytes were collected, the pregnancy rate was double that of a matched control group (i.e., both groups of patients received the same mean number of embryos at transfer).[32] Plasma E_2 levels in the patients producing more than seven oocytes were significantly higher than in the control group, from which it is possible to conclude that higher plasma E_2 levels do not compromise the prospects of pregnancy, and may even be beneficial.

In the second study,[34] follicular E_2 responses were categorized in 175 cycles (33 pregnancies) from patients receiving HMG alone for ovarian stimulation. Pregnancy rates varied from 27% for the most favorable E_2 pattern to 0% for the least. Once again, it is not possible to draw any conclusions about the influence of these E_2 profiles on uterine receptivity, since it is possible that they just reflect better follicle development and oocyte quality, and are not acting preferentially on endometrial preparation for implantation.

B. THE NEED FOR LUTEAL SUPPORT

Many IVF centers use P_4 supplementation in the luteal phase of stimulated cycles in the hope that uterine receptivity will be improved. In reviewing the effectiveness of this strategy, it is necessary to consider different stimulation protocols separately.

The majority of studies published to date have looked at luteal support following CC/HMG stimulation. While it is possible to find a limited number of reports claiming improved pregnancy rates following luteal support in CC/HMG treated patients,[35] the bulk of the data has failed to confirm any improvement in pregnancy rates.[36] These studies have included luteal support with oral and intramuscular P_4, as well as with human chorionic gonadotrophin (hCG), and have looked at supplementation commencing from before oocyte retrieval to after embryo transfer. More recently, our group has failed to show any improvement in pregnancy rate following the administration of vaginal P_4 in a prospective randomized controlled trial involving 245 women undergoing routine IVF or GIFT.[37] In this study, P_4 was given as 100 mg pessaries twice a day, commencing the evening before oocyte retrieval and continuing for 14 days.

The rationale for giving vaginal rather than oral or intramuscular P_4 in this last study[37] was based on the following evidence: anatomical studies in the rhesus[38] and human[39,40] have clearly established the basis for a counter current exchange mechanism between the veins and arteries of the ovarian pedicle. That this counter current exchange is of physiological significance has been proven in the rhesus, where the plasma P_4 levels in the blood entering the uterus have been shown to be at least tenfold those found in the general circulation.[41] Other limited studies have also demonstrated counter current exchange from the ovarian vein into the uterine artery in the human.[42,43] Although less well studied, the lymphatics draining the corpus luteum also provide a major source of P_4[44] that may possibly find its way back into the uterine circulation by counter current exchange. Taken together, these observations strongly suggest that local pathways play an important role in moving ovarian P_4 directly to the uterus, rather than allowing it to pass through the systemic circulation. While the biological significance of these increased uterine P_4 levels is unclear at present, it is not unreasonable to assume that they play a significant role in the preparation of the endometrium for implantation. Thus, if luteal support is going to be effective in mimicking normal ovarian P_4 delivery, we believe that consideration should be given to local rather than systemic administration. Indeed, there have been reports of improved pregnancy rates[45] and endometrial maturation[46,47] following the vaginal administration of P_4 in patients without ovarian function, suggesting that this may be the most efficacious route of administration.

The conclusion from these results, and the treatment strategy most commonly followed by those IVF groups still using CC/HMG for ovarian stimulation, is that luteal support offers no advantage to this group of patients.

By contrast to CC/HMG stimulation, IVF patients receiving GnRH-a down regulation clearly require luteal support to prevent premature luteolysis. This has been demonstrated by significant improvements in pregnancy rates in clinical trials,[48] as well as by studies of corpus luteum function in women receiving GnRH-a down regulation.[49] In this latter study, serum E_2 and P_4 levels were reduced by 88% and 80%, respectively by 10 to 12 days after oocyte retrieval in patients not receiving luteal support with hCG compared to those that were. Furthermore, the establishment of pregnancy failed to restore E_2 and P_4 secretion to the levels observed in women who had received luteal support with hCG, indicating that the corpus luteum had undergone irrevocable regression by this time.

Undoubtedly the endocrinological parameters necessary for uterine receptivity will become more clearly defined as studies such as those described above continue. Unfortunately, interpretation of results will always be plagued by the wide natural variation in uterine response to E_2 and P_4 that occurs in the human.[50]

V. MORPHOLOGICAL STUDIES: THE SEARCH FOR A RECEPTIVE ENDOMETRIUM

Identification of one or more endometrial parameters that definitely indicate receptivity for implantation remains a much sought after and elusive goal. An ability to readily identify receptive human endometrium would be of major clinical value in both infertility and contraceptive medicine. For this reason, there have been numerous studies describing and quantifying morphological and histological changes in the endometrium during the menstrual cycle in an attempt to identify markers for uterine receptivity. Some of these studies are reviewed below. Unfortunately, despite many well-documented endometrial changes around the time of implantation, it appears unlikely that obligatory markers for uterine receptivity will be conclusively established in the near future. The primary reason for this revolves around the ethical dilemma that prevents endometrial sampling from a uterus known to contain peri-implantation stage embryos. As a consequence, it is not possible to plan studies where given endometrial parameters can be correlated with the success of the implantation process. Despite this problem, significant progress has been made in establishing endometrial changes that do occur in both normal and abnormal menstrual cycles during the peri-implantation period, and from this information a picture is developing of features presumed to be desirable for receptivity.

A. ENDOMETRIAL MORPHOLOGY AND THE LUTEAL PHASE DEFECT

It is well documented that the endometrium undergoes a cyclical series of changes in histological appearance under the influence of estrogen and progesterone during the menstrual cycle.[51] Many similar studies have also been made using scanning and transmission electron microscopy.[52,53] The functional importance of these morphological changes with respect to uterine receptivity for implantation remains unclear, as was highlighted in recent work from our laboratory where endometrial biopsies from patients receiving hormone replacement therapy for premature ovarian failure were examined using scanning electron microscopy.[50] In this study, semiquantitative morphometric analysis of seven variables was used to identify an endometrial appearance that we and others[52-54] predicted would be implantation receptive. However, a single biopsy taken inadvertently from a conception cycle in one of these patients produced an endometrium that rated as relatively nonreceptive by morphometric analysis,[55] throwing doubt on the overall conclusion that receptivity could be assumed from the histological variables that were being measured.

Logically then, if it is not yet possible to identify an endometrium that is receptive for implantation, it cannot be possible to identify one that is not receptive for implantation. Thus, the importance of the luteal phase defect (LPD) in infertility, as assessed by endometrial histology, is, at best, questionable. LPD is defined as a defect of corpus luteum progesterone output, either in amount or duration, which results in inadequate stimulation of the endometrium for implantation of the blastocyst.[56] While some authors claim significant success from treating patients diagnosed as having LPD,[57] others claim that the incidence of LPD among the fertile population is no different than that among infertile women.[58] The observation by Wentz et al.,[59] from a study of 54 biopsies taken inadvertently during conception cycles, that the endometrium was on average dated significantly earlier than expected, clearly proves that delayed endometrial maturation to a degree consistent with the definition of LPD does not necessarily preclude implantation.

One explanation for this variability in opinion about LPD is the original method of back-calculating the predicted day of the luteal phase from the day of onset of the next menstrual period. This method was originally adopted because of the problems associated with obtaining an accurate estimate of the time of ovulation. In a recent study,[60] it has been clearly shown that endometrial dating has a significantly better correlation to the date of the luteinizing hormone (LH) surge than to the onset of the next menstrual period. This observation is hardly surprising, since calculations based on the start of the next menstrual period assume a luteal phase of 14 days, whereas in reality the luteal phase can vary considerably in length, with one study reporting 31% of women having luteal phases of either less than 12 or more than 16 days.[61]

Further error in the dating of endometrial biopsies also arises from interobserver variability. There can be little doubt that judgments based on the subjective evaluation of histologic patterns is likely to introduce some degree of error in experimental data. A more appropriate method of dating endometrial biopsies utilizes objective morphometric analysis. In a study of 70 biopsies, Li et al.[62] measured 17 quantitative and semiquantitative endometrial parameters before deriving a regressions equation utilizing five of the parameters to predict chronological dating of the endometrial biopsy. Using this new morphometric approach, predicted vs. actual endometrial dates correlated more accurately than using the original criteria of Noyes et al.[51] ($r = 0.98, p < 0.0001$ using morphometry; $r = 0.88, p < 0.001$ by Noyes et al. criteria).

In summary, studies on LPD that use date of onset of next menstrual period or that rely on qualitative assessment of histological appearance have an inherent degree of inaccuracy that is sufficiently large to throw doubt on the validity of their conclusions. That this is indeed the case is supported by the continuing lack of agreement over the role of LPD in infertility (for review see[63]).

B. THE EFFECTS OF OVARIAN STIMULATION ON ENDOMETRIAL MORPHOLOGY

There have been numerous publications dealing with endometrial histopathology following ovarian stimulation.[64-69] A comparison of results from these papers presents a confusing picture, due in part to the many significant methodological differences between each study. Factors that can influence endometrial histology in this type of work include stimulation regimen, endocrine response, patient age and cause of infertility, timing of the endometrial biopsy, and the subjective nature of histopathological classification of the biopsy. A brief review of recently published information on endometrial response to ovarian stimulation is provided below.

In patients given CC/HMG and biopsied 2 to 4 d after oocyte retrieval, 8 out of 15 had hypotrophic endometrium that was thought to be unsuitable for nidation,[64] and 9 out of 24 still had proliferative endometrium.[65] By contrast, biopsies taken during the proliferative phase 24 to 48 h after the end of CC administration showed advanced secretory changes in 10 out of 19 cases.[66] In another study, a variety of endometrial defects were identified 2 d after oocyte retrieval in 84% of patients receiving CC/HMG and in 52% of patients receiving HMG only.[67] The same study reported that normal endometrial histology was only found in women less than 36 years of age. A study of patients receiving HMG without CC and biopsied 1 to 3 d after the LH surge found 11 out of 22 to have advanced endometrium,[68] while in 18 patients receiving buserelin/HMG and biopsied on day 21 of the cycle, the average delay in endometrial maturation was 2.6 d, a delay which was not influenced by the administration of luteal support.[69]

In general terms, these results do not agree with our own experience of the endometrial response to ovarian stimulation,[70] where we have found that subjective histopathology does not identify abnormalities or structural changes that can be detected using other methods. In a study of 17 women (12 received CC/HMG and 5 received buserelin/HMG) biopsied 2 d after oocyte retrieval, 15 had histopathological dating that agreed exactly with the chronological age of the endometrium. By contrast, both morphometric analysis and ultrasound imaging techniques demonstrated significant differences in endometrial structure between women receiving the two different stimulation protocols. The major conclusion from this study was a highlighting of the importance of morphometry and ultrasound in the evaluation of endometrial structure, both in identifying features that may be missed by routine histopathology and in providing standardized measurements that can be objectively compared from one study to the next.

C. ULTRASOUND STUDIES OF THE ENDOMETRIUM

When ultrasound-guided follicle aspiration replaced laparoscopy as the method of choice for IVF, it became inevitable that ultrasound imaging would also be used to assess the endometrium. A number of studies have now been published,[71,72] some of which show a good correlation between endometrial thickness and the stage of the follicular phase. It has also been reported that endometrial thickness and pattern on the day before oocyte retrieval may be indicators of the likelihood of achieving pregnancy.[73]

We have found that ultrasound imaging can be used to differentiate between the endometrial response to CC/HMG versus buserelin/HMG, and that these different ultrasound images reflect real morphological differences in the endometrium.[70] The value of ultrasound for assessing endometrial appearance is that the results are immediate, that it can be performed repeatedly to follow serial changes in the same patient, and that because it is noninvasive, it can be used on patients known to have an embryo in their uterus. This flexibility of ultrasound as a technique for investigating the endometrium, coupled with the promise of new information already shown by early observations, opens the exciting possibility that ultrasound imaging may provide an avenue for significantly improving our understanding of endometrial features that are important for uterine receptivity.

The recent incorporation of color Doppler processing in transvaginal transducer/probes has provided a completely new clinical mode for investigating utero-ovarian physiology. While it is too early to conclude anything with certainty, there are already reports in the literature that an increased uterine artery pulsatility index at the time of embryo transfer is associated with a reduced implantation rate.[74]

D. HUMAN UTERINE EPITHELIAL TIGHT JUNCTIONS

Tight junctions are important ultrastructural features of epithelial cells, playing a significant role in joining adjacent cell walls closely together and thus maintaining the integrity of the epithelium. It has been suggested that endometrial epithelial integrity plays a major role in determining uterine receptivity for implantation, since removal of the epithelium from a non-progestational rat uterus will overcome the block to implantation that normally occurs.[8] For implantation to occur in the human, the embryo must breach the epithelium, raising the possibility that, in the receptive uterus, mechanisms may exist to reduce the integrity of the epithelial barrier. Recent studies in our group[75] using freeze-fracture followed by morphometry to study endometrial biopsies from premature ovarian failure patients receiving hormone replacement therapy have shown that epithelial tight junctions are regulated in a controlled manner during the peri-implantation period. This work demonstrated a significant decrease in tight junction area between days 13 and 23 of the menstrual cycle, as well as a reduction in geometrical complexity. These data support the hypothesis that sex steroid conditioning of the human uterus for implantation causes a reduction in epithelial integrity. In a related study,[76] the surprising observation was made that in 9 out of 11 biopsies from six Turner's syndrome patients, there were no tight junctions, while in the remaining two biopsies, tight junctions were greatly reduced. Two of these Turner's patients subsequently had successful pregnancies. This observation that an apparently compromised epithelium does not appear to interfere with implantation is consistent with the hypothesis that the uterine epithelium normally acts as a barrier to the embryo, only becoming receptive for implantation when appropriately conditioned with E_2 and P_4. Certainly, it would appear that the absence of uterine epithelial tight junctions does not prevent successful pregnancy.

VI. THE CONTRIBUTION OF STUDIES WITH AGONADAL WOMEN RECEIVING HORMONE REPLACEMENT THERAPY FOR IVF TO OUR UNDERSTANDING OF UTERINE RECEPTIVITY IN THE HUMAN

The reporting of the world's first donor oocyte pregnancy in a woman with premature ovarian failure[77] opened a valuable experimental avenue for further exploring the E_2 and P_4 levels required for implantation.[78] In these patients, exogenous E_2 and P_4 are given solely to create a receptive uterine environment, since there is no need to manipulate the follicular phase of the cycle to produce oocytes.

A. FIXED AND VARIABLE LENGTH HORMONE REPLACEMENT CYCLES

The first steroid replacement regimens developed were based very closely on the standardized 28 d menstrual cycle, with increasing levels of E_2 reaching 6 mg daily during the first half of the cycle and P_4 commencing mid cycle.[77-79] A number of pregnancies were achieved using this type of hormone replacement protocol, although there are problems associated with the very short period of time during the 28 d cycle in which the recipient can be synchronized with a donated oocyte or embryo.

More recently, successful hormone replacement regimes have been developed that use a constant dose of E_2 over a variable length of time up to the moment that the donor oocyte is obtained.[80,81] Progesterone is then given to the patient from either the day before or the day of oocyte collection from the donor. This new approach has the advantage of allowing a much wider time span in which the donor and the recipient can be synchronized. To date we have found no difference in pregnancy rates per embryo transfer between the fixed and the variable length protocols;[82] however, far more patients receive transfers with the variable length protocol compared to the fixed one, resulting in more patients overall becoming pregnant. Using the variable length schedule, we have achieved pregnancies with follicular phases ranging from 10 to 24 d.[82] Histological and ultrastructural studies of endometrial morphology currently underway suggest that these limits may well be extended further. Indeed, other workers in this field have reported pregnancies following fixed follicular phases ranging from 5 to 35 d.[83] This raises the possibility that, as with some animal species,[3] follicular phase E_2 might not be necessary for the development of uterine receptivity in the human. However, reports that a short follicular phase of 5 d results in significantly increased early pregnancy wastage[83] may be an indication that this is approaching the physiological minimum for the human.

It is interesting to note that many IVF centers performing donor oocyte transfers report higher success rates for their oocyte recipients than for the patients undergoing ovarian stimulation for IVF.[79-95] This observation, where oocytes and embryos of similar quality are placed in uteri that have seen very different endocrine environments, provides strong evidence that either the drugs used for or the large changes in circulating estrogen and progesterone that result from ovarian stimulation are acting to reduce uterine receptivity. Identification of structural and functional differences between endometria from women in each of these groups may identify parameters that can eventually be used to measure uterine receptivity.

B. THE HUMAN IMPLANTATION WINDOW

Prior to the advent of IVF and associated procedures, knowledge of the human implantation window could only be conjectural. Two IVF-related procedures, freezing and donation, now provide an opportunity whereby developing embryos can be replaced into the uterus outside the normal obligatory uterus-embryo developmental time frame. This ability to study asynchronous embryo transfers provides an avenue whereby the length of the human implantation window may soon be clearly established.

In previous reviews of published pregnancies established in patients receiving donated oocytes for premature ovarian failure,[90,91] it was estimated that successful implantation occurred when the embryo was anywhere from 39 h in

TABLE 2
Summary of Data on Embryonic-Uterine Synchrony Based on Patients with Ovarian Failure Receiving Hormone Replacement Therapy for Donor Oocyte and Embryo Transfers

Source	Pregnancies reported	Uterus ahead of embryo (hours)	Uterus behind embryo (hours)
Monash donor oocyte[92] (Fixed cyclical protocol)	11		18–39
Monash donor oocyte[45,82] (Variable length protocol)	40		20–36
Salat-Baroux et al.[93]	4		36
Feichtinger and Kemeter[84]	1		18
Asche et al.[81]	6		18
Rosenwaks[85]	8	0–48(?)	0–24
Junca et al.[88]	4	0(?)	
Devroey et al.[94,95]	11	0–12(?)	
Navot et al.[79]	2	4–28	
Serhal and Craft[80,86]	18	12	
Abdalla et al.[96]	8	12	
{Formigli et al.[87]	8	0–96	0–72}

(Not all ovarian failure recipients)

Note: The synchrony calculations in Table 2 are based on the two assumptions that in the natural cycle (a) significant P_4 secretion starts 12 h before ovulation and (b) fertilization occurs 6 h after ovulation. (For more detail on embryo-uterine developmental synchrony see Rogers et al.[90]). Where it has not been possible from the published information to estimate accurately the timing of embryonic development relative to the point in time that the uterus first received P_4, a (?) has been placed next to the calculated synchrony.

front to 48 h behind the uterus. These calculations give an implantation window of at least 3.5 d. A summary of these two reviews and a large amount of additional new data, representing more than 120 pregnancies, is given in Table 2. The calculations in Table 2 are based on the assumption that, as in animals,[3,4] the commencement of P_4 in the human will initiate a "clock" that results in the uterus passing through a receptive phase or window. Uterine age is thus calculated as the time from when the uterus first received P_4, and embryonic age is taken from the time of ovulation.

Of particular interest in Table 2 is the work of Formigli et al.[87] These workers used embryos lavaged from the uteri of donors 5 d postovulation, and report pregnancies in cases where the recipient was anywhere from 4 d in front to 3 d behind the donor at the time of ovulation. However, there may be possible sources of error in the calculations of timing in this study. For example, ovulation was only assessed by daily ultrasound of the ovaries, monitoring for disappearance of the follicle, and could therefore be up to 24 h out. More importantly, it was not possible to exclude the possibility of spontaneous pregnancy in five out of six patients with ovarian function. Accepting these limitations, this study suggests that the human implantation window may be up to 7 d, twice that previously demonstrated by donor oocyte and embryo results.

In the only major study published to date where embryo-uterine synchrony has been systematically varied to explore the length of the implantation window,[83] pregnancies were achieved over a 6 d window that equated to implantation occurring anywhere from days 18/19 through to 23/24. Numbers were not large enough in this study to determine whether differences in success rate existed within this time frame. It may also be possible to artificially widen the implantation window by manipulating the pre- and peri-implantation endocrine environment. In one study, it has been reported that ovarian stimulation with GnRH-a/HMG compared with HMG alone appears to widen the implantation window.[97] In this work, the time of implantation was estimated by regression analysis of serial hCG measurements between 7 and 16 d after embryo transfer.

Knowledge of the length of the human implantation window is of critical significance to all future studies aimed at identifying endometrial markers for uterine receptivity. Unless we can identify when the uterus is receptive to the implanting embryo, it will never be possible to correlate changing endocrine, biochemical, and morphological endometrial parameters with receptivity.

VII. STRATEGIES FOR IMPROVING UTERINE RECEPTIVITY

Broadly speaking, there are two strategies that can be utilized for improving uterine receptivity. The first is to develop ovarian stimulation protocols that cause a minimum reduction in uterine receptivity (or may even increase it), and the second is to avoid the endometrium altogether during stimulated cycles by freezing the embryos and replacing them in subsequent natural cycles.

Avoiding a reduction in endometrial receptivity as a result of ovarian stimulation will have to remain a largely theoretical exercise until an objective way of assessing uterine receptivity is developed. Despite this, there are still a number of factors which we know from animal and human studies can influence endometrial receptivity, and which should be taken into account when planning ovarian stimulation for IVF. There is statistical evidence from the human,[24] and experimental evidence from mouse work,[98,99] that CC impairs endometrial receptivity. A number of IVF programs, including ours at Monash, are now recognizing this fact and moving to ovarian stimulation protocols that do not use CC. This strategy has been helped by the recent development of a number of new ovarian stimulation protocols based on GnRH-a that do not utilize CC. As of yet, however, consensus has not been reached that elimination of CC results in higher pregnancy rates,[100] although reports are suggesting it.[101]

The strategy of freezing all embryos produced from a stimulated cycle and replacing them in subsequent natural cycles, when the endometrium has not been subjected to abnormal levels of E_2 and P_4, has been available for many years now. That it has not become a commonly used approach suggests that at present most IVF groups, either correctly or incorrectly, do not consider it advantageous. This may be for a number of reasons. The foremost of these is the belief that currently available freezing protocols cause a loss in embryo viability that will negate any beneficial effect that may accrue from the increase in uterine receptivity. This belief is supported by the results of a study comprising 40 cycles of oocyte donation to patients receiving hormone replacement therapy.[102] Of 162 embryos, 17/76 (24%) that were transferred fresh implanted, compared with only 7/91 (7.7%) that were frozen. However, these results do not take into account any deleterious effect that the process of superovulation may have had on the endometrium, since all transfers were to women receiving hormone replacement schedules known to support high implantation rates. In the donors from this same study, all of whom had undergone superovulation, only 9/144 (6.25%) of the same cohort of embryos implanted. In a study at The Royal Women's Hospital IVF Unit in Melbourne, designed to test the relative merits of fresh transfers in stimulated cycles versus frozen transfers in unstimulated cycles,[103] it was found that 48/880 (5.5%) fresh transfers resulted in live births compared with 98/1336 (7.3%) for frozen transfers. When these figures were corrected for embryo quality, and a 15% loss rate included for embryo freezing, it was estimated that freezing would still give 62 live births per 1,000 freezable embryos, compared with 55 live births if the same embryos were transferred fresh in the original stimulated cycle.

There are also a number of practical and financial considerations revolving around the increased number of embryos requiring freezing and storage, as well as the need for patients to return for subsequent tracking cycles prior to frozen embryo replacement. Despite this, there is still a clear need for more studies to address the issue of fresh versus frozen embryo transfers, and thus to provide some consensus on the relative merits of each course of action.

Another approach that has been used to avoid the reduced uterine receptivity that undoubtedly occurs following ovarian hyperstimulation is to return to natural cycle IVF, as was practiced when human IVF first started. While this strategy clearly avoids any reduction in uterine receptivity associated with hyperstimulation, the disadvantages of working with a single developing follicle would seem to outweigh any advantage gained. There is clear evidence that IVF pregnancy success rates improve with the number of embryos transferred, at least up to a total of 3.[104] Thus, an optimal superovulation strategy should aim to produce at least three high quality transferable embryos, to maximize the chances of success.

REFERENCES

1. **Finn, C. A. and Porter, D. G.,** Implantation of ova, in *The Uterus, Handbooks in Reproductive Biology,* Vol. 1, Finn, C. A., Ed., Elek Science, London, 1975, 57.
2. **Sherman, M. I. and Wudl, L. R.,** The implanting mouse blastocyst, *Cell Surface Rev.,* 1, 81, 1976.
3. **Humphrey, K. W.,** Induction of implantation of blastocysts transfered to ovariectomized mice, *J. Endocrinol.,* 44, 299, 1969.
4. **De Feo, V. J.,** Determination of the sensitive period for the induction of deciduomata in the rat by different inducing procedures, *Endocrinology,* 73, 488, 1963.
5. **Psychoyos, A. and Casimiri, V.,** Factors involved in uterine receptivity and refractoriness, *Prog. Reprod. Biol.,* 7, 143, 1980.
6. **Weitlauf, H. M.,** Factors in mouse uterine fluid that inhibit the incorporation of ^{3}H-uridine by blastocysts in vitro, *J. Reprod. Fertil.,* 52, 321, 1978.
7. **Psychoyos, A., Roche, D., and Gravanis, A.,** Is cholic acid responsible for embryotoxicity of the post-receptive uterine environment?, *Hum. Reprod.,* 4, 832, 1989.
8. **Cowell, T. P.,** Implantation and development of mouse eggs transferred to the uteri of non-progestational mice, *J. Reprod. Fertil.,* 19, 239, 1969.
9. **Runner, M. N.,** Development of mouse eggs in the anterior chamber of the eye, *Anat. Rec.,* 98, 1, 1947.
10. **Rogers, P. A. W., Macpherson, A. M., and Beaton, L. A.,** Vascular response in a non-uterine site to implantation-stage embryos in the rat and guinea-pig: in vivo and ultrastructural studies, *Cell Tissue Res.,* 254, 217, 1988.
11. **Fawcett, D. W.,** The development of mouse ova under the capsule of the kidney, *Anat. Rec.,* 108, 71, 1950.
12. **Kirby, D. R. S.,** The development of mouse blastocysts transplanted to the scrotal and cryptorchid testis, *J. Anat.,* 97, 119, 1963.
13. **Kirby, D. R. S.,** Development of the mouse blastocyst transplanted to the spleen, *J. Reprod. Fertil.,* 5, 1, 1963.
14. **Macpherson, A. M., Rogers, P. A. W., and Beaton, L. A.,** Vascular response in a non-uterine site to implantation stage embryos following interspecies transfers between the rat, mouse and guinea-pig, *Cell Tissue Res.,* 258, 417, 1989.
15. **Ombelet, W., Vandermerwe, J. V., and Van Assche, F. A.,** Advanced extrauterine pregnancy: description of 38 cases with literature survey, *Obstet. Gynecol. Surv.,* 43, 386, 1988.
16. **Sandell, M.,** The evolution of seasonal delayed implantation, *Q. Rev. Biol.,* 65, 23, 1990.
17. **Lundkvist, Ö. and Nilsson, B. O.,** Endometrial ultrastructure in the early uterine response to blastocysts and artificial deciduogenic stimuli in rats, *Cell Tissue Res.,* 225, 355, 1982.
18. **Garrett, J. E., Geisert, R. D., Zavy, M. T., and Morgan, G. L.,** Evidence for maternal regulation of early conceptus growth and development in beef cattle, *J. Reprod. Fertil.,* 84, 437, 1988.
19. **Leridon, H.,** *Human Fertility,* University of Chicago Press, Chicago, 1977.
20. **Wood, J. W.,** Fecundity and natural fertility in humans, in *Oxford Reviews of Reproductive Biology,* Vol. 11, Milligan, S. R., Ed., Oxford University Press, Oxford, 1989, 61.
21. **Hertig, A. T., Rock, J., and Adams, E. C.,** A description of 34 human ova within the first 17 days of development, *Am. J. Anat.,* 98, 435, 1956.
22. **Boué, J., Boué, A., and Lazar, P.,** Retrospective and prospective epidemiological studies of 1500 karyotyped spontaneous human abortions, *Teratology,* 12, 11, 1975.
23. **Leeton, J., Shaw, G., and Short, R. V.,** Twin ovulations, dizygotic twins and human fecundability, *Br. J. Obstet. Gynaecol.,* in press, 1993.
24. **Rogers, P. A. W., Milne, B. J., and Trounson, A. O.,** A model to show human uterine receptivity and embryo viability following ovarian stimulation for in vitro fertilization, *J. In Vitro Fertil. Embryo Transfer,* 3, 93, 1986.

25. **Walters, D. E., Edwards, D. G., and Meistrich, M. L.,** A statistical evaluation of implantation after replacing one or more human embryos, *J. Reprod. Fertil.,* 74, 557, 1985.
26. **Speirs, A. L., Lopata, A., Gronow, M. J., Kellow, G. N., and Johnston, W. I. H.,** Analysis of the benefits and risks of multiple embryo transfer, *Fertil. Steril.,* 39, 468, 1083.
27. **Navot, D., Bergh, P. A., Williams, M. A., Garrisi, G. J., Guzman, I., Sandler, B., and Grunfeld, L.,** Poor oocyte quality rather than implantation failure as a cause of age-related decline in female fertility, *Lancet,* 337, 1375, 1991.
28. **Abdalla, H. I., Baber, R., Kirkland, A., Leonard, T., Power, M., and Studd, J. W. W.,** A report on 100 cycles of oocyte donation; factors affecting the outcome, *Hum. Reprod.,* 5, 1018, 1990.
29. **Landgren, B. M., Unden, A. L., and Diczfalusy, E.,** Hormonal profile of the cycle in 68 normally menstruating women, *Acta Endocrinol.,* 94, 89, 1980.
30. **Morris, J. M. and Van Wagenan, G.,** Interception: the use of post-ovulatory estrogens to prevent implantation, *J. Am. Obstet. Gynecol.,* 115, 101, 1973.
31. **Sharp, N. C., Anthony, F., Willams, J., Masson, G. M., and Miller, J. F.,** Oestradiol and progesterone levels at the time of implantation and their effect upon its success in a subfertile population, in Proceedings of the Sixth Scientific Meeting of the Fertility Society of Australia, 1987, 43.
32. **Healy, D. L., Okamoto, S., Morrow, L., Thomas, A., Jones, M., McLachlan, V., Besanko, M., Martinez, F., and Rogers, P.,** Contributions of in vitro fertilization to knowledge of the reproductive endocrinology of the menstrual cycle, in *Bailliére's Clinical Endocrinology and Metabolism,* Vol. 1, No. 1, Burger, H. G., Ed., 1987, 133.
33. **Okamoto, S., Healy, D. L., Howlett, D. T., Rogers, P. A. W., Leeton, J. F., Trounson, A. O., and Wood, E. C.,** An analysis of plasma estradiol concentrations during clomiphene citrate–human menopausal gonadotropin stimulation in an in vitro fertilization-embryo transfer program, *J. Clin. Endocrinol. Metab.,* 63, 736, 1986.
34. **Jones, H. W., Acosta, A., Andrews, M. C., Garcia, J. E., Jones, G. S., Mantzarinos, T., McDowell, J., Sandow, B., Veeck, L., Whibley, T., Wilkes, C., and Wright, G.,** The importance of the follicular phase to success and failure in in vitro fertilization, *Fertil. Steril.,* 40, 317, 1983.
35. **Ben-Nun, I., Ghetler, Y., Jaffe, R., Siegal, A., Kaneti, H., and Fejgin, M.,** Effect of preovulatory progesterone administration on the endometrial maturation and implantation rate after in vitro fertilization and embryo transfer, *Fertil. Steril.,* 53, 276, 1990.
36. **Daya, S.,** Efficacy of progesterone support in the luteal phase following in vitro fertilization and embryo transfer: meta-analysis of clinical trials, *Hum. Reprod.,* 3, 731, 1988.
37. **Polson, D. W. and Rogers, P. A. W.,** unpublished data, 1990.
38. **Ginther, O. J., Dierschke, D. J., Walsh, S. W., and Del Campo, C. H.,** Anatomy of arteries and veins of uterus and ovaries in rhesus monkeys, *Biol. Reprod.,* 11, 205, 1974.
39. **Bendz, A.,** The anatomical basis for a possible counter current exchange mechanism in the human adnex, *Prostaglandins,* 13, 355, 1977.
40. **Bendz, A., Hansson, H. A., Svendsen, P., and Wigvist, N.,** On the extensive contact between veins and arteries in the human ovarian pedicle, *Acta Physiol. Scand.,* 114, 611, 1982.
41. **Riesen, J. W., Koering, M. J., Meyer, R. K., and Wolf, R. C.,** Origin of ovarian venous progesterone in the rhesus monkey, *Endocrinology,* 86, 1212, 1970.
42. **Bendz, A., Einer-Jensen, N., Lundgren, O., and Janson, P. O.,** Exchange of krypton-85 between the blood vessels of the human uterine adnexa, *J. Reprod. Fertil.,* 57, 137, 1979.
43. **Bendz, A., Lundgren, O., and Hamberger, L.,** Counter current exchange of progesterone and antipyrine between human utero-ovarian vessels, and of antipyrine between the femoral vessels in the cat, *Acta Physiol. Scand.,* 114, 611, 1982.

44. **Hein, W. R., Shelton, J. N., Simpson-Morgan, M. W., Seamark, R. F., and Morris, B.,** Flow and composition of lymph from the ovary and uterus of cows during pregnancy, *J. Reprod. Fertil.,* 83, 309, 1988.
45. **Leeton, J., Rogers, P., Cameron, I., Caro, C., and Healy, D.,** Pregnancy results following embryo transfer in women receiving low-dosage variable-length estrogen replacement therapy for premature ovarian failure, *J. In Vitro Fertil. Embryo Transfer,* 6, 232, 1989.
46. **Bourgain, C., Devroey, P., Van Waesberghe, L., Smitz, J., and Van Steirteghem, A. C.,** Effects of natural progesterone on the morphology of the endometrium in patients with primary ovarian failure, *Hum. Reprod.,* 5, 537, 1990.
47. **Critchley, H. O. D., Buckley, C. H., and Anderson, D. C.,** Experience with a "physiological" steroid replacement regimen for the establishment of a receptive endometrium in women with premature ovarian failure, *Br. J. Obstet. Gynaecol.,* 97, 804, 1990.
48. **Smith, E. M., Anthony, F. W., Gadd, S. C., and Masson, G. M.,** Trial of support treatment with human chorionic gonadotrophin in the luteal phase after treatment with buserelin and human menopausal gonadotrophin in women taking part in an in vitro fertilisation programme, *Br. Med. J.,* 298, 1483, 1989.
49. **McClure, N., Laya, J., Radwanska, E., Rawlings, R., and Haning R. V.,** Luteal phase support and ovarian hyperstimulation syndrome, *Hum. Reprod.,* 7, 758, 1992.
50. **Rogers, P., Murphy, C., Cameron, I., Leeton, J., Hosie, M., Beaton, L., and Macpherson, A.,** Uterine receptivity in women receiving steroid replacement therapy for premature ovarian failure: ultrastructural and endocrinological parameters, *Hum. Reprod.,* 4, 349, 1989.
51. **Noyes, R. W., Hertig, A. T., and Rock, J.,** Dating the endometrial biopsy, *Fertil. Steril.,* 1, 3, 1950.
52. **Lawn, A. M.,** The ultrastructure of the endometrium during the sexual cycle, in *Advances in Reproductive Biology,* Vol. 6, Bishop, M. H. W., Ed., Elek, London, 1973, 61.
53. **Martel, D., Malet, C., Gautray, J. P., and Psychoyos, A.,** Surface changes of the luminal uterine epithelium during the human menstrual cycle: a scanning electron microscope study, in *The Endometrium: Hormonal Impacts,* de Brus, J., Martel, J., and Gautray J. P., Eds., Plenum, New York, 1981, 15.
54. **Murphy, C. R., Rogers, P. A. W., Leeton, J., Hosie, M., Beaton, L., and Macpherson, A.,** Surface ultrastructure of uterine epithelial cells in women with premature ovarian failure following steroid hormone replacement, *Acta Anat.,* 130, 348, 1987.
55. **Rogers, P. A. W., Murphy, C. R., Leeton, J., Hosie, M., Beaton, L., and Macpherson, A.,** An ultrastructural study of human uterine epithelium from a patient with a confirmed pregnancy, *Acta Anat.,* 135, 176, 1989.
56. **Jones, G. S.,** Luteal phase defects, in *Progress in Infertility,* 2nd ed., Behram, S. J. and Kistner, R. W., Eds., Little, Brown, Boston, 1975, 316.
57. **Witten, B. I. and Martin, S. A.,** The endometrial biopsy as a guide to the management of luteal phase defect, *Fertil. Steril.,* 44, 460, 1985.
58. **Glazener, C. M. A., Kelly, N. J., and Hull, M. G. R.,** Luteal deficiency not a persistent cause of infertility, *Hum. Reprod.,* 3, 213, 1988.
59. **Wentz, A. C., Herbert, C. M., Maxson, W. S., Hill, G. A., and Pittaway, D. E.,** Cycle of conception endometrial biopsy, *Fertil. Steril.,* 46, 196, 1986.
60. **Li, T.-C., Rogers, A. W., Lenton, E. A., Dockery, P., and Cooke, I.,** A comparison between two methods of chronological dating of human endometrial biopsies during the luteal phase, and their correlation with histologic dating, *Fertil. Steril.,* 48, 928, 1987.
61. **Lenton, E. A., Langdren, B.-M., and Sexton, L.,** Normal variation in the length of the luteal phase of the menstrual cycle: identification of a short luteal phase, *Br. J. Obstet. Gynaecol.,* 91, 685, 1984.

62. **Li, T.-C., Rogers, A. W., Dockery, P., Lenton, E. A., and Cooke, I. D.**, A new method of histologic dating of human endometrium in the luteal phase, *Fertil. Steril.*, 50, 52, 1988.
63. **Balasch, J. and Vanrell, J. A.**, Corpus luteum insufficiency and fertility: a matter of controversy, *Hum. Reprod.*, 2, 557, 1987.
64. **Cohen, J. J., Debache, C., Pigeau, F., Mandelbaum, J., Plachot, M., and de Brux, J.**, Sequential use of clomiphene citrate, human menopausal gonadotropin, and human chorionic gonadotropin in human in vitro fertilization. II. Study of luteal phase adequacy following aspiration of the preovulatory follicles, *Fertil. Steril.*, 42, 360, 1984.
65. **Abate, V., de Corato, R., Cali, A., and Stinchi, A.**, Endometrial biopsy at the time of embryo transfer: correlation of histological diagnosis with therapy and pregnancy rate, *J. In Vitro Fertil. Embryo Transfer*, 4, 173, 1987.
66. **Birkenfeld, A., Navot, D., Levij, I. S., Laufer, N., Beier-Hellwig, K., Goecke, J. G., Schenker, J. G., and Beier, H. M.**, Advanced secretory changes in the proliferative human endometrial epithelium following clomiphene citrate treatment, *Fertil. Steril.*, 45, 462, 1986.
67. **Sterzik, K., Dallenbach, C., Schneider, V., Sasse, V., and Dallenbach-Hellweg, G.**, In vitro fertilization: the degree of endometrial insufficiency varies with the type of ovarian stimulation, *Fertil. Steril.*, 50, 457, 1988.
68. **Garcia, J. E., Acosta, A. A., Hsiu, J.-G., and Jones, H.-W.**, Advanced endometrial maturation after ovulation induction with human menopausal gonadotropin/human chorionic gonadotropin for in vitro fertilization, *Fertil. Steril.*, 41, 31, 1984.
69. **Van Steirteghem, A. C., Smitz, J., Camus, M., Van Waesberghe, L., Deschacht, J., Khan, I., Staessen, C., Wisanto, A., Bourgain, C., and Devroey, P.**, The luteal phase after in-vitro fertilization and related procedures, *Hum. Reprod.*, 3, 161, 1988.
70. **Rogers, P. A. W., Polson, D., Murphy, C. R., Hosie, M., Susil, B., and Leoni, M.**, Correlation of endometrial histology, morphometry, and ultrasound appearance after different stimulation protocols for in vitro fertilization, *Fertil. Steril.*, 55, 583, 1991.
71. **Randall, J. M., Fisk, N. M., McTavish, A., and Templeton, A. A.**, Transvaginal ultrasonic assessment of endometrial growth in spontaneous and hyperstimulated cycles, *Br. J. Obstet. Gynaecol.*, 96, 954, 1989.
72. **Lenz, S. and Lindenberg, S.**, Ultrasonic evaluation of endometrial growth in women with normal cycles during spontaneous and stimulated cycles, *Hum. Reprod.*, 5, 377, 1990.
73. **Gonen, Y. and Casper, R. F.**, Prediction of implantation by the sonographic appearance of the endometrium during controlled ovarian stimulation for in vitro fertilization, *J. In Vitro Fertil. Embryo Transfer*, 7, 146, 1990.
74. **Fleischer, A. C.**, Ultrasound imaging–2000: assessment of utero-ovarian blood flow with transvaginal color Doppler sonography; potential clinical applications in infertility, *Fertil. Steril.*, 55, 684, 1991.
75. **Murphy, C. R., Rogers, P. A. W., Hosie, M. J., Leeton, J., and Beaton, L.**, Tight junctions of human uterine epithelial cells change during the menstrual cycle: a morphometric study, *Acta Anat.*, 144, 36, 1992.
76. **Rogers, P. A. W., Murphy, C. R., Leeton, J., Hosie, M. J., and Beaton, L.**, Turner's syndrome patients lack tight junctions between uterine epithelial cells, *Hum. Reprod.*, 7, 883, 1992.
77. **Lutjen, P., Trounson, A., Leeton, J., Findlay, J., Wood, C., and Renou, P.**, The establishment and maintenance of pregnancy using in vitro fertilization and embryo donation in a patient with primary ovarian failure, *Nature*, 307, 174, 1984.
78. **Cameron, I. T., Rogers, P. A. W., Salamonsen, L. A., and Healy, D. L.**, The endocrine requirements for implantation and early embryogenesis, *J. Reprod. Fertil.*, Suppl. 36, 17, 1988.

79. **Navot, D., Laufer, N., Kopolovic, J., Rabinowitz, R., Birkenfeld, A., Lewin, A., Granat, M., Margalioth, E. J., and Schenker, J. G.**, Artificially induced endometrial cycles and establishment of pregnancies in the absence of ovaries, *N. Engl. J. Med.*, 314, 806, 1986.
80. **Serhal, P. and Craft, I.**, Simplified treatment for ovum donation, *Lancet*, I, 687, 1987.
81. **Asche, R. H., Balmoceda, J. P., Ord, T., Borrero, C., Cefalu, E., Gastaldi, C., and Rojas, F.**, Oocyte donation and gamete intrafallopian transfer in premature ovarian failure, *Fertil. Steril.*, 49, 263, 1988.
82. **Leeton, J., Rogers, P., King, C., and Healy, D.**, A comparison of pregnancy rates for 131 donor egg transfers using either a sequential or fixed regime of steroid replacement therapy, *Hum. Reprod.*, in press, 1991.
83. **Navot, D., Bergh, P. A., Williams, M., Garrisi, G. J., Guzman, I., Sandler, B., Fox, J., Schreiner-Engel, P., Hofmann, G. E., and Grunfeld, L.**, An insight into early reproductive processes through the in vivo model of ovum donation, *J. Clin. Endocrinol. Metab.*, 72, 408, 1991.
84. **Feichtinger, W. and Kemeter, P.**, Pregnancy after total ovariectomy achieved by ovum donation, *Lancet*, II, 722, 1985.
85. **Rosenwaks, Z.**, Donor eggs; their application in modern reproductive technologies, *Fertil. Steril.*, 47, 895, 1987.
86. **Serhal, P. and Craft, I.**, Oocyte donation in 61 patients, *Lancet*, I, 1185, 1989.
87. **Formigli, L., Formigli, G., and Roccio, C.**, Donation of fertilised uterine ova to infertile women, *Fertil. Steril.*, 47, 162, 1987.
88. **Junca, A.-M., Cohen, J., Mandelbaum, J., Alnot, M.-O., Debache, C., Plachot, M., and Pez, J. P.**, Anonymous and non-anonymous oocyte donation: preliminary results, *Hum. Reprod.*, 3, 121, 1988.
89. **Paulson, R. J., Sauer, M. V., and Lobo, R. A.**, Embryo implantation after human in vitro fertilization: importance of endometrial receptivity, *Fertil. Steril.*, 53, 870, 1990.
90. **Rogers, P., Leeton, J., Cameron, I. T., Murphy, C., Healy, D., and Lutjen, P.**, Oocyte donation, in *Clinical In Vitro Fertilization and Embryo Transfer*, 2nd ed., Wood, C. and Trounson, A. O., Eds., Springer-Verlag, Berlin, 1988, 143.
91. **Rogers, P. A. W. and Murphy, C. R.**, Uterine receptivity for implantation: human studies, in *Blastocyst Implantation*, Yoshinaga, K., Ed., Serono Symposia, Adams Publishing Group, Boston, 1989, 231.
92. **Cameron, I. T., Rogers, P. A. W., Caro, C., Harman, J., Healy, D. L., and Leeton, J. F.**, Oocyte donation: a review, *Br. J. Obstet. Gynaecol.*, 96, 839, 1989.
93. **Salat-Baroux, J., Cornet, D., Alvarez, S., Antoine, J. M., Tibi, C., Mandelbaum, J., and Plachot, M.**, Pregnancies after replacement of frozen-thawed embryos in a donation program, *Fertil. Steril.*, 49, 817, 1988.
94. **Devroey, P., Wisanto, A., Camus, M., Van Waesberghe, L., Bourgain, Cl., Liebaers, I., and Van Steirteghem, A. C.**, Oocyte donation in patients without ovarian function, *Hum. Reprod.*, 3, 699, 1988.
95. **Devroey, P., Camus, M., Van Den Abbeel, E., Van Waesberghe, L., Wisanto, A., and Van Steirteghem, A. C.**, Establishment of 22 pregnancies after oocyte and embryo donation, *Br. J. Obstet. Gynaecol.*, 96, 900, 1989.
96. **Abdalla, H. I., Baber, R. J., Kirkland, A., Leonard, T., and Studd, J. W. W.**, Pregnancy in women with premature ovarian failure using tubal and intrauterine transfer of cryopreserved zygotes, *Br. J. Obstet. Gynaecol.*, 96, 1071, 1989.
97. **Tur-Kaspa, I., Confino, E., Dudkiewicz, A. B., Myers, S. A., Friberg, J., and Gleicher, N.**, Ovarian stimulation protocol for in vitro fertilization with gonadotropin-releasing hormone agonist widens the implantation window, *Fertil. Steril.*, 53, 859, 1990.
98. **Nelson, L. M., Hershlag, A., Kurl, R. S., Hall, J. L., and Stillman, R. J.**, Clomiphene citrate directly impairs endometrial receptivity in the mouse, *Fertil. Steril.*, 53, 727, 1990.

99. **Dziadek, M.,** Preovulatory administration of clomiphene citrate to mice causes fetal growth retardation and neural tube defects (exencephaly) by an indirect maternal effect, *Teratology,* in press, 1993.
100. **Ferrier, A., Rasweiler, J. J., Bedford, J. M., Prey, K., and Berkeley, A. S.,** Evaluation of leuprolide acetate and gonadotropins versus clomiphene citrate and gonadotropins for in vitro fertilization or gamete intrafallopian transfer, *Fertil. Steril.,* 54, 90, 1990.
101. **Abdalla, H. I., Ahuja, K. K., Leonard, T., Morris, N. N., Honour, J. W., and Jacobs, H. S.,** Comparative trial of luteinizing hormone-releasing hormone analog/human menopausal gonadotropin and clomiphene citrate/human menopausal gonadotropin in an assisted conception program, *Fertil. Steril.,* 53, 473, 1990.
102. **Levran, D., Dor, J., Rudak, E., Nebel, L., Ben-Shlomo, I., Ben-Rafael, Z., and Mashiach, S.,** Pregnancy potential of human oocytes — the effect of cryopreservation, *New Engl. J. Med.,* 323, 1153, 1990.
103. **Hales, L. and McBain, J.,** personal communication, 1991.
104. **Jones, H. W. and Rogers, P. A. W.,** Results from in vitro fertilization, in *Clinical In Vitro Fertilization and Embryo Transfer,* 2nd ed., Wood, C. and Trounson, A. O., Eds., Springer-Verlag, Berlin, 1988, 51.

Chapter 14

ETHICAL ASPECTS OF IVF AND HUMAN EMBRYO RESEARCH

Karen Dawson

TABLE OF CONTENTS

I. Introduction 288
    A. The Increasing Applications of IVF 288
    B. Increasing Debate about Human Embryo Research 289
    C. The Scope of This Chapter 289

II. The Major Opposition to IVF and Human Embryo Research 289
    A. The Right-to-Life View 289
    B. The Official Vatican View 290
        1. What is Fertilization? 291
    C. The Radical Feminist View 292

III. Views in Support of IVF and Human Embryo Research 293
    A. Public Support 293
    B. The Stage of Development as the Determinant
       of Moral Status 293
        1. The Use of These Views in Legislation 294

IV. Should an Upper Limit for Human Embryo Research
be Legislated? 295

V. Where Will the Embryos Used for Research
Come From? 296
    A. "Spare" or Intentionally-Created Embryos
       for Research? 296

VI. Some Issues Relevant to Current Research 297
    A. Embryo/Oocyte Freezing 297
    B. *In Vitro* Oocyte Maturation 298
    C. Embryo Biopsy 298

VII. Conclusion 299

References 300

I. INTRODUCTION

The birth of Louise Brown in 1978 laid the foundations for the technique of *in vitro* fertilization to become important in the treatment of infertility. It was also in 1978 that the ongoing debate about the ethics of IVF and *in vitro* human embryo research began.

It would have been impossible then to predict the rapid growth of reproductive technology that was to follow during the 1980s. It also would have been impossible to foretell the establishment of the many committees* that would be formed to inquire into the legal, ethical, and social implications of IVF and human embryo research[1] and to estimate the amount of legislation that would be enacted by governments around the world to regulate these areas.[2] What was apparent in 1978, however, was that both the clinical use of IVF and any human embryo research required for the development of further IVF procedures raised many ethical concerns.

Some warning of these problems had been provided by a few scientists when human *in vitro* fertilization was achieved, prior to the establishment of any clinical IVF programs.[3] But there was little attempt to identify and analyze the theological, ethical, legal, and social implications of the issues raised until after the first IVF baby had been born.

A. THE INCREASING APPLICATIONS OF IVF

The uses of IVF have continued to increase since 1978. Devised initially as a procedure for bypassing infertility caused by blockages in the fallopian tubes which prevented the sperm from reaching the oocyte for fertilization,[4] IVF is now being used clinically with sperm microinjection to overcome male infertility,[5] for the alleviation of the infertility of couples who need donor gametes,[6] and sometimes for the formation of embryos to be donated to another couple or to be transferred to a surrogate for gestation when a woman is unable to carry a pregnancy.[7]

Each new use of IVF has raised specific ethical questions and has precipitated widespread, and at times heated, community debate about the ethics of assisted reproduction.

B. INCREASING DEBATE ABOUT HUMAN EMBRYO RESEARCH

There has been extensive community debate about the use of *in vitro* human embryos for research. Whether the research is being undertaken to improve or to formulate new fertilization methods,[8] to develop techniques for the analysis of the chromosomal or genetic constitution of the embryos from a couple at risk of having a child affected by a serious genetic or chromosomal disorder prior to transfer,[9] to improve procedures for freezing embryos not transferred in the current cycle of treatment,[10] or to provide information about fertilization,[11] the central question of what moral status should properly be accorded to the early human embryo continues to be raised and disputed. Some consideration of this question is essential for the formation of any opinion about whether human

---

* By 1987, over 70 reports had been produced by more than 50 committees around the world.

Ethical Aspects of IVF and Human Embryo Research **289**

embryo research is ethical and for the formation of any policies or legislation to regulate the area.

C. THE SCOPE OF THIS CHAPTER

This chapter is an examination of some of the ethical issues raised by reproductive technology and *in vitro* human embryo research. The major positions for and against reproductive technology and human embryo research will be outlined, and some of the questions that have arisen in relation to some developments in IVF and human embryo research will be discussed. The legislative responses to these problems in some jurisdictions around the world also will be considered.

II. THE MAJOR OPPOSITION TO IVF AND HUMAN EMBRYO RESEARCH

The main opposition to the use of reproductive technology and to human embryo research comes from three sources: right-to-life organizations, religious groups, and radical feminist groups. Although these positions share the conclusion that reproductive technology and human embryo research are unacceptable, the reasoning underlying each is quite distinct.

A typical form of each of these views will be outlined. It is important at the outset to recognize the limitations of this approach and to be aware that there are gradations within each of these main views. For instance, the official Vatican view, which is outlined below, does not reflect the range of views about IVF and human embryo research that exists among Roman Catholic scholars and theologians.[12] As considered here, the official Vatican view is merely an example of one of the opinions in opposition to IVF and human embryo research that has been forwarded by a religious body.

A. THE RIGHT-TO-LIFE VIEW

The right-to-life view is the most uniform of the three positions to be considered. The principle underlying this view is that human life is to be protected at all stages.

No explicit reason for why the human embryo is deserving of absolute protection is provided. The defense of this position rests on the assumption that from fertilization the human embryo is a human person (in the same sense that you and I are persons), and is deserving of all the rights and moral considerations that accompany our interactions with other persons. According to right-to-lifers, the early human embryo has full moral status, which includes an absolute right to life. Therefore, no human embryo should be created unless it is transferred to a woman, and no human embryo should be used in destructive research.

Pro-life organizations worldwide have gained the reputation of being among the most militant participants in debates about abortion, euthanasia, reproductive technology, and human embryo research because of their adherence to the basic principle of protecting human life at all stages. However, this belief has been used at times to present a misinformed and exaggerated view of the aims and intentions of reproductive technology and human embryo research that more accurately reflects misunderstanding and a fear of science and technology than establishes a reasoned case for why IVF and human embryo research are undesirable.[13]

B. THE OFFICIAL VATICAN VIEW

In initial protests from the churches, it was claimed that the scientists and clinicians involved in IVF were "playing God," effectively usurping the role of the Creator. The use of IVF, therefore, was an unacceptable way to reproduce. A more sophisticated restatement of this point of view is central to a document produced by the *Congregation for the Doctrine of the Faith,* which presents the official Vatican opinion on matters relating to procreation and human embryo research.[14] The essence of this view is that the use of reproductive technology is unacceptable because of the separation of the unity of the conjugal act in marriage from its procreative function. The creative role of the scientist in reproductive technology is an unacceptable intrusion into this relationship.

In contrast to IVF, the use of GIFT (gamete intra-fallopian transfer) is allowable under the official Vatican view, provided that certain conditions are met in the collection of the sperm used and in the transfer of the male and female gametes to the woman. The sperm used must be collected in a specially-designed condom, which does not rule out the possibility of *in vivo* fertilization occurring. Because fertilization must occur within the body of the woman, the gametes are separated by an air bubble in the catheter used for transfer.

The official Vatican view on human embryo research is based on the notion that a human being is formed at fertilization — implicitly, at the formation of the zygote. Fertilization is the determinant of full moral status for this position. Various features of fertilization may be highlighted as the specific determinant of moral status. For some proponents, fertilization is important to determining moral status because it is when the genotype of a new human being is formed.[15] Others contend that fertilization is important because the change from two gametes to a single zygote at fertilization is the only discrete stage in development at which it might be contended that a new human entity begins to exist.[16] Still other claims are that fertilization is important because it marks the formation of a new human individual,[17] or because fertilization results in the formation of a new human entity with the internal potential to develop into an adult.[18]

Each of these assertions has been examined elsewhere and has been found to be inadequate in its present form for supporting the claim that fertilization determines the moral status of the human embryo,[19] particularly the moral status of the *in vitro* human embryo.[20]

According to the official Vatican view, human embryo research is acceptable only if the research is therapeutic to the embryo on which it is carried out. There must also be a certainty of success of the research before it is attempted.

Ethical Aspects of IVF and Human Embryo Research 291

These requirements make most current human embryo research unacceptable and overlook completely the intentions of conducting this kind of research.

1. What is Fertilization?

When the technique of sperm microinjection was proposed, the claim that fertilization is the determinant of moral status led to legal and ethical debate over the question "What is fertilization?". This debate continued for more than a year in the Australian state of Victoria.

This episode shows some of the general dilemmas raised by the interaction among developments in reproductive technology, legislation in this area, and an alternative Roman Catholic view of the immorality of *in vitro* human embryo research. Some of the difficulties that have been raised by the use of terminology in the debate about human embryo research in the context of legislation and moral beliefs are also highlighted.

Until the advent of clinical IVF and *in vitro* human embryo research, it was reasonable for nonscientists to consider fertilization as an event which resulted in the formation of the embryo. This reasoning underpins the opinions of some philosophers and Roman Catholic theologians in their claims that fertilization determines the moral status of the human embryo. Their emphasis is on the formation of the zygote at syngamy — the final stage of fertilization when the genetic contributions of the sperm and oocyte come together to form the zygote.

Many legislators have adopted a view similar to this when enacting legislation to outlaw human embryo research. The Norwegian legislation of 1987, for example, prohibits any research on human embryos formed by artificial procreation.[21]

Victorian legislators also seem to have adopted this line of thinking in 1984 when they passed legislation to regulate clinical IVF and *in vitro* human embryo research.[22] Neither *embryo* nor *fertilization* was defined in the Act.

In vitro fertilization has confirmed that fertilization is a process made up of stages which include the penetration of the zona pellucida and membrane of the oocyte by a sperm, and pronuclear formation by the oocyte and sperm before the coming together of the male and female genetic contributions to form the zygote. This knowledge made it feasible for sperm microinjection to be attempted as a method of treating male infertility.

Attempts to gain approval to begin research aimed to test the efficiency and reliability of sperm microinjection, however, raised a legal problem for the Standing Review and Advisory Committee on Infertility (SRACI), the committee established by the Act to consider and approve research proposals. Specifically, the proposal to test sperm microinjection initiated debate about what was intended by the use of the terms *embryo* and *fertilization* in the Act.

In an attempt to more precisely define the significant stage of fertilization that determined the moral status of the embryo, it was claimed by some Roman Catholic philosophers that a new human individual begins to exist when the sperm enters the oocyte, a much earlier stage of fertilization than syngamy.[23]

The claim was that once a sperm enters the oocyte, the oocyte gains the potential to develop into a new human being. The implications of this assertion are that an oocyte undergoing fertilization has the moral status of the zygote. Therefore, no research should be carried out on oocytes that have been penetrated by a sperm. In terms of this claim, the oocyte has been *fertilized*, and by default the embryo has come into existence.

However, this claim is unconvincing: it demonstrates little understanding of the biological events which occur during fertilization.[24]

On the recommendations of SRACI, the Victorian Parliament amended the *Infertility (Medical Procedures) Act* to allow oocytes not intended for transfer in an IVF cycle to be fertilized in approved research up until the stage of syngamy. *Syngamy* is defined in the Amendment as "the alignment on the mitotic spindle of the chromosomes derived from the pronuclei."[25] No explicit definition of either *fertilization* or *embryo* was offered in the amendment. When this amendment is considered in relation to the Act, which forbids the fertilization of oocytes without the intention to transfer the resulting embryo to a woman, the implication is that an embryo is formed at the completion of fertilization, that is at the completion of syngamy.

The passage of this amendment cleared the way for sperm microinjection to be tested and its safety investigated prior to its introduction as a clinical treatment.

C. THE RADICAL FEMINIST VIEW

Radical feminists, such as the members of FINRRAGE (Feminist International Network of Resistance to Reproductive And Genetic Engineering), hold the view that the use of reproductive technology is an unacceptable means of having children, alleging that the abuses to the woman's body in undergoing the treatment far outweigh any possible benefits of the treatment. To a radical feminist, reproductive technology is an unsuccessful technology that threatens the freedom of women. It is also claimed that reproductive technology is a male-dominated area of medicine in which women's bodies are used for experimental purposes, as "living laboratories."[26] For this view, a woman's participation in a reproductive technology program is the result of coercion from males, not an expression of her desire or her free choice to have a child.

Of particular concern to radical feminists are the possibilities that IVF is seen to provide for genetic engineering and for sex selection of the early human embryo.[27] Human embryo research is unacceptable because of these possibilities, and more importantly because women must undergo IVF treatment to provide the oocytes from which the embryos used for research are formed. Any benefits that might come from human embryo research are considered unimportant when compared with the risks to which these women have been exposed.[28]

Not all feminists share these opinions, and claim instead that properly informed women are able to decide autonomously whether or not they will participate in a reproductive technology program.[29] In feminist writings about reproductive technology, there is commonly some concern about whether women are being informed properly about the treatments to be undertaken. Providing that this is the case, according to alternative feminist viewpoints, a woman should be free to participate in a reproductive technology program if she so chooses and to donate embryos for research.

The existence of these disparate viewpoints within the feminist movement has underscored both the obligation of clinicians to inform women adequately, so that they might give genuine informed consent for the treatment being undertaken, and the obligation of the scientists involved in human embryo research to present a clear explanation of the research project in which any embryo donated for research will be used.

III. VIEWS IN SUPPORT OF IVF AND HUMAN EMBRYO RESEARCH

The views expressed by the Vatican, right-to-life groups, and radical feminists represent the range of arguments used in opposition to clinical reproductive technology programs and human embryo research. It cannot be maintained validly that these views are widely held within the community.

A. PUBLIC SUPPORT

Since the early 1980s, public opinion polls in Britain[30] and in Australia have indicated consistently that there is substantial community support for the use of IVF and IVF-related procedures to overcome infertility.[31]

The results of a 1991 opinion poll in Australia showed that 81% of the Australian population are in favor of IVF being used as a treatment to overcome infertility.[32] There was also surprising community support for human embryo research, with 58% of those polled approving of human embryo research. Public support was increased further when the purpose of the research was specified: 70% of the sample approved of human embryo research for the improvement of infertility treatment, 68% supported human embryo research for the prevention of genetic disease, and 67% supported the use of human embryos in research aimed at overcoming the problems of pregnancy. In this sample of more than 1,200 people, only 21% of the population polled thought that human embryo research was never justified.

It might be contended that the introduction of legislation to regulate, rather than outlaw, clinical reproductive technology programs is a response to this kind of public support. It is also evident from this survey that scientists need to specify the goals of their research.

B. THE STAGE OF DEVELOPMENT AS THE DETERMINANT OF MORAL STATUS

The official Vatican view about reproductive technology and human embryo research is a claim that the earliest stage of human development, fertilization, is the determinant of the moral status of the embryo. This position allows research on gametes, but no human embryo research, unless the research is certain to be therapeutic for the embryo used in the research. Later landmarks in prenatal development have also been nominated as the determinant of moral status. These include, for instance, the time when segmentation (twinning or chimera formation) becomes no longer possible, at about 14 d after fertilization;[33] the attainment of human form at 4[34] or 13 weeks after fertilization;[35] the beginning of brain function at between 40 d[36] and 12 weeks after fertilization;[37] and the development of sentience at about 20 weeks after fertilization.[38]

With each of these claims, human embryo research is acceptable at any stage of development prior to that nominated as the determinant of moral status. Most of the stages of development mentioned above, however, were claimed to be the determinant of moral status during the debate about abortion in the 1970s and would have little application to regulating current technically possible *in vitro* human embryo research. The claim that moral status is acquired when segmentation ceases to be a possibility, the earliest developmental landmark nominated as the determinant of moral status after fertilization, however, may have been important in the formulation of legislation to regulate clinical IVF and human embryo research.

1. The Use of These Views in Legislation

The recommendations of the British Warnock Committee, which were the basis of the recently passed *Human Embryology and Fertilisation Act 1989*, and the recommendations of the Victorian Waller Committee, which were the basis of the *Infertility (Medical Procedures) Act 1984* were that approved human embryo research be permitted for up to 14 d after fertilization.[39,40] This upper limit to human embryo research has also been adopted in legislation enacted in Sweden,[41] Spain,[42] and some states of the U.S.[43]

The British and Victorian committees were reluctant to specifically nominate a limit to human embryo research. Although both committees stated that the early human embryo should be accorded some respect, their recommendations that human embryo research be permitted within 14 d after fertilization is a denial of the claim that the early human embryo is a person to whom moral status can be attributed or even a potential person to whom full moral status applies. The legislative sanctioning of human embryo research during the first 14 d after fertilization has not been without controversy.[44]

One justification for this limit to human embryo research was that the knowledge that might be obtained from this research potentially outweighed the wrong of using the early embryo in research. It also was appreciated that beyond 14 d after fertilization (the end of what has become known as the *pre-embryo* stage of development), the primitive streak is formed, twinning can no longer occur, and an individual embryo begins to develop.

The importance of the beginning of the development of the *individual* from about 14 d after fertilization sometimes has been proposed by some philosophers and theologians of different Christian[45] and non-Christian religions,[46] including Roman Catholicism[47] as the determinant of the moral status of the human embryo, and therefore the upper limit to acceptable human embryo research.

One question that seems to have been overlooked in these considerations, however, is whether a fourteen day old *in vitro* human embryo can be considered as analogous to the same age *in vivo* embryo, and whether it is deserving of the moral status that might be accorded to the *in vivo* embryo. Present knowledge and technical possibility would answer this question in the negative.[48]

IV. SHOULD AN UPPER LIMIT FOR HUMAN EMBRYO RESEARCH BE LEGISLATED?

The recommendation of the Warnock Committee that approved human embryo research up to 14 d following fertilization was adopted in the British legislation. The Victorian legislation, however, did not nominate a specific time limit to approved human embryo research, although 14 d following fertilization was recommended by the Waller Committee. Instead, the stipulation of the time limit for each research project approved became the responsibility of the Standing Review and Advisory Committee on Infertility created by the legislation, when considering each research proposal for approval. In an amended plain English version of the *Infertility (Medical Procedures) Act* released in October 1991, which is due to be considered by Parliament early in 1992, the need to specify 14 d as the upper limit for approved human embryo research has been proposed.[49]

It makes sense, from the view of allaying community anxiety, to nominate a specific limit for approved human embryo research. It is clear, however, that this approach to legislation may be fraught with problems.

On the one hand, it might be argued that it is preferable to have a project-specific limit to any approved research.[50] The aim of any research project should be to terminate the research at the earliest possible stage at which answers to the question being addressed can be gained. In this respect, a limit of 14 d may be too generous, allowing scientists to continue to grow embryos for curiosity rather than to obtain only the specific answers sought. Any solution to this problem rests on the systems for approval of the research and on the integrity of the scientists conducting the research.

On the other hand, it might be argued that the imposition of an absolute limit may, in some cases, interfere with the conduct of some clinically important research from which the answers being sought may not become available until day 15 after fertilization, or later. Should this research be undertaken illegally? Or should research into solving some of the problems of development not be pursued? Will any allowance be made for the importance of the questions being addressed by such research and the answers it may provide? How absolute is the limit being imposed? These are important questions that need to be considered when a limit to human embryo research is being legislated.

It is possible that the 14 d limit will be tested when it becomes possible to grow *in vitro* human embryos that develop normally for 14 d or longer.

V. WHERE WILL THE EMBRYOS USED FOR RESEARCH COME FROM?

Sanctioning human embryo research raises the question, "Where will the embryos to be used for research come from?". There are three possible sources: "spare" embryos not transferred to the woman, embryos produced solely for the purposes of research from donated gametes, and embryos produced in the course of research. The question of the origin of the embryos to be used for research has been considered by government committees formulating recommendations for legislation. Different resolutions of this question have been incorporated into legislation in different jurisdictions.[51,52]

A. "SPARE" OR INTENTIONALLY-CREATED EMBRYOS FOR RESEARCH?

With the use of superovulants in IVF, more embryos than can be safely transferred in one treatment cycle are sometimes formed. The options for couples with "spare" or excess embryos were to donate these embryos to another couple unable to achieve fertilization, to discard the embryos, or to donate the embryos for research. In 1983, the additional option of having the embryos stored by freezing for use in a later cycle of treatment became available.[53] The excess embryos could be used in a later cycle of treatment if the current cycle were unsuccessful or kept in storage for future family planning if the treatment was successful.

The use of donated "spare" embryos in research may not be a realistic expectation in future if reproductive technology optimizes oocyte freezing and oocyte maturation. Moving toward a reproductive technology based on the use of frozen and possibly *in vitro* matured oocytes that would produce fewer "spare" embryos for research brings several questions into sharper focus. Should embryos formed as a result of research be used for other research? Should embryos be created from donated gametes solely for research? Are these embryos morally different from spare embryos created with the intention of being transferred and then donated for research?

At present there does not appear to be any consensus among scientists or legislators on these questions. It seems that the only distinction that might be drawn among these three categories of embryos is one based on the legal notion of intention, which has resulted in these different types of embryos being considered differently in various pieces of legislation.

There is no simple answer to these questions; the answers decided by people depend on personal beliefs about what respect should be accorded to the human embryo and what status the embryo is considered to have. These questions may need to be reexamined at some time in the future.

VI. SOME ISSUES RELEVANT TO CURRENT RESEARCH

A question that might be raised reasonably in relation to the procedures to be discussed in this section is whether these techniques should be restricted to being used by infertile couples or individuals. These recent developments also offer particular advantages to fertile couples and individuals who are prepared to undergo IVF treatment to establish a family.[54]

A. EMBRYO/OOCYTE FREEZING

The introduction of embryo freezing makes more options available to the infertile couple and has also created several legal dilemmas that have demonstrated the present inability of the legal systems in some states of the U.S.A. and Australia to deal with such problems. Law-makers and couples wishing to use the option of having embryos stored by freezing need to address questions such as "What is to happen to the embryos if the 'parents' die?"[55] and "Who gets the embryos in the case of a divorce?".[57]

One solution would be for the State to have possession of the frozen embryos in these circumstances and for the embryos to be either discarded, donated to another couple, or used for approved research under State direction. Discarding embryos would be a misuse of this discretion if it were invoked when infertile couples unable to produce an embryo were waiting for an embryo to be donated or when valid research projects were being held up because of a lack of embryos.

The State having this power could possibly facilitate research in jurisdictions where only spare embryos can be used for this purpose. This facilitation, however, would involve taking away any right to make a decision about the future disposition of embryos from the parties whose gametes were used to form them.

A preferable approach, which would not take away this discretion of the gamete donors, would be to introduce an enforceable agreement about the fate of any frozen embryos in the case of divorce or the possibility of death. This agreement would need to be entered into before any embryos could be frozen. The drawing up of these agreements would not be easy; neither would the provision of the appropriate counselling that would be required to enable the couples involved to enter into these agreements in a properly informed way.

One solution to these quandaries, at least as far as divorce is concerned, would be the introduction of oocyte freezing. The death of a woman with oocytes frozen may still raise questions about the fate of the oocytes, unless stipulated previously. The choice of the oocytes going to research, being used for donation, or being discarded, however, would be an easier issue to discuss with the couple or the woman.

This choice would need to be made only in jurisdictions which do not allow the use of gametes in fertilization after the death of the gamete donor. A further possibility would be for gamete donors to specify that the oocytes or sperm are to go to research or be donated in the event of their death; otherwise the gametes would be discarded. Some amendment of current legislation would be required to make this a possible option.

B. *IN VITRO* OOCYTE MATURATION

In vitro oocyte maturation potentially offers several advantages to infertile and fertile women. To reduce the incidence of chromosomal abnormalities likely to affect any child born, a woman could have immature oocytes collected during her early 20s, the optimal years for child bearing. The immature oocytes then could be stored frozen until she wished to start a family. At that time, the oocytes could be removed from storage, matured in the laboratory, and fertilized *in vitro* before the resulting embryos were transferred. The results from the use of oocyte donation by younger to older women suggest that the IVF treatment involved may have a higher success than for older women using "older" oocytes.[57]

The use of *in vitro* oocyte maturation could contribute substantially to providing reassurance to women who have delayed childbearing because of a career and the opportunity of creating a secure future for their proposed family. Its use would reduce the risk of having a child affected by a chromosomal abnormality, such as Down's Syndrome, which is known to increase with increasing maternal age. The need for any decision about whether to terminate a pregnancy following prenatal diagnosis would be minimized, and the instances of disappointment and heartbreak experienced by older parents having a child affected by an age-related chromosomal disorder would be diminished. The use of *in vitro* oocyte maturation also has the potential to reduce the costs to the public that are presently allocated to the provision of care and accommodation for babies affected by chromosomal disorders.

In vitro oocyte maturation could also be used by women of childbearing age who require radiotherapy treatment. Any risk of chromosomal damage to their oocytes caused by the treatment could be avoided by the collection of immature oocytes before treatment.

Few babies have as yet resulted from the use of *in vitro* oocyte maturation. Further research is needed to make these possibilities a reality.

C. EMBRYO BIOPSY

The use of embryo biopsy by a couple at risk of having a child affected by a serious genetic or chromosomal disorder may in the future replace the anxiety and stress experienced by these couples when waiting for the results from prenatal diagnosis testing during pregnancy. Only embryos unaffected by the disorder for which the couple is at risk would be transferred to the woman to establish a pregnancy. The difficult decision of whether to terminate a pregnancy affected by the condition could thus be avoided by the use of embryo biopsy, provided that the couple is prepared to undergo a cycle of

IVF treatment. The success of IVF in these couples, therefore, may be an important determinant of their choosing to use this option.

The clinical use of embryo biopsy has so far been limited to the detection of the sex of the embryos of couples at risk of having a child affected by a serious sex-linked disorder.[58] This use of embryo biopsy and its potential to be used for the diagnosis of single gene disorders, however, have raised several questions which need to be considered.

Many of these questions are unanswerable at present. Among them are concerns such as "Who will have access to use of this technology?", "Will embryo biopsy come to be used as a method of sex selection?", "For detecting what traits other than genetic diseases might embryo biopsy come to be used in the future?". These questions also raise complex issues that need to be kept in mind as research on embryo biopsy continues.

VII. CONCLUSION

Reproductive technology has come a long way since 1978; it has helped thousands of couples worldwide overcome their infertility. However, reproductive technology still has a long way to go before infertile couples can be assured of a successful treatment that will overcome their childlessness, and, regardless of the substantial public support, before its critics will be satisfied.

The points of contention continue to increase as IVF advances. Many of the debates, such as those surrounding IVF surrogacy, oocyte donation, patient access to reproductive technology programs, recordkeeping in reproductive technology programs, the role of counselling for the patients, and other topics which would be unique to different jurisdictions have not been considered here. Nevertheless, the complexity of the debate, as evidenced by the range of views about IVF and human embryo research within the community, has been shown, and the possibility of the need for the reassessment of enacted legislation in the future, particularly in regard to different aspects of *in vitro* human embryo research, has been discussed.

The constant controversy that has accompanied any developments in clinical treatments and in *in vitro* human embryo research has changed the problems of infertility from being a personal matter between a couple and their physician into being a matter of social concern, debate, and legal regulation. This change has expanded the role of the clinician involved in a reproductive technology program and the scientist involved in human embryo research. In many countries, the clinician and the scientist now are expected to be part philosopher, part lawyer, and part public relations officer and educator.

The important point to be remembered in these circumstances is that, through continued research, reproductive technology, although not perfect at present, does have the potential to provide an understanding of normal and abnormal human development and to help infertile and fertile couples to have healthy much-wanted children. This is after all its *raison d'etre*.

REFERENCES

1. **Walters, L.** Ethics and new reproductive technologies: an international review of committee statements, *Hastings Center Report*, 17[3], (Special Suppl.), 1, 1987.
2. **Gunning, J.**, *Human IVF, Embryo Research, Fetal Tissue for Research and Treatment, and Abortion: International Information*, Her Majesty's Stationery Office, London, 1990.
3. **Edwards, R. G.**, Fertilisation of human eggs *in vitro:* morals, ethics and the law, *Q. Rev. Biol.*, 49, 3, 1974.
4. **Steptoe, P.C. and Edwards, R. G.**, Birth after the reimplantation of a human embryo, *Lancet*, II, 366, 1978.
5. **Laws-King, A., Trounson, A., Sathananthan, H., and Kola, I.**, Fertilization of human oocytes by microinjection of a single spermatozoon under the zona pellucida, *Fertil. Steril.*, 48, 395, 1987.
6. **Cameron, I. T., Rogers, P. A., Caro, C., Harman, J., Healy, D. L., and Leeton, J. F.**, Oocyte donation: a review, *Br. J. Obstet. Gynaecol.*, 96, 893, 1989.
7. **Kirkman, M.**, *My Sister's Child*, Penguin Books, Ringwood, Australia, 1988.
8. **Laws-King, A., Trounson, A., Sathananthan, H., and Kola, I.**, Fertilization of human oocytes by microinjection of a single spermatozoon under the zona pellucida, *Fertil. Steril.*, 48, 395, 1987.
9. **Handyside, A. H., Kontogianni, E. H., Hardy, K., and Winston, R. M. L.**, Pregnancies from biopsied human preimplantation embryos sexed by Y-specific DNA amplification, *Nature*, 344, 768, 1990.
10. **Trounson, A. O., Peura, A., and Kirby, C.**, Ultra-rapid freezing: a new low-cost and effective method of embryo cryopreservation, *Fertil. Steril.*, 48, 843, 1987.
11. **Kola, I., Trounson, A. O., Dawson, G., and Rogers, P.**, Tripronuclear human oocytes: altered cleavage patterns and subsequent karyotypic analysis of embryos, *Biol. Reprod.*, 37, 395, 1987.
12. **Dawson, K.**, *Human Embryo Experimentation: A Background Paper and Select Bibliography*, National Bioethics Consultative Committee, Adelaide, 1990.
13. **Right to Life**, *The Opaque World of In Vitro Fertilisation*, Right to Life, Brunswick, Victoria, 1990.
14. **Congregation for the Doctrine of the Faith**, *Instruction on Respect for Human Life in its Origins and on the Dignity of Procreation: Replies to Certain Questions of the Day*, Polyglot Press, Vatican City, 1987.
15. **Werner, R.**, Abortion: the moral status of the unborn, *Soc. Theor. Pract.*, 3, 201, 1974.
16. **Quinn, W.**, Abortion: identity and loss, *Philos. Publ. Aff.*, 13, 24, 1984.
17. **Iglesias, T.**, *In vitro* fertilization: the major issues, *J. Med. Ethics*, 10, 32, 1984.
18. **Pluhar, W.**, Abortion and simple consciousness, *J. Philos.*, 74, 167, 1977.
19. **Dawson, K.**, Fertilisation and moral status: a scientific perspective, *J. Med. Ethics*, 13, 173, 1987.
20. **Singer, P. and Dawson, K.**, IVF technology and the argument from potential, *Philos. Pub. Aff.*, 17, 87, 1988.
21. Norwegian legislation, Act No. 628 of 1987.
22. **Parliament of Victoria**, *Infertility (Medical Procedures) Act 1984*, Victorian Government Printer, Melbourne, 1984.
23. **Anonymous**, Identifying the origin of a human life, *St. Vincent's Bioeth. Newsl.*, 5, 4, 1987.
24. **Buckle, S., Dawson, K., and Singer, P.**, The syngamy debate: when precisely does a human life begin?, *Law, Med. Health Care*, 14, 174, 1989.
25. **Parliament of Victoria**, *Infertility (Medical Procedures) (Amendment) Act 1987*, Victorian Government Printer, Melbourne, 1987.
26. **Rowland, R.**, Technology and motherhood: reproductive choice reconsidered, *Signs: J. Women Cult. Soc.*, 12, 512, 1987.
27. **Holmes, H. B. and Hoskins, B. B.**, Prenatal and preconception sex choice technologies: a path to femicide? in *Man-made Women*, Corea, G., Duelli-Klein, R., Hanmer, J., Holmes, H. B., Hoskins, B., Kishwar, M., Raymond, J., Rowland, R., and Steinbacher, R., Eds., Indiana University Press, Bloomington, 1987, 15.

28. **Rowland, R.,** Making women visible in the embryo experimentation debate, *Bioethics*, 1, 1, 1987.
29. **Warren, M. A.,** Is IVF research a threat to women's autonomy? in *Embryo Experimentation,* Singer, P., Kuhse, H., Buckle, S., Dawson, K., and Kasimba, P., Eds., Cambridge University Press, Melbourne, 1990, 125.
30. **NOP Market Research Limited,** *A Report on a Survey: Embryos,* unpublished, London, 1989.
31. **Brumby, M.,** Australian community attitudes to in vitro fertilization, *Med. J. Aust.,* 1984.
32. **Roy Morgan Research Centre,** *Survey on Human Embryo Research Conducted for the Department of Community Services and Health,* Adelaide, 1991, unpublished.
33. **Ward, K.,** An irresolvable dispute?, in *Experiments on Embryos,* Dyson, A. and Harris, J., Eds., Routledge, London, 1990, 106.
34. **Ramsey, P.,** Reference points in deciding about abortion, in *The Morality of Abortion,* Noonan, J. T., Jr., Ed., Harvard University Press, Cambridge, 1970, 60.
35. **Grobstein, C.,** *From Chance to Purpose: an Appraisal of External Human Fertilization,* Addison-Wesley, Reading, 1981, 102.
36. **Haring, B.,** A theological evaluation, in *The Morality of Abortion,* Noonan, J. T., Jr., Ed., Harvard University Press, Cambridge, 1970, 123.
37. **Goldenring, J. M.,** The brain-life theory: towards a consistent biological definition of humanness, *J. Med. Ethics,* 10, 5, 1985.
38. **Singer, P.,** Animals and the value of life, in *Matters of Life and Death: New Introductory Essays in Moral Philosophy,* Regan, T., Ed., Random House, New York, 1980, 218.
39. **Warnock, M.,** *A Question of Life: the Warnock Report on Human Fertilisation and Embryology,* Basil Blackwood, Oxford, 1985.
40. **The Committee to Consider the Social, Ethical and Legal Issues Arising from *In Vitro* Fertilization,** *Report on the Disposition of Embryos Produced by in vitro Fertilization,* Victorian Government Printer, Melbourne, 1984.
41. **Sweden,** *In vitro Fertilisation Act,* Law No. 711 of 1988.
42. **Spain,** *Health: Assisted Reproduction Techniques,* Law No. 35 of 1988.
43. **Gunning, J.,** *Human IVF, Embryo Research, Fetal Tissue for Research and Treatment, and Abortion: International Information,* Her Majesty's Stationery Office, London, 1990.
44. **Holland, A.,** A fortnight of my life is missing: a discussion of the status of the human `pre-embryo', *J. Appl. Philos.,* 7, 25, 1990.
45. **Dunstan, G. R.,** In the name of human dignity: a denial of human liberty, in *Procreation Artificielle: Ou Sont L'Ethique et le Droit?,* Byk, C., Ed., Alexandre Lacassagne, Paris, 1989.
46. **Fisher, A.,** *IVF: the Critical Issues,* Collins Dove, Melbourne, 1989.
47. **Ford, N.,** *When Did I Begin?,* Cambridge University Press, Cambridge, 1988.
48. **Dawson, K.,** Segmentation and moral status *in vivo* and *in vitro*: a scientific perspective, *Bioethics,* 2, 1, 1988.
49. **Standing Review and Advisory Committee on Infertility,** *Report to the Minister for Health on Matters Related to the "Review of `Post-Syngamy' Embryo Experimentation. Part III: Recommendations for Amendment to the Infertility (Medical Procedures) Act 1984,* Victorian Government Printer, Melbourne, 1991.
50. **Edwards, R. G.,** Discussion, in *Human Embryo Research: Yes or No?,* Ciba Foundation, Tavistock Press, London, 1986, 196.
51. **Warnock, M.,** *A Question of Life: the Warnock Report on Human Fertilisation and Embryology,* Basil Blackwood, Oxford, 1985.
52. **Gunning, J.,** *Human IVF, Embryo Research, Fetal Tissue for Research and Treatment, and Abortion: International Information,* Her Majesty's Stationery Office, London, 1990.
53. **Mohr, L. and Trounson, A.,** Human pregnancy following cryopreservation, thawing and transfer of an eight-cell embryo, *Nature,* 305, 707, 1983.
54. **Dawson, K. and Singer, P.,** Should fertile people have access to in vitro fertilisation? *Brit. Med. J.,* 300, 167, 1990.
55. **Fisher, A.,** *IVF: the Critical Issues,* Collins Dove, Melbourne, 1989, 190.
56. **Robertson, J. A.,** Ethical and legal issues in the cryopreservation of human embryos, *Fertil. Steril.,* 47, 371, 1987.

57. **Leeton, J., Rogers, P., King, C., and Healy, D.,** A comparison of pregnancy rates for 131 donor oocyte transfers using either a sequential or fixed regime of steroid replacement therapy, *Hum. Reprod.,* 6, 299, 1991.
58. **Handyside, A. H., Kontogianni, E. H., Hardy, K., and Winston, R. M. L.,** Pregnancies from biopsied human preimplantation embryos sexed by Y-specific DNA amplification, *Nature,* 344, 768, 1990.

Chapter 15

FUTURE PROSPECTS

Karen Dawson and Alan Trounson

TABLE OF CONTENTS

I. Introduction 304

II. Improving Pregnancy Rate and Outcome 304
    A. Simplifying the Treatment 304
    B. Understanding Fertilization 305
    C. Reducing Embryo Loss and Miscarriage 306
    D. Reducing Ectopic Pregnancy 307
    E. Reducing Multiple Births 307
    F. Bettering Perinatal Outcome 308

III. Developing New Technologies 309
    A. Oocyte Maturation and Cryopreservation 309
    B. Treating Severe Male Infertility 310

IV. Conclusion 310

References 311

I. INTRODUCTION

The figures from the World Collaborative Report released at the *7th World Congress on IVF and Assisted Procreations* in Paris in 1991,[1] affirm that IVF and other techniques of assisted reproduction are widespread, established medical procedures for the treatment of infertility. The more than 55,000 babies around the world born as a result of this technology are also a demonstration of its success.

It is clear from the chapters in this book, however, that assisted reproductive technologies have not yet been optimized. It is possible for the outcome of the technology to be bettered through clinical studies to improve the outcome of treatment and scientific research to provide new techniques and a fuller understanding of the biology of fertilization and early human embryo development *in vitro*. Through solving the problems of embryo loss, spontaneous abortion, ectopic pregnancy, and multiple births, and improving perinatal outcome, reproductive technology for the infertile may become, in all respects, comparable with *in vivo* conception in the fertile population.

This chapter is an examination of some of the clinical aspects of IVF technology that may be improved by further studies and also of some of the scientific research that may contribute to the broader application and to the optimization of the technology. In conclusion, the possibility of these goals being realized is addressed.

II. IMPROVING PREGNANCY RATE AND OUTCOME

A. SIMPLIFYING THE TREATMENT

Some of the past problems of reproductive technology have been that the treatment has been costly, in terms of both money and time. Infertile couples wishing to undergo reproductive technology (especially the woman) have needed to assess whether their lifestyle can contend with the stresses and disruption caused by the treatment. The implementation of public funding for IVF procedures in some countries[2] has relieved the economic burden for patients to some extent. On a more global scale, the demands for time and the resulting stresses induced by the treatment[3] are also being reduced.

The improvement in the drugs used for ovarian stimulation and an improved understanding of the predictability of response to these drugs have led to fewer treatment cycles being cancelled because of a failure to respond (see Chapter 1). With the development of the use of vaginal ultrasound for oocyte collection,[4] it is possible for the collection of oocytes to be a procedure performed in a day care center, with sedation, but without a general anesthetic (see Chapter 2). No overnight hospital stay is required for oocyte collection, and the transfer of gametes[5] and embryos can be carried out using day care facilities. Further improvements may lead to oocyte collection and gamete and embryo transfer being carried out within well-equipped doctors' surgeries.

Future Prospects 305

These changes in the clinical management of infertility mean that beginning a cycle of treatment has become more reliable (thus increasing the chances of a successful outcome for any cycle of treatment) and that the treatment is less disruptive of normal lifestyle.

The disadvantages of the stimulated cycle include the prospect of multiple pregnancy (to be discussed below) and the possibility of adverse responses to the drugs used, particularly for women who have polycystic ovaries or other conditions for which the use of these drugs is contraindicated (see Chapter 1).

The use of natural cycle IVF avoids these risks and also has the advantage of being less demanding in terms of time. The success rates reported for the use of natural cycle IVF range from about 20% per treatment[6] to about 7%.[7] The use of natural cycle IVF to date has not been very successful in many clinics, nor have the problems of using this procedure yet been thoroughly investigated.

By restricting the patients undergoing natural cycle IVF to under 35 years of age, repeating treatments in consecutive menstrual cycles if required, and by using day care facilities and minimal monitoring to time the oocyte pick-up, however, the natural cycle may be acceptable to many younger women and also have an improved chance of success.[8]

The current success rate of natural cycle IVF makes it an unsuitable treatment for use by women of the age when fertility starts to decline. Until the success of natural cycle IVF is improved, for these cases, the use of the stimulated cycle continues to offer a more reliable treatment for achieving pregnancy in a shorter time.

B. UNDERSTANDING FERTILIZATION

Despite the rapid increase in the number and types of procedures used for treating infertility in the female and the male, the fertilization rate obtained in IVF has not improved since its beginning. Aspects of the interaction between the oocyte and the sperm throughout fertilization have been documented by the use of electronmicroscopy (see Chapter 12), but the reasons for fertilization failure *in vitro* remain poorly understood. There is some evidence that most fertilization failure is attributable to the characteristics of the sperm used (see Chapter 3).

The many tests developed for assessing the morphological and biochemical characteristics of the sperm prior to fertilization currently seem to provide little capacity for predicting IVF success. Further research is needed to correct this situation and to improve the rate of fertilization. A more complete understanding of the biochemical interactions between the gametes prior to fertilization should allow for the development of a test or battery of tests which would enable improved selection of the sperm being used for fertilization and, possibly, better prediction of the success of fertilization.

Methods for achieving fertilization, such as fusion of sperm and oocyte membranes, techniques of micromanipulation including the laser manipulation of sperm, and the direct injection of the sperm head into the ooplasm of an activated oocyte are being further developed and refined. These technologies, when applied, may contribute to an increase in the rate of *in vitro* fertilization.

C. REDUCING EMBRYO LOSS AND MISCARRIAGE

Patients undergoing IVF and GIFT have a spontaneous abortion rate of more than 20%,[1,9] with by far most of these abortions occurring before the 12th week of pregnancy.[1] Some of these abortions are related to the duration of infertility, to advanced maternal age, or to genetic or chromosomal abnormalities in the fetus.[9] The majority of spontaneous abortions and early losses of the embryo in IVF and GIFT however, are from unknown causes. The role of the effects of the superovulatory drugs used in IVF in changing the receptivity of the uterus for implantation needs to be further studied and should not be completely discounted (see Chapter 13).

The success of IVF pregnancies using donor oocytes has focused attention on and attached more importance to the quality of the oocyte or embryo being used for transfer in the outcome of pregnancy. There are several avenues of research involving the development of both noninvasive and invasive techniques for the assessment of the embryo that have the potential to contribute to a reduction in this incidence of spontaneous abortion.

The inexplicability of the frequency of pregnancy loss emphasizes the importance of developing appropriate and accurate noninvasive scoring systems for assessing the quality of gametes and embryos to be transferred (see Chapters 2 and 3). A fuller understanding of metabolism and metabolic requirements of the *in vitro* embryo during the stages prior to transfer may provide some insight into differentiating between embryos likely to develop to birth and those embryos likely to result in a later spontaneous abortion (see Chapter 10). Understanding embryo metabolism may facilitate the formulation of specific culture media which will increase the viability of the embryos to be transferred (see Chapter 5), and may explain the enhanced viability obtained by the use of co-culture techniques (see Chapter 12).

Embryo biopsy is an invasive technique for assessing the genotype of the IVF embryo at the 4-cell stage or later (see Chapter 6); this process provides a powerful method of prenatal diagnosis for detecting genetic defects (see Chapter 8) or chromosomal abnormalities (see Chapter 9) prior to transfer. The use of embryo biopsy by an infertile couple at risk of having a child affected by a serious genetic or chromosomal disorder may reduce the occurrence of spontaneous abortions or still-births in assisted reproduction from these causes. The anxiety and stress experienced by these couples during the time of waiting for the results from prenatal diagnosis during pregnancy would also be alleviated. Only embryos unaffected by the disorder for which the couple is at risk would be transferred to the woman to initiate a pregnancy, and the difficult decision of whether or not to terminate a pregnancy affected by the condition could thus be avoided.

If it becomes possible to detect more genetic defects and chromosomal disorders reliably by the use of embryo biopsy, and if the success of IVF is improved, it would become feasible for the use of embryo biopsy to be considered by all couples at risk of having a child affected by a genetic or chromosomal disorder.[10] It is as yet unknown whether the success of IVF would be higher in these couples.

The future possibility of embryo biopsy being performed using laser microbeams should also add to the precision of the present technique (see Chapter 8). For the present, however, it is crucial that these techniques undergo thorough development by research to establish their reliability before entering widespread clinical use.[11]

D. REDUCING ECTOPIC PREGNANCY

Ectopic pregnancy (pregnancy in the fallopian tube) occurs in about 5 to 7% of IVF and GIFT pregnancies, compared with an incidence of about 3% in the general population.[1,9] The increase in ectopic pregnancies in IVF patients implies that the embryos transferred to the uterus must move after the transfer of the embryos to the uterus is confirmed by ultrasound. There is some evidence that the increase in ectopic pregnancies may be related to the causes of infertility: the equivalent incidence of ectopic pregnancy has been found in more than 100 spontaneous pregnancies in infertile women on an IVF waiting list (Carl Wood, personal communication). A greater understanding of the reasons for the increased incidence of ectopic pregnancy in infertile patients is required. Perhaps this understanding may come from more knowledge of fertilization and early embryo development (see Chapters 4, 10, and 12).

For now, it is important that the occurrence of an ectopic pregnancy be detected at the earliest possible stage. It has been suggested that all women having assisted reproduction treatments should undergo ultrasound scanning at between 4 and 6 weeks after the treatment to eliminate the possibility of an ectopic pregnancy, and that women who are at risk of ectopic pregnancy, or who are symptomatic of this condition, should be more closely monitored from an earlier stage.[12]

E. REDUCING MULTIPLE BIRTHS

The incidence of multiple births from IVF and GIFT is about 20%, (see Table 1)[1,9,14] and is a product of both the number and quality of the oocytes or embryos transferred.[13] Multiple births, especially of a high order, need to be reduced to decrease the possibility of adverse perinatal outcomes.

Most IVF programs in Australia have already reduced the number of embryos transferred in IVF (to three) and the number of oocytes transferred in GIFT (to three) in response to the need to reduce the incidence of multiple births. A similar recommendation has also been made by the Human Fertilisation and Embryology Authority in Britain.[15] It is also possible to reduce the risk of high-order multiple births by taking into account the quality of the oocytes or embryos to be transferred (see Chapter 2).

The uniform adoption of a limit to the number of embryos or oocytes to be transferred provides a preferable solution to the occurrence of multiple births than the practice of fetal reduction. Although fetal reduction may have a valid

TABLE 1
Percentage of Multiple Pregnancies >20 Weeks Gestation for IVF and GIFT in Australia and Internationally in 1989 and in Britain in 1990[a]

		Twins	Triplets	Quadruplets
International	IVF	21.1	4.2	0.4
	GIFT	21.5	5.0	0.4
Australia	IVF	19.4	2.4	0.3
	GIFT	22.8	4.8	0.7
Britain	IVF	21.9	3.6	0.1
	GIFT	16.4	3.6	0.4

[a] Based on data from references 1, 9, and 15.

TABLE 2
Percentage of Low Birth Weight (<2500 g) in IVF and GIFT Infants in Australia in 1989 in Relation to the Plurality of the Pregnancy[a]

	Singleton	Twin	Triplet	Overall
IVF	15.5	56.8	94.5	34.8
GIFT	15.6	56.4	90.5	35.7

[a] Based on data from references 9.

place in treatment for eliminating an inviable fetus from a multiple pregnancy, the use of the practice to overcome an error which could have been avoided by transferring fewer oocytes or embryos may be problematic.

F. BETTERING PERINATAL OUTCOME

The incidence of genetic and congenital malformations in babies born from reproductive technology is 1.5%, comparable with the incidence in the general population.[1] However, the occurrence of low birth weight infants, pre-term labor, and miscarriage are more frequent from the use of reproductive technology. The incidence of infants born with low birth weight (<2500 g) from IVF and GIFT in Australia in 1989 in relation to the plurality of the pregnancy is given in Table 2. The cumulative incidence of pre-term births from IVF and GIFT in Australia in relation to the plurality of the pregnancy is given in Table 3. Although these aspects are each related to some extent to the occurrence of multiple pregnancies, the duration of infertility of the woman and the maternal age at the time of delivery also have some influence.[9]

The contribution of multiple births to these problems and to the increase in perinatal mortality may be expected to decline as the incidence of multiple births decreases from the adoption of upper limits to the number of eggs and embryos to be transferred in each treatment cycle. The outcome of infants born from single and multiple IVF and GIFT pregnancies in Australia is given in

TABLE 3
Percentage of Pre-Term Births from IVF Pregnancies in Australia 1979–1989 and GIFT Pregnancies 1985–1989 in Relation to Plurality of Pregnancy

	Singleton	Twin	Triplet	Total
IVF	17.8	55.1	97.4	27.8
GIFT	14.7	58.3	95.5	27.5

TABLE 4
Outcome of Infants Born from Single and Multiple IVF (1979–1989) and GIFT (1985–1989) Pregnancies in Australia (per/1000 births)[a]

		Singleton	Twin	Triplet	Other[b]	Total
IVF	Still-birth	29.0	36.1	51.3	—	32.6
	Neonatal death	7.6	18.4	51.1	81.1	14.7
	Perinatal death	36.4	53.8	99.7	81.1	46.9
GIFT	Still-birth	21.3	35.2	39.8	27.8	27.6
	Neonatal death	6.7	42.6	51.8	171.4	25.0
	Perinatal death	27.8	76.2	89.6	194.4	51.9

[a] Based on data from reference 9.
[b] Births from quadruplet and quintuplet pregnancies.

Table 4. These figures demonstrate clearly the effect of multiple births on this outcome. The contributions of advanced maternal age and the effects of the underlying causes of infertility to these outcome problems, however, have yet to be understood properly.

III. DEVELOPING NEW TECHNOLOGIES

A. OOCYTE MATURATION AND CRYOPRESERVATION

The success of assisted reproduction procedures currently is related to the number of mature oocytes that are collected. For this reason, the oocytes collected at pick-up are allowed time in culture prior to their use to ensure maturity (see Chapter 2). Immature oocytes have a reduced potential to fertilize, although immature oocytes can be matured in the laboratory, fertilized, and result in a successful pregnancy and birth. The collection and maturation of immature oocytes *in vitro* provides an alternative to stimulated cycles for women who respond poorly to ovarian stimulants, or for whom the use of these drugs is contraindicated (see Chapter 1).

The use of *in vitro* oocyte maturation potentially offers several other advantages. A young woman could have immature oocytes collected and cryopreserved for future use when required. The results from the use of oocyte donation by younger to older women suggest that IVF in these cases may have a higher success than for older women using "older" oocytes. The storage of immature oocytes as compared to the established practice of cryopreserving embryos (see Chapter 11) would avoid the problems raised in the courts by a couple divorcing or dying without previously deciding upon or leaving instructions as to the disposition of the embryos in storage.

The cryopreservation of immature oocytes may be safer than cryopreserving the mature oocyte. The chromosomes in the immature oocyte are more stable than in the mature oocyte; as a result, cryopreservation of the mature oocyte may result in an increased risk of aneuploidy after thawing. Few babies have as yet resulted from *in vitro* oocyte maturation (see Chapter 2). There is yet no tested, reliable method for cryopreserving the human oocyte. However, the technique of oocyte cryopreservation has been developed in the mouse (see Chapter 11), and further research is needed to make the possibility of reliably storing immature human oocytes for future use by cryopreservation a reality.

B. TREATING SEVERE MALE INFERTILITY

The treatment of severe male factor infertility, in which the number of motile sperm produced is insufficient for IVF or GIFT, has given rise to the techniques of microdrop insemination and various micromanipulation techniques which have attempted to promote the chances of fertilization occurring by bypassing penetration of the zona pellucida by the sperm (see Chapter 7). The zona pellucida may be perforated, torn with microneedles, or digested by acid Tyrode's solution, with differing effects on the resulting developmental potential of the zygote formed.

Mechanical methods of disrupting the zona pellucida seem to provide better results than acid digestion. The microinjection of sperm into the perivitelline space of the oocyte has a higher fertilization rate than other methods of mechanical disruption of the zona pellucida and is in widespread clinical use for males with severe infertility. In the future, the present mechanical methods of micromanipulation may be replaced by the use of laser microbeam technology, which will improve the precision of the techniques and provide a potent technology for the correction of fertilization abnormalities *in vitro*.

IV. CONCLUSION

Since 1978, assisted reproduction has been a rapidly developing and successful area of medical science. Probably more than any other branch of medicine, the advances, progress, and successes of the technology have depended on the support of the community and on some understanding of what the community is prepared to accept as useful research (see Chapter 14). Consistent with the range of expertise available in this area, there are many aspects of the technology that will be improved in the future. Although the use of reproductive technology has come a long way since its inception, whether or not many of the possible developments will occur in the future depends not only on the available clinical and scientific expertise, but also on the continued support and acceptance of the technology by the community.

REFERENCES

1. **Testart, J., Plachot, M., Mandelbaum, J., Salat-Baroux, J., Frydman, R., and Cohen J.,** World collaborative report on IVF-ET and GIFT: 1989 results, *Hum. Reprod.*, 7, 362–369, 1992.
2. **Gunning, J.,** *Human IVF, Embryo Research, Fetal Tissue for Research and Treatment and Abortion: International Information,* Department of Health, London, 1990.
3. **Newman, N. E. and Zouves, C. G.,** Emotional experiences of in vitro fertilization, *J. In Vitro Fertil. Embryo Transfer,* 8, 321–328, 1991.
4. **Wikland, M., Hamberger, L., Enk, L., Hammarberg, K., and Nilsson, L.,** Use of a vaginal transducer for oocyte retrieval in IVF/ET program, *J. Clin. Ultrasound,* 15, 245–251, 1987.
5. **Jansen, R. P. S., Anderson, J. C., Birrell, W. S. R., Lyneham, R. C., Sutherland, P. D., Turner, M., Flowers, D., and Ciancaglini, E.,** Outpatient gamete intrafallopian transfer: a clinical analysis of 710 cases, *Med. J. Aust.,* 153, 182, 1990.
6. **Dubnisson, J. B., Foulot, H., Ranoux, C., Aubriot, F. X., Poirot, C., Halouani, L., and Salesses, A.,** IVF without ovarian stimulation: a simplified protocol applied in 90 cycles, Proceedings VI World Congress on In Vitro Fertilization and Alternate Assisted Reproduction, Jerusalem, Israel, 1989, 7.
7. **Lenton, E. A., Cooke, I. D., Hooper, M. A. K., King, H., Kumar, A., Mellows, H. J., Monks, N. J., and Osborn, J. C.,** Natural Cycle IVF Results Obtained During More than 200 Treatment Cycles, Proc. VI World Congress In Vitro Fertilization and Alternate Assisted Reproduction, Jerusalem, Israel, 1989, 12.
8. **Paulson, R. J., Sauer, M. V., Francis, M. M., Macaso, T. M., and Lobo, R. A.,** In vitro fertilization in unstimulated cycles: the University of Southern California experience, *Fertil. Steril.,* 57, 290–293, 1992.
9. **AIH National Perinatal Statistics Unit,** *Assisted Conception: Australia and New Zealand 1989,* Fertility Society of Australia, Sydney, Australia, 1991.
10. **Dawson, K. and Singer, P.,** Should fertile people have access to in vitro fertilization? *Br. Med. J.,* 300, 167–169, 1990.
11. **Trounson, A. O.,** Preimplantation diagnosis — counting chickens before they hatch?, *Hum. Reprod.,* 7, 583–584, 1992.
12. **Guirgis, R. R. and Craft, I. L.,** Ectopic pregnancy resulting from gamete intra-fallopian transfer and in vitro fertilization. Role of ultrasonography in diagnosis and treatment, *J. Reprod. Med.,* 36, 793–796, 1991.
13. **Staessen, C., Camus, M., Bollen, N., Devroey, P., and Van Steirtegham, A. C.,** The relationship between embryo quality and the occurrence of multiple pregnancies, *Fertil. Steril.,* 57, 626–630, 1992.
14. **Interim Licensing Authority,** *Statistical Analysis of the United Kingdom IVF and GIFT Data 1985–1990,* London, 1992.
15. **Human Fertilization and Embryology Authority,** *Annual Report,* London, 1992.

INDEX

A

Abortion, 65, 306–307
Abstinence, 37
Acrosomal status in sperm, 40–41, 46, 58, 132
  cryopreservation and, 243
  microinjection and, 139–140
  oocytes and, 145
  transmission electron microscopy in analysis of, 240–241
β-Actin genes, 162, 163
Adenosine, 50, 95
Adoption, 35
Aging oocytes, 248
Agonadal women, 275–278
Alanine, 93, 201
Albumin, 47
Allele-specific oligonucleotide probing, 167
"All or none" phenomenon, 190
Amino acids, 93–94, see also specific types
Aminobutyric acid, 199
Ammonium, 94
Amplification refractory mutation system (ARMS), 167–168
Ampullary cells, 63, 106, 254
Androgen deficiency, 35
Aneuploidies of chromosomes, 188
Antibiotics, 36, 37, see also specific types
Anti-estrogens, 267, see also specific types
Antioxidants, 46, 108
ARMS, see Amplification refractory mutation system
Asparagine, 94
Aspartate, 94
Aspiration embryo biopsy method, 120, 125
Autocrine factors, 87
Autoimmunity of sperm, 35, 36, 45
Automated polymerase chain reaction, 158
Autosomal recessive genetic conditions, 147
Azoospermia, 34, 35

B

Bicarbonate, 96
Biochemical microassays, 118
Bioluminescence assays, 201
Biopsy, 86, 116
  embryo, see Embryo biopsy
Bipronucleate oocytes, 76

Blastocele, 126
Blastocysts, 73, 74, 76
  embryo biopsy of, 116–118, 124, 125
  embryo cultures in, 86, 92, 94–96, 255
  expansion of, 94
  formation of, 96
  growth of, 78
  hatching of, 254, 255
  implantation of, 256
  partial zone dissection oocytes and, 133
  reduced numbers of, 119
  trophectoderms in, 120
  uterine receptivity and, 264
  viability of, 198
Blastomeres
  analysis of after embryo biopsy, 188–189
  biopsy of, 116
  cytogenetic analysis of, 178
  cytoplasm of, 71
  extrusion of, 116
  lysosomal activity in, 253–254
  minimal number of, 117
  multinucleate, 74
  pinocytotic activity in, 253–254
Blastulation timing, 119
Boveri's theories, 174, 251–252
Buffer systems, 96–97
Buserelin, 274

C

Caffeine, 50
Calcium ionophore A23187, 41
Cancer, 174
Capacitation of sperm, 46
Capillary tubes, 59–60
Carbon dioxide, 97
Catholic view of IVF, 290–292
CC, see Clomiphene citrate
Cell dissociation, 23
Cell lysate preparation, 155
Cellsoft computer system, 40
Cellular mass reduction, 119–120
Centrifugation, 46, 47, 50, 240
Centrioles, 146, 147, 251–252, 254
Centrosomes, 252
Cervical mucus, 36
CES, see Cummulative embryo score
CG, see Cortical granules
Chelators, 108, see also specific types
Chemotherapy, 45

313

Chlorpromazine, 198
Chromatids, 58, 178–179
Chromatins, 67, 140
Chromosomes
  aberrations in, 190, 219
  analysis of, see Cytogenetic analysis of embryos
  aneuploidies of, 188
  loss of, 180
  overspreading of, 175, 180
  spreading of, 175, 176, 180
Chymotrypsin, 133
Citrate, 95
Cleavage
  arrest of, 93
  division in, 68, 73, 119
  early events in, 69–71
  embryo, 145
  embryo biopsy at stages of, 118–119
  patterns of, 183–184
  rate of, 73, 197
  retardation of, 74
  stimulation of, 95
Clinical analysis of male, 34–37
Clomid, see Clomiphene citrate
Clomiphene citrate
  cumulus cell removal and, 25
  endocrinology and, 4, 7–8
  protocol for, 7–8
  uterine receptivity and, 267, 269, 270, 271, 273, 274
Co-culture systems, 63, 105–107, 254–257
Coital disorders, 35
Coitus interruptus, 45
Colloidal silica particles, 47
Corona cells, 23, 63
Cortical granules (CG), 244, 248, 251
Coupling enzymes, 201, see also specific types
Cryopreservation, 213–234, see also Cryoprotectants
  of donor sperm, 45
  of embryos, 116, 214
    ethics of, 297–298
    rapid cooling in, 226–230
    slow cooling in, 224–225
  equipment for, 220–223
  ethics of, 297–298
  freezing straws and tubes in, 221–222
  future of, 309–310
  history of, 214–215
  of husband's sperm, 45
  oocyte maturation and, 309–310
  of oocytes, 45, 214
    ethics of, 297–298
    rapid cooling in, 232–233
    slow cooling method in, 230–231
  of pre-embryos, 36
  protocols for, 223–233
    general guidelines for, 223–224
    propanediol slow cooling and, 224–225
    rapid cooling and, 226–230
    slow cooling and, 230–231
    vitrification and, 226, 231–232
  rapid cooling method in, see Rapid cooling method
  seeding and, 215–217
  of semen, 49
  slow cooling method in, 215–218, 224–225, 230–231
  of sperm, 46, 241–243
  ultrarapid cooling in, 219
Cryoprotectants, 214, 217–220, 222, 243, see also Cryopreservation; specific types
Culture systems, see also specific types
  co-, 63, 105–107, 254–257
  embryo, see Embryo culture systems
  embryo development and, 76–78
Cummulative embryo score (CES), 71, 73
Cumulus cells
  dissociation of, 23
  microdrops and, 62
  morphology of, 244
  oocyte interactions with, 244
  oocyte mass and, 21, 28
  removal of, 25–27, 176
  spreading of, 23–25
  zona proteins secreted by, 247
Cycle monitoring, 9–11
Cyclophosphamide, 190
Cysteine, 50, 94
Cystic fibrosis, 168
Cytogenetic analysis
  of blastomeres, 178
  of embryos, 173–191, see also Genetic analysis of embryos
    applications of, 183–190
    data interpretation in, 179–182
    embryo developmental biology and, 183–184
    sister chromatid exchanges and, 178–179
    techniques used for, 175–179
Cytokines, 78
Cytokinesis, 74
Cytoplasm, 24, 58, 71, 74, 144
Cytotoxic drugs, 45, see also specific types

D

Degenerated oocytes, 66
Dehydration, 215, 217, 239
Delayed implantation, 265
Deletion disorders, 166–167, see also specific types
2-Deoxyadenosine, 50, 137
Desmosomes, 244
Diploid embryos, 252
Direct sequencing, 168
Dispermic embryos, 252
Dispermy, 184
Displacement embryo biopsy method, 120, 125
Dizygotic twins, 266
DMD, see Ducheme muscular dystropy
DNA, 161, 164
  analysis of, 116
  damage of, 179
  heteroduplex, 168
  morphology of, 174
  recombinant, 152
  sequences of, 163
  synthesis of, 154
  template of, 154, 155, 159, 166
DNA polymerases, 154
DNAses, 166
Donor insemination, 35
Donor Rescue, 66
Donor sperm, 45
Donor viral testing, 48
Doppler processing, 274
Doxycycline, 37
Drug-induced perturbation of embryo development, 189–190
Ducheme muscular dystrophy (DMD), 166–168
Dye exclusion, 197

E

Ectopic implantation, 265
Ectopic pregnancy, 307
EDR, see Embryo development ratio
EDTA, see Ethylenediaminetetraacetic acid
EGF, see Epidermal growth factor
Electron microscopy (EM), 142
  scanning, 245, 246, 272
  transmission, see Transmission electron microsopy (TEM)
Electrophoresis, 158, 164, 168
EM, see Electron microscopy

Embryo biopsy, 115–127
  at blastocyst stage, 116–118, 124, 125
  blastomere analysis and, 178, 188–189
  cellular mass reduction and, 119–120
  cleavage stages and, 118–119, 125
  ethics of, 298–299
  methods of, 116, 120–121, 124–126, see also specific methods
  optimal embryo stage for, 117–119
Embryo culture systems, 85–108, see also specific types
  blastocysts and, 86, 92, 94–96, 255
  co-culture systems, 105–107, 254–257
  cytogenetic analysis and, 175
  development of, 87–89
  future of, 107–108
  glassware in, 98–99
  improvement in, 86
  media for, 86–89
    amino acids in, 93–94
    buffer system in, 96–97
    collecting of, 100–101
    complex type, 100
    energy substrates in, 87, 92–93
    flushing of, 100–101
    gas phase, 97
    growth factors in, 96
    hormones in, 96
    ions in, 92
    nucleic acid precursors in, 94–95
    pH of, 101, 102
    preparation of, 98–102
    proteins in, 95–96, 101–102
    screening of, 102–104
    simple type, 99–100
    vitamins in, 94
    water in, 90–92
  problems associated with, 87
  ultrastructure and, 254–257
Embryo development ratio (EDR), 69, 70, 73
Embryos, 57–80
  biopsy of, see Embryo biopsy
  cleavage of, 145
  cryopreservation of, 116, 214, see also Cryopreservation
    ethics of, 297–298
    rapid cooling in, 226–230
    slow cooling in, 224–225
  cytogenetic analysis of, see Cytogenetic analysis of embryos
  cytological characteristics of, 74
  debate about research on, 288–289
  development of, 69–80
    biopsy and, 125

in culture, 197, see also Embryo culture
    systems
culture systems and, 76–78
cytology and, 74
drug-induced perturbation of, 189–190
early, 252–254
early cleavage events and, 69–71
errors in, 74
impaired, 86
morphology and, 71–74
nuclear characteristics and, 74
stage of and ethics, 293–295
ultrastructure in, see Ultrastructure
developmental biology of, 183–184
diapause of, 265
diploid, 252
dispermic, 252
drug-induced perturbation of development
    of, 189–190
early cleavage-stage, 177, 252
early development of, 252–254
ethics of research on, see Ethical aspects
    of IVF
fertilization event timing and, 67–68
genetic analysis of, see Genetic analysis
    of embryos
genetic diseases in, 116
genetic errors in, 74
incubation of, 202–203
intentionally created, 296
late preimplantation, 76
loss of viability of, 86
manipulation of, 119
metabolism in, 206–208
    assessment of, 202–208
        fluorometric assays in, 199–202
        metabolite assays in, 199–202
micromanipulation of, 116
monospermic, 252
morphology of, 71–74, 76, 196
mortality of, 266, 306–307
nuclear characteristics of, 74
nutrient uptake in, 199, 202–208
oocyte insemination and, 58–63
opposition to research on, 289–293
optimal stage for biopsy of, 117–119
polypronuclear, 64
pre-, 36
pronuclear, 68–69
pronucleate single cell, 71
propanediol slow cooling for, 224–225
protectants for, 108
rapid cooling of, 226–230
reduction in mortality of, 306–307

reinseminated, 66
sexing of, 159, 292
"spare", 296
spreading of, 176
transfer of, see Embryo transfer (ET)
transmission electron microscopy of, 239
triploid, 252
tripronuclear, 183
uterine replacement of, 79
viability of, 87, 116, 206–208
    assessment of, 196–199
    defined, 196
    uterine receptivity and, 266–267
vitrification of, 226
Embryo transfer (ET), 2, 64–65, 79–80
clinical indications for, 4
multiple, 266
pronuclear, 68–69
tubal, 79, 144
Endocrine evaluation, 3–4, 268–271, see
    also Endocrinology of IVF
Endocrinology of IVF, 1–13, see also
    Endocrine evaluation
cycle monitoring and, 9–11
endocrine evaluation and, 3–4
folliculogenesis and, 2–3
growth hormone and, 9
luteal phase support and, 12–13
natural cycle and, 9–11
ovarian hyperstimulation syndrome and,
    11–12
polycystic ovarian syndrome and, 12
stimulation protocols and, 4–9
Endometrial cells, 254
Endometrium, 271–275
Energy metabolism, 87
Energy requirements, 92, 199, 202
Energy sources, 93
Energy substrates, 87, 92–93, see also
    specific types
Enzymes, 200, 201, see also specific types
Eosin Y, 197
Epidermal growth factor (EGF), 2, 96
Epididymal sperm aspiration, 35
Epididymis, 34
Epidilymal obstruction, 35
Epidymal sperm, 36
Epithelial cells, 106, 274–275
Epithelial tight junctions, 274–275
Erythromycin, 37
Estradiol, 3, 269–270
Estrogen priming, 264
ET, see Embryo transfer
Ethical aspects of IVF, 287–299

Index

cryopreservation and, 297–298
embryo biopsy and, 298–299
feminist view of, 292–293
legislation and, 294–296
religious views of, 289–293
right-to-life view of, 289–290
stage of development and, 293–295
supportive view of, 293–295
Ethylenediaminetetraacetic acid (EDTA), 95, 108
Exocytosis, 142
Extrusion embryo biopsy method, 116, 120

F

Fallopian tube epithelial cells, 106
Fallopscopy, 79
FDA, see Fluorescein diacetate
Feminist view of IVF, 292–293
Fertility prediction, 38
Fertilization
  abnormalities of, 64–66
  Boveri's theories of, 174
  checking for, 63–64
  debate over definition of, 291–292
  micro-, 251
  micromanipulation techniques for, see Micromanipulation
  polyspermic, 27, 251
  timing of events in, 67–68
  ultrastructure in, see Ultrastructure
  understanding of, 304–306
Fetal bovine fibroblasts, 106
Fibroblasts, 106
Ficoll method, 47, 139
Fluorescein diacetate (FDA), 198
Fluorescence, 197–198, 200, 202, 241
Fluorescence microscopy, 202
Fluorescent metabolites, 198
Fluorochromes, 42, 202
Fluorometric assays, 199–202
Follicle flushing, 18, 20
Follicle stimulating hormone (FSH), 2–5, 8, 35
Follicle stimulating hormone (FSH) receptors, 2
Folliculogenesis, 2–4
Free oxygen species, 46, 47
Freezing, see Cryopreservation
FSH, see Follicle stimulating hormone
Fusion
  gamete, 67
  gamete membrane, 249
  plasma membrane-oocyte, 58

sperm-oocyte, 58, 67, 140–142, 145, 248
Future of IVF, 303–310

G

Gamete intrafallopian transfer (GIFT), 18, 20, 308, 310
  clinical indications for, 4
  ectopic pregnancy and, 307
  embryo development and, 79, 80
  embryo mortality and, 306
  ethics of, 290
  IVF vs., 28, 68
  miscarriage and, 306
  multiple births and, 307
  oocyte preparation for, 28–29
Gametes, 67, 247–249
  intrafallopian transfer of, see Gamete intrafallopian transfer (GIFT)
Gap junctions, 244
Gel electrophoresis, 158, 168
Genetic abortions, 65
Genetic analysis of embryos, 151–169, see also Cytogenetic analysis of embryos
  allele-specific oligonucleotide probing in, 167
  amplification refractory mutation system in, 167–168
  cell lysate preparation and, 155
  clinical application of, 168–169
  controls in, 155–158
  deletion disorders and, 166–167
  direct sequencing in, 168
  embryo sexing and, 159
  heteroduplex analysis in, 168
  methods of, 155–159, see also specific methods
  multiplex, 168
  one-step PCR assay and, 159–161
  polymerase chain reaction in, see Polymerase chain reaction (PCR)
  problem solving in, 164–166
  sample contamination and, 164
  single gene detection in, 161
  two-step polymerase chain reaction and, 162–164
Genetic conditions, 147
Genetic disorders, 116, 120, 152, 153, 166–167, see also specific types
Genetic engineering, 152, 292
Germ cell arrest, 35
Germinal vesicle (GV), 21, 24, 25, 244
Germinal vesicle breakdown (GVBD), 21

GIFT, see Gamete intrafallopian transfer
Glassware, 98–99
α-Globin genes, 162
β-Globin genes, 163
Globozoospermia (round-headed sperm syndrome), 145
Glucocorticoids, 36, see also specific types
Glucose, 91, 92, 93, 205
　consumption of, 203
　requirements for, 202
　uptake of, 199–201, 205
Glucose 6-phosphate, 200, 201
Glutamate, 93
Glutamine, 93, 201
Glutathione, 108
Glycine, 93, 94, 108
Glycolysis, 93
Glycoproteins, 246, see also specific types
GnRH, see Gonadotrophin releasing hormone
Golgi membranes, 244
Gonadotrophin, 35, 196
　human chorionic, see Human chorionic gonadotrophin (HCG)
　human menopausal, see Human menopausal gonadotrophin (HMG)
Gonadotrophin releasing hormone (GnRH), 4, 5, 267
Gonadotrophin releasing hormone (GnRH) agonist, 5, 6
Gradient separation procedures, 47
Growth factors, 2, see also specific types
　in embryo culture system media, 96
　embryo development and, 78
　epidermal, 2, 96
　folliculogenesis and, 2
　insulin-like, 2, 96
　male pronucleus, 58
　production of, 78
　transforming, 96
Growth hormone, 9
GV, see Germinal vesicle
GVBD, see Germinal vesicle breakdown

H

Hamilton-Thron computer system, 40
Hamster egg-penetration test, 145
HCG, see Human chorionic gonadotrophin
Hemizona assay (HZA), 42
Hepatitis, 48, 106
Herniation embryo biopsy method, 116, 120, 124

Heteroduplex, 168
Hexokinase, 200
High-speed centrifugation, 240
Histidine, 94
History of IVF, 2–3
HIV, see Human immunodeficiency virus
HMG, see Human menopausal gonadotrophin
Hormone replacement therapy, 272, 275–278
Hormones, see also specific types
　in embryo culture system media, 96
　follicle stimulating, 2–5, 8, 35
　gonadotrophin releasing, 4–6, 267
　growth, 9
　luteinizing, 2–6, 272
　steroid, 36
HOS, see Hypoosmotic swelling
HTF, see Human tubal fluid
Human ampullary cells, 63, 106
Human chorionic gonadotrophin (HCG), 5, 6
　embryo biopsy and, 126
　insemination timing and, 27
　luteal phase support and, 13
　mouse bioassays and, 104
　oocyte maturation and, 22, 25
　production of, 76, 126
　uterine receptivity and, 270, 271, 278
Human immunodeficiency virus (HIV), 48
Human menopausal gonadotrophin (HMG)
　cumulus cell removal and, 25
　dosage of, 8, 12
　luteal phase support and, 13
　ovarian hyperstimulation syndrome and, 12
　protocol for, 5–8
　stimulation by, 9
　uterine receptivity and, 269, 271, 273, 274, 278
Human tubal fluid (HTF), 99–101
Hyalinized tubules, 35
Hyaluronidase, 23, 25–27
Hybridization, 125, 159, 161
Hybridoma cells, 103
Hydatidiform moles, 65
Hyperstimulation syndrome, 11–12
Hypoosmotic swelling (HOS), 43, 44
Hypospermatogenesis, 35
Hypoxanthine, 94, 95
Hysteroscopy, 79
HZA, see Hemizona assay

Index

I

ICM, see Inner cell mass
IGFs, see Insulin-like growth factors
Immotile cilia syndrome, 248–249
Immotile sperm, 243
Immunobead test, 36
Immunofluorescence, 241
Immunoglobulins, 36, 61
Implantation, 256, 264, 265
Implantation window, 264, 265, 276–278, see also Uterine receptivity
Incident light fluorescence, 202
Inhibin, 2, 3
Inner cell mass (ICM) cells, 116, 120, 124
Inosine, 95
Insemination
  in capillary tubes, 59–60
  in coculture systems, 63
  donor, 35
  efficacy of, 62
  in embryo cryopreservation straws, 59–60
  in microdrops, 60–63
  number of sperm for, 46
  of oocytes, 58–63
  re-, 66
  timing of, 27
In situ hybridization, 125
Insulin, 96
Insulin-like growth factors (IGF), 2, 96
Isoleucine, 94

K

Kallikrein, 50
Kartegener's syndrome, 147
Karyotypes, 134, 142
  metaphase spreads and, 175–178
  prediction of, 189
  status of, 183

L

Lactate, 77, 91, 93, 205
  concentrations of, 203
  uptake of, 199–201, 205
Lactate dehydrogenase, 200
Laparoscopy, 79
Late preimplantation embryos, 76
Legislation on IVF, 294–296
Leucine, 94
Leukocytes, 46
LH, see Luteinizing hormone
Light microscopy (LM), 240, 241, 252
LM, see Light microscopy
LPD, see Luteal phase defect
Luteal phase defect (LPD), 272–273
Luteal phase progesterone, 10
Luteal phase support, 12–13
Luteal support, 270–271
Luteinizing hormone (LH), 2–6, 272

M

Malate, 201
Male factor sperm, 63
Male infertility, 34–36, 62, 310
Male pronucleus growth factor, 58
Male subfertility, 36–37
Maximum human fecundability, 266
Maximum likelihood logistic regression analysis, 43
MD, see Muscular dystrophy
Mechanical division embryo biopsy method, 116, 120, 124
Meiosis, 3, 25
Mental retardation, 152
Metabolite assays, 203–205
Metal ions, 95
Methylprednisolone, 133
MF, see Microfilaments
Microchemical techniques, 199
Microdrops, 60–63
Microfertilization, 251
Microfilaments, 244
Microfluorometric techniques, 199
Microinjection, 36
  ethics of, 292
  quality of sperm and success of, 138
  sperm acrosomal status and, 139–140
  of sperm into oocytes, 145–147
  of sperm into ooplasm, 143–147
  of sperm into perivitelline space, 133–142, 145–147
    acrosomal status and, 139–140
    sperm-oocyte fusion and, 140–142
    sperm quality and, 138
    techniques in, 135–138
  sperm-oocyte fusion and, 140–142, 248
  success of, 138
Micromanipulation, 131–147, see also specific types
  classification of, 132
  of embryos, 116
  of oocytes, 34, 36
  ooplasm and, 143–147
  sperm acrosomal status and, 139–140
  sperm-oocyte fusion and, 140–142, 145

sperm quality and, 138
zona fellucida disruption and, 132–133
Microscopy, see also specific types
  electron, 142
  fluorescence, 202
  light, 240, 241, 252
  Nomarski, 255
  phase, 255
  quantitative fluorescence, 202
  scanning electron, 245, 246, 272
  transmission electron, see Transmission electron microscopy (TEM)
Microspectrofluorometry, 202
Microtubules, 247
Mini-Percoll method, 47, 49, 50
Miscarriage, 65, 306–307
Mitotic division, 184
Monospermic embryos, 252
Monospermic oocytes, 142
Morality, see Ethical aspects of IVF
Morphometry, 274
Mouse embryo bioassays, 102–104
Multinucleate blastomeres, 74
Multiple births, 266, 307–308
Multiple embryo transfer, 266
Multiple folliculogenesis, 4
Multiple oocytes, 196
Multiplex analysis, 168
Multipronucleate oocytes, 76
Muscular dystrophy (MD), 166–168

N

Narcotics, 36
Natural cycle, 9–11, 266, 305
Necrospermia, 37
Nitrofurantoin, 37
Nomarski interference, 24
Nomarski microscopy, 255
Nomarski optics, 244
Nonhysteroscopic fallopscopy, 79
Noroxin, 37
Nuclear envelope vesiculation, 140
Nucleic acid precursors, 94–95
Nucleokinesis, 74
Nucleotides, 201, 205, see also specific types
Nutrients, 87, 92, 93, 199
Nycodenz, 47

O

OAM, see Outer acrosomal membrane
Obstructive azoospermia, 35

OHSS, see Ovarian hyperstimulation syndrome
Oligoasthenozoospermia, 58
Oligonucleotide primers, 160, 167
Oligonucleotide probing, 167
One-step polymerase chain reaction assays, 159–161
Oocytes, 4, 17–29
  abnormal features of, 247
  activation of, 67
  aging, 142, 248
  bipronucleate, 76
  chemotactic signals between sperm and, 51
  co-incubation of, 137
  collection of, 18–19
  cryopreservation of, 45, 214, see also Cryopreservation
    ethics of, 297–298
    rapid cooling in, 232–233
    slow cooling method in, 230–231
  cumulus cell interactions with, 244
  cumulus cell removal and, 25–27
  cytoplasm of, 58
  degenerated, 66
  donation of, 267–268
  donor, 275, 279
  follicle flushing and, 18, 20
  fusion of plasma membrane with, 58
  fusion of sperm with, 58, 67, 140–142, 145, 248
  identification of, 20–21
  immature, 23, 25
  injection of sperm into, 145–147
  insemination of, 58–63
  insemination timing and, 27
  masses of, 21, 28
  maturation of, 21–23, 298
    cryopreservation and, 309–310
    nuclear, 23–27
    ultrastructure and, 243–247
    zona protein secretion during, 247
  meiosis in, 3
  in metaphase II, 124–125
  microinjection and fertilization of, 134
  micromanipulation of, 34, 36
  monospermic, 142
  morphology of, 138
  multiple, 196
  multipronucleate, 76
  nuclear maturity in, 23–27
  one-cell fertilized, 76
  partial zona dissection, 133
  plasma membrane of, 132, 144

Index

polypronuclear, 64
polyspermic, 67, 126
postmature, 142, 248
preparation of for GIFT, 28–29
pronuclear, 183
pronucleate, 74, 76
quality of, 267–268, 270
rapid cooling of, 232–233
recovery of, 61, 68, 133, 196
sperm direct access to, 132
sperm suspensions with, 60
spreading of, 176
superovulated, 188
surface microvilli loss in, 248
temperature and, 19–20
transmission electron microscopy of, 239
tripronuclear, 183, 184
unfertilized, 66, 142, 214
vacuolated, 66
variability of, 42
viability of, 125
vitrification of, 185, 231–232
zona-free, 67, 68
zona proteins secreted by, 247
Ooplasm, 143–147
Osmiophilic centrosomes, 252
Osmolarity, 92, 100
Osmolytes, 108
Outer acrosomal membrane (OAM), 240, 243
Ovarian hyperstimulation syndrome (OHSS), 11–12
Ovarian stimulation, 273–274, 304
Overspreading of chromosomes, 175, 180
Oxygen, 97

P

PAF, see Platelet activating factor
Paracrine factors, 87
Partial zona dissection (PZD), 132–134, 138
Partial zona dissection (PZD) oocytes, 133
Paternal centrioles, 251–252
PCOS, see Polycystic ovarian syndrome
PCR, see Polymerase chain reaction
Pentoxifylline, 50, 137
Percoll method, 47, 49, 50
Pergonal, see Human menopausal gonadotrophin (HMG)
Perivitelline space, sperm injection into, see under Sperm
Phagocytosis, 67
Phase-contrast optics, 244

Phase microscopy, 255
pH of embryo culture system media, 101, 102
Phenylalanine, 94
6-Phosphogluconate, 201
Plasma membrane, 58, 132, 144, 240, 243
Platelet activating factor (PAF), 198
Platelet activating factor (PAF) antagonists, 198
PM, see Plasma membrane
Polycystic ovarian syndrome (PCOS), 12
Polymerase chain reaction (PCR), 125, 152
  amplification of, 159, 164–165
  automated, 158
  diagnostic assays using, 166–168
  mixture of, 155
  one-step, 159–161
  principles of, 152–154
  products of, 158–159, 165–168
  sensitivity of, 162–164
  two-step, 162–164
  visualization of products of, 158–159
Polypronuclear embryos, 64
Polypronuclear oocytes, 64
Polyspermic fertilization, 27, 251
Polyspermic oocytes, 67
Polyspermy, 46, 133, 142
Polyvinyl alcohol (PVA), 95, 96
Polyvinylpyrollidone, 47
Postmature oocytes, 248
Potassium, 92
Pre-embryos, 36
Pregnancy rate improvement, 304–309
Progesterone, 3, 4, 10, 264
Prolactin, 4, 50
Pronuclear embryos, 68–69
Pronuclear oocytes, 183
Pronuclear stage tubal transfer (PROST), 68
Pronucleate oocytes, 74, 76
Pronucleate single cell embryos, 71
Propanediol slow cooling, 224–225
PROST, see Pronuclear stage tubal transfer
Prostaglandins, 3, see also specific types
Protectants for embryos, 108, see also specific types
Proteins, see also specific types
  concentrations of, 46
  in embryo culture system media, 95–96, 101–102
  glyco-, 246
  supplementation of, 101–102
  uptake of, 254
  zona, see Zona proteins (ZP)

Public funding, 304
Public support for IVF, 293
Push embryo biopsy method, 125
PVA, see Polyvinyl alcohol
Pyridine nucleotides, 201, 205
Pyruvate, 77, 91–93, 199, 203–205
 uptake of, 200, 205, 206
PZD, see Partial zona dissection

Q

Quantitative fluorescence microscopy, 202

R

Radical feminist view of IVF, 292–293
Radiotherapy, 45
Rapid cooling method, 215, 218–220
 for embryos, 226–230
 for oocytes, 232–233
Reactive oxygen molecules, 190
Recessive genetic conditions, 147
Recombinant DNA, 152
Regression analysis, 43
Regulation of IVF, 294–296
Rehydration of cells, 215
Reinsemination, 66
Relaxin, 50
Religious opposition to IVF, 289–293
Restriction fragment length polymorphisms (RFLPs), 152, 167
RFLPs, see Restriction fragment length polymorphisms
Right-to-life view of IVF, 289–290
Roman Catholic view of IVF, 290–292
Round-headed sperm syndrome (globozoospermia), 145

S

Safety of IVF, 185–188
Salazopyrin, 36
Sample contamination, 164
Scanning electron microscopy (SEM), 245, 246, 272
Seeding, 215–217
Semen, see also Sperm
 analysis of, 34–44
  clinical examination of male and, 34–37
  future of, 50–51
  male infertility and, 34–35
  variability of results of, 37
 aspiration of, 34
 collection of, 36, 37, 45, 48

cryopreservation of, 49
 donor, 35
 infection in, 37
 preparation of for IVF, 44–50
  principles of, 45–46
  procedures in, 46–50
SER, see Smooth endoplasmic reticulum
Serine, 93, 94
Sertoli cell only syndrome, 35
Sexing of embryos, 159, 292
Shorr method, 38
Simplification of IVF, 304–305
Single gene detection, 161
Sister chromatid exchanges, 178–179
Slow cooling method, 215–218, 224–225, 230–231
Smooth endoplasmic reticulum (SER), 248
Somatic cells, 76
Sonication, 98, 144
Southern blotting, 159
Sperm, see also Semen
 abnormal, 36, 138, 143, 145
 acrosomal status in, see Acrosomal status in sperm
 autoimmunity of, 35, 36, 45
 capacitation of, 46
 chemotactic signals between oocytes and, 51
 collection of, 45
 concentration of, 38, 43, 132
 cryopreservation of, 46, 241–243
 cytoplasmic, 144
 damage of, 46
 decondensation of nucleus of, 67
 defective, 36, 138, 143, 145
 direct access to oocytes for, 132
 donor, 45
 epidymal, 36
 frozen, see Cryopreservation of sperm
 function of, see Sperm function tests
 fusion of oocyte membrane with, 248
 fusion of oocytes with, 58, 67, 145
 immotile, 243
 incompetence of, 66
 injection of into ooplasm, 143–147
 injection of into perivitelline space, 133–142, 145–147
  acrosomal status and, 139–140
  sperm-oocyte fusion and, 140–142
  sperm quality and, 138
  techniques in, 135–138
 insemination of, see Insemination
 isolation of, 139
 male factor, 63

Index **323**

microinjection of, see Microinjection
morphology of, 36, 38–39, 43, 44, 46, 132
  microinjection success and, 138
  transmission electron microscopy in analysis of, 240–243
motility of, 38–40, 43, 50, 132, 243
nuclear maturity of, 44
number of, 46
oocyte suspensions with, 60
plasma membrane of, 240, 243
preparation of for IVF, 44–50
  principles of, 45–46
  procedures in, 46–50
preparation of for TEM, 238
problems in collection of, 45
quality of, 138
stimulation of motility of, 50
viability of, 243
Sperm function tests, 34, 38–44
  IVF rates and, 42–44
  transmission electron microscopy as, 240–243
Sperm-zona pellucida binding, 42
Spindle defects, 142
Spreading, 175–178, 180
Steroid hormones, 36, see also specific types
Stitch and pull embryo biopsy method, 120, 125
Stimulation protocols, 4–9
Subfertility, 36–37
Substrates, 87, 92–93, see also specific types
Superovulation procedures, 188
Superoxide dismutase, 108
Superoxide radicals, 97, 108
Surfactants, 96, see also specific types
Swim-up procedure, 47–49, 50
Synchrony, 265
Syngamy, 58, 292

T

Taq polymerase, 154, 165
Taurine, 50, 93
TE, see Trophectoderm
TEM, see Transmission electron microscopy
TEST, see Tubal embryo transfer
Testicular atrophy, 34
Tetracycline, 133
α-Thalassemia, 166
β-Thalassemia, 167

Threonine, 93, 94
Toxins, 35
Transfer
  embryo, see Embryo transfer (ET)
  gamete intrafallopian, see Gamete intrafallopian transfer (GIFT)
  pre-embryo, 36
  pronuclear embryo, 68–69
  pronuclear stage tubal, 68
  tubal embryo, 79
  zygote intrafallopian, 68, 69
Transferrin, 108
Transforming growth factor (TGF), 96
Transmission electron microscopy (TEM), 183, 184
  of embryos, 239
  endometrial morphology and, 272
  fluorescence combined with, 241
  of oocytes, 239
  in sperm function analysis, 240–243
  in sperm morphology analysis, 240–243
  sperm preparation for, 238
  in ultrastructure analysis, 238–244, 248
    co-cultures and, 254–256
    zona proteins and, 245
Triploid embryos, 252
Triploid infants, 65
Tripronuclear embryos, 183
Tripronuclear oocytes, 183, 184
Trophectoderm biopsy, 86
Trophectoderm herniation embryo biopsy method, 116, 120, 124
Trophectoderms, 117, 120
Trophoblasts, 76
Trypan blue, 197
Tuarine, 94
Tubal embryo transfer (TEST), 79, 144
Tumors, 174
Two-cell test, 104
Two-step polymerase chain reaction, 162–164

U

Ultrarapid cooling, 219
Ultrasonography, 79, 274
Ultrastructure, 237–256
  co-culture systems and, 254–257
  early embryonic development and, 252–254
  embryo culture systems and, 254–257
  of gametes, 247–248
  oocyte maturation and, 243–247

paternal centriole inheritance and, 251–252
transmission electron microscopy in analysis of, 238–244, 248
co-cultures and, 254–256
Ultraviolet irradiation, 164
Unfertilized oocytes, 66
Uterine receptivity, 263–279, see also Implantation window
agonadal women and, 275–278
animal studies on, 264–265
embryo viability and, 266–267
endocrine requirements for, 268–271
endometrial morphology and, 272–274
hormone replacement therapy and, 272, 275–278
importance of, 267–268
improvement in, 278–279
luteal support and, 270–271
morphological studies and, 271–275
natural cycle and, 266
ovarian stimulation and, 273–274
strategies for improvement in, 278–279
theoretical calculations of, 266–268

V

Vacuolated oocytes, 66
Valine, 94
Varicoceles, 37
Vasectomy reversals, 35
Vasoepididymostomies, 35
Vasovasostomies, 35
Vatican view of IVF, 290–292
Vero cells, 106–107

Vesiculation of nuclear envelope, 140
Viability
of blastocysts, 198
of embryos, 87, 116, 206–208
assessment of, 196–199
defined, 196
uterine receptivity and, 266–267
of oocytes, 125
of sperm, 243
Viruses, 48, 106, see also specific types
Vitamins, 94, 108
Vitelline membrane, 142
Vitrification, 185, 219, 226, 231–232

X

X-linked disorders, 120, 152, see also specific types

Z

Zona-free oocytes, 67, 68
Zona pellucida, 40–41, 46, 67, 76
disruption of, 132–133
embryo biopsy and, 120
sperm binding to, 42
Zona perforation, 78
Zona proteins (ZP), 41–43, 244
maturation of, 245
origin of, 247
surface architecture of, 246
ZP, see Zona proteins
Zygote intrafallopian transfer (ZIFT), 68–80
Zygote test, 104